"An important book."

MEMORY
RESCUE

SUPERCHARGE YOUR BRAIN, REVERSE MEMORY LOSS, AND REMEMBER WHAT MATTERS MOST

THE OFFICIAL PROGRAM OF THE AMEN CLINICS

DANIEL G. AMEN, MD

This is an incredibly helpful book for anyone who wants to increase their brain capacity and strengthen their memory. I want to stay sharp, and that's why I read everything Dr. Amen writes, and you should too!

PASTOR RICK WARREN
Author of *The Purpose Driven Life* and *The Daniel Plan*

Rescue your memory with Dr. Amen's embraced habits that will brighten your mind.

MEHMET OZ, MD
Professor of surgery, New York-Presbyterian/Columbia University Medical Center

Memory Rescue is such an important book if you want to strengthen and keep your memory strong for the rest of your life. Millions of people find themselves victims of memory loss and have no idea that there are simple interventions to help keep their memory strong. I deeply believe this approach can help you or your loved ones.

TONY ROBBINS
#1 *New York Times* bestselling author, philanthropist, and America's #1 life and business strategist

While there's no pharmaceutical fix for memory decline, research now validates the powerfully therapeutic role of lifestyle choices in recovering and preserving memory. Dr. Amen's *Memory Rescue* eloquently embraces this science and presents it to the reader in a wonderfully user-friendly format.

DAVID PERLMUTTER, MD, FACN
Author of the *New York Times* #1 bestsellers *Grain Brain* and *The Grain Brain Whole Life Plan*

Memory Rescue is a powerful new book that shows you step-by-step how to improve your memory and overall health. The information is smart, simple, research-based, and effective. It's your road map to the best brain possible.

MARK HYMAN, MD
Physician and bestselling author

This is an insanely simple guide for preventing and possibly reversing memory loss and dementia, based on Dr. Amen's 25-plus years of clinical experience treating thousands of brain-injured patients. *Memory Rescue* is a must-read, not only for patients fearful of memory loss, but also for physicians who too often take a fatalistic approach to this epidemic. Dr. Amen provides scientifically based measures that can prevent or slow dementia. This book is the most current and succinct source to date on "how to do it."

JOSEPH MAROON, MD
Clinical professor and vice chairman, Department of Neurosurgery, University of Pittsburgh Medical Center; team neurosurgeon, the Pittsburgh Steelers

Dr. Amen's work continues to break ground. All cultures put great value in living a long life, but what if we can't take our memories with us? Now we have a choice. The sage wisdom and scientific advances taught in this book are the secret to living a long, healthy, and fulfilling life.

PEDRAM SHOJAI, OMD
Founder of Well.org; *New York Times* bestselling author of *The Urban Monk*

Dementia with aging is the sad new normal, but it is neither natural nor inevitable—if you follow Dr. Amen's brilliant guidance. Keeping and even improving your brain is really quite simple: Get nutrients in; keep toxins out; and use it or lose it.

JOSEPH PIZZORNO, ND
Author of 12 books, including *The Toxin Solution*; editor-in-chief, *Integrative Medicine: A Clinician's Journal*

Your mind is everything that makes you human. Your memory is the most important part of your mind. My friend and mind mentor, Dr. Daniel Amen, is the master's master of memory. In his page-turning book, you will discover the wisdom, insights, and understanding to optimize and maximize your mind and memory. It is a must-read for everyone with a mind.

MARK VICTOR HANSEN
Cocreator of the Chicken Soup for the Soul series; cochairman of Metamorphosis Energy, LLC

Memory Rescue is an important book that shows you how to keep your memory strong. If you want to protect your most important organ and keep it healthy, you'll find a clear, simple path in this book.

DAVID S. LUDWIG, MD, PhD
Professor, Harvard Medical School; author of the #1 *New York Times* bestseller *Always Hungry?*

Our ability to remember is a precious gift, one that makes us human. Until reading *Memory Rescue*, I had not realized how much I could do for and with my memory. In this warm and very accessible book, Dr. Daniel Amen uses brain scans and science-based insights to help protect our precious asset. The book does more than help us boost our memories—it promises and delivers a program for healthy aging and a happier life. I highly recommend it.

MICHAEL GURIAN
Author of *The Wonder of Aging* and *Lessons of Lifelong Intimacy*

Dr. Amen has done it again with *Memory Rescue*, the quintessential book on how to get your brain healthy and how to keep it that way. It is full of essential information, based on the latest research, that everyone needs to keep their brain working at optimum health. Its easy-to-read format will allow everyone to find what they need for their individual brain. The brain scan data is second to none in showing how people can fully engage ways of keeping their brain happy and healthy for a long lifetime.

ANDREW NEWBERG
Bestselling author of *How Enlightenment Changes Your Brain*

As a heart researcher, I'm amazed at how many of Dr. Amen's BRIGHT MINDS factors apply to cardiac as well as brain health. Following his clear plan will slow the aging of both your ticker and your thinker.

WILLIAM S. HARRIS, PhD
Professor of medicine, Sanford School of Medicine, University of South Dakota; president of OmegaQuant, LLC

I have known Daniel for more than 25 years. He has been amazingly consistent in his journey, not only to describe neurological conditions from a more physiological basis, but also to promote a structured dietary program to improve brain function. This book carries on his explorations to build a better brain. As with each of his books, I always find new and provocative information. *Memory Rescue* is no exception. I highly recommend it to everyone.

BARRY SEARS, PhD
Author of *The Zone*

Memory is critical to success in every area of life. For more than a decade, Dr. Amen has been my go-to guy for all things related to memory, the brain, and performance. This terrific book is a complete manual for making your brain better now and into the future.

JONNY BOWDEN, PhD, CNS
Board-certified nutrition specialist; editorial advisory board (emeritus) for *Men's Health* magazine; columnist for *Clean Eating, Better Nutrition, Amazing Wellness*; author of *The 150 Healthiest Foods on Earth, Living Low Carb*, and *The Great Cholesterol Myth*

Without healthy brains with healthy memories, we suffer significant losses in the quality of our lives. Dr. Amen's book is a highly valuable resource on how to not only stop the degeneration, but reverse it. Highly recommended, and well worth the reading.

JOHN TOWNSEND, PhD
New York Times bestselling author, psychologist, and founder of the Townsend Institute for Leadership and Counseling

At a time when memory loss is increasing at epidemic rates, Dr. Amen leads the way to better health. *Memory Rescue* is easy to read and simple to implement, and it will definitely help protect your brain.

STEVEN MASLEY, MD, FAHA, FACN, CNS
Bestselling author of *The Better Brain Solution*

Following the protocol in Dr. Daniel Amen's new book will not only renew your memory, it will renew your very life. You know enough to tune your car—experience what happens when you tune your brain!

CHRIS PRENTISS
Cofounder and codirector of Passages Malibu and coauthor of *The Alcoholism and Addiction Cure*

Dr. Amen helped to rescue my memory and brain, which changed my life. *Memory Rescue* will give you strategies to quickly improve your memory and brain now and for the rest of your life too. I highly recommend it.

DAVE ASPREY
Founder and CEO of Bulletproof 360

Memory Rescue will empower you to take charge of your life by embracing simple habits and strategies that will boost your memory. I am eager to recommend it to my patients.

FREDERICK ROBERT CARRICK, DC, PhD, MS-HPEd
Senior research fellow, Bedfordshire Centre for Mental Health Research in association with the University of Cambridge

A SAMPLE OF OTHER BOOKS BY DANIEL AMEN

The Brain Warrior's Way, with Tana Amen, New American Library, 2016

The Brain Warrior's Way Cookbook, with Tana Amen, New American Library, 2016

Change Your Brain, Change Your Life (revised), Harmony Books, 2015, *New York Times* Bestseller

Healing ADD (revised), Berkley, 2013, *New York Times* Bestseller

The Daniel Plan, with Rick Warren, DMin, and Mark Hyman, MD, Zondervan, 2013, #1 *New York Times* Bestseller

Unleash the Power of the Female Brain, Harmony Books, 2013

Use Your Brain to Change Your Age, Crown Archetype, 2012, *New York Times* Bestseller

The Amen Solution, Crown Archetype, 2011, *New York Times* Bestseller

Unchain Your Brain, with David E. Smith, MD, MindWorks, 2010

Change Your Brain, Change Your Body, Harmony Books, 2010, *New York Times* Bestseller

Magnificent Mind at Any Age, Harmony Books, 2008, *New York Times* Bestseller

The Brain in Love, Three Rivers Press, 2007

Making a Good Brain Great, Harmony Books, 2005, Amazon Book of the Year

How to Get Out of Your Own Way, MindWorks, 2005

ADD in Intimate Relationships, MindWorks, 2005

Preventing Alzheimer's, with William R. Shankle, MS, MD, Perigee, 2005

Healing Anxiety and Depression, with Lisa Routh, MD, Putnam, 2003

Healing the Hardware of the Soul, Free Press, 2002

New Skills for Frazzled Parents, MindWorks, 2000

The Most Important Thing in Life I Learned from a Penguin!?, MindWorks, 1995

MEMORY

MEMORY

MEMORY

RESCUE

SUPERCHARGE YOUR BRAIN,
REVERSE MEMORY LOSS, AND
REMEMBER WHAT MATTERS MOST

THE OFFICIAL PROGRAM OF THE AMEN CLINICS

DANIEL G. AMEN, MD

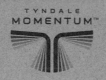

TYNDALE
MOMENTUM™

The nonfiction imprint of
Tyndale House Publishers, Inc.

TYNDALE, *Tyndale Momentum*, and Tyndale's quill logo are registered trademarks of Tyndale House Publishers, Inc. The Tyndale Momentum logo is a trademark of Tyndale House Publishers, Inc. Tyndale Momentum is the nonfiction imprint of Tyndale House Publishers, Inc., Carol Stream, Illinois.

Memory Rescue: Supercharge Your Brain, Reverse Memory Loss, and Remember What Matters Most

Copyright © 2017 by Daniel G. Amen, MD. All rights reserved.

Author photograph by Lesley Bohm, copyright © 2013. All rights reserved.

Interior photographs, including brain scans, and illustrations provided by author and used with permission. All rights reserved.

Designed by Dan Farrell and Dean H. Renninger

Published in association with the literary agency of WordServe Literary Group, www.wordserveliterary.com.

Unless otherwise indicated, all Scripture quotations are taken from the *Holy Bible*, New Living Translation, copyright © 1996, 2004, 2015 by Tyndale House Foundation. Used by permission of Tyndale House Publishers, Inc., Carol Stream, Illinois 60188. All rights reserved.

Scripture quotations marked NASB are taken from the New American Standard Bible,® copyright © 1960, 1962, 1963, 1968, 1971, 1972, 1973, 1975, 1977, 1995 by The Lockman Foundation. Used by permission.

Scripture quotations marked NCV are taken from the New Century Version.® Copyright © 2005 by Thomas Nelson, Inc. Used by permission. All rights reserved.

Scripture quotations marked NIV are taken from the Holy Bible, *New International Version*,® *NIV*.® Copyright © 1973, 1978, 1984, 2011 by Biblica, Inc.® Used by permission. All rights reserved worldwide.

For information about special discounts for bulk purchases, please contact Tyndale House Publishers at csresponse@tyndale.com, or call 1-800-323-9400.

Library of Congress Cataloging-in-Publication Data

Names: Amen, Daniel G., author.
Title: Memory rescue : supercharge your brain, reverse memory loss, and remember what matters most / Daniel G. Amen, MD.
Description: Carol Stream, Illinois : Tyndale Momentum, the nonfiction imprint of Tyndale House Publishers, Inc., [2017] | The official program of Amen Clinics. | Includes bibliographical references and index.
Identifiers: LCCN 2017030617 | ISBN 9781496425607 (hc) | ISBN 9781496429551 (international trade paper edition)
Subjects: LCSH: Memory disorders—Prevention—Popular works. | Mental health—Popular works. | Brain—Diseases—Nutritional aspects—Popular works.
Classification: LCC RC394.M46 A43 2017 | DDC 616.8/3—dc23 LC record available at https://lccn.loc.gov/2017030617

ISBN 978-1-4964-2561-4 (sc)

Printed in the United States of America

23   22   21
6   5   4   3   2

To my mother and father, who, at the ages of 86
and 88, still inspire me every day.
This book is also dedicated to you, my dear reader.
You are the reason I wrote Memory Rescue.

Contents

The Problem . . .
the Promise . . . the Program

THE PROBLEM

Memory problems are common at every stage of life, and they can impair learning, working, relationships, and even self-reliance. Memory problems clearly get worse as we age, with 75 percent of older adults complaining about them. No problem is more closely associated with memory loss than Alzheimer's disease (AD), one of the most feared and devastating illnesses of all. With the aging population, experts expect the incidence of AD to triple in the next 30 years, and there is no cure on the horizon. The Centers for Disease Control and Prevention report that the US death rate from AD rose by 55 percent between 1999 and 2014.[1] If you live until age 85, you have a nearly 50 percent chance of being diagnosed with AD or another form of dementia; and these illnesses start in the brain *decades* before any symptoms appear.

THE PROMISE

Your brain's history is *not* its destiny. Even if you have brain fog or trouble remembering now, it doesn't mean you always will. You can start having a better memory today by engaging in the Amen Clinics' simple Memory Rescue: BRIGHT MINDS program. What's more, the same plan will help your energy, mood, anxiety, sleep, weight, and overall success in life. The plan will also help you decrease your risk of developing Alzheimer's disease and other forms of dementia. Scientists have estimated that delaying the onset of AD by as little as one year could reduce the number of cases worldwide by as many as 9,200,000 by 2050![2] Of course, we must do much better than that—and you can and will.

THE PROGRAM

Memory Rescue is based on an insanely simple idea: The best way to sharpen your memory, reverse brain aging, and prevent AD is to *eliminate*, *prevent*, or *treat* all of the risk factors that steal your mind, represented by the mnemonic (a memory device) BRIGHT MINDS.

B – Blood flow: hypertension or prehypertension, stroke, cardiovascular disease, cholesterol problems, erectile dysfunction, infrequent exercise (less than twice a week)

R – Retirement/Aging: risk increases with age (over 50); lack of new learning—when you stop learning, your brain starts dying

I – Inflammation: gum disease, high homocysteine or C-reactive protein (CRP) levels in your blood, low omega-3 fatty acids

G – Genetics: a family member with Alzheimer's disease, any other form of dementia, or Parkinson's disease; having the e4 version of the *APOE* gene

H – Head Trauma: a history of head injuries with or without loss of consciousness; playing contact sports, even without a concussion

T – Toxins: alcohol or drug abuse, exposure to toxins in the environment (mold, pollution) or personal products, cancer chemotherapy, etc.

M – Mental Health: chronic stress, depression, attention deficit disorder/ attention deficit hyperactivity disorder, post-traumatic stress disorder, bipolar disorder, schizophrenia

I – Immunity/Infection Issues: chronic fatigue syndrome; autoimmune issues, such as rheumatoid arthritis or multiple sclerosis; untreated infections, such as Lyme disease, syphilis, or herpes

N – Neurohormone Deficiencies: low levels of thyroid, testosterone (males and females), estrogen and progesterone (females), DHEA (dehydroepian-drosterone); high cortisol levels

D – Diabesity: diabetes, prediabetes, and obesity

S – Sleep Issues: chronic insomnia and sleep apnea

The good news is that almost all of these risk factors are either preventable or treatable. Even those that aren't, such as a family history of dementia, can be ameliorated with the right strategies.

YOU NEED THIS BOOK IF:

- Your memory has never been good and now it's getting worse.
- Your memory is not as sharp as it was 10 years ago.
- You're having trouble remembering to take medications or supplements consistently.
- You frequently misplace your keys or phone.
- You often wonder why you came into a room.
- You're embarrassed by forgetting appointments.
- You read a book or an article but don't remember much of it.
- You struggle with brain fog.
- You notice that a loved one's failing memory is interfering with everyday tasks.
- You are concerned about a family member who has been diagnosed with dementia.
- You wonder what you can do to avoid Alzheimer's, which has been diagnosed in one or more of your close relatives.

As you read *Memory Rescue*, keep an eye out for the icon on the following page. It will accompany many BRIGHT MINDS tips that will help keep your memory strong and reverse problems that may be present. Rest assured, you don't have to do everything at once! Most people are successful when they make one simple change at a time. Once they see how easy it is and how much better they feel, they often make scores of other healthy changes.

BRIGHT MINDS TIP

Loving your brain means treating it with respect and care.

Preface

Memory is the treasury and guardian of all things.
MARCUS TULLIUS CICERO

Can you relate to any of these people?

- Steve, a 60-year-old father and CEO, lost both his father and grandfather to Alzheimer's disease. Steve was terrified he'd get it too, because he noticed his own memory was slipping.

- Joelle, 42, had no filter. She just said whatever came to her mind, which tended to hurt other people's feelings.

- Jim, 61, was a very successful businessman who had overcome addictions, as well as growing up with attention deficit disorder and dyslexia. After he got into a bad car accident, his memory became worse, his behavior changed, and he started to engage in habits that nearly cost him his family.

- Sherman, 71, had been under a great deal of work-related stress for years and had started to struggle with memory, decision making, and anxiety. He frequently woke up in the middle of the night.

- Todd, 53, a busy, stressed-out executive, was really struggling with his memory. He frequently misplaced things and hoped it was just part of normal aging. Secretly, he suspected something might be wrong.

- Sarah, a 62-year-old grandmother of six, worried because her memory had started to fail. Several months before she came to Amen Clinics, she had a ministroke that left her transiently paralyzed on her right side. Her faith was critically important to her, and she wanted to pass it on to her grandchildren. However, she was concerned that she wouldn't be able to if she lost her memory.

- Bud, 52, was concerned about his memory, focus, and energy. His mother had died of Alzheimer's disease, and he had a wife 20 years younger than he was and two children, ages five and seven.

- Jasmine, 26, couldn't get out of the funk she had been in for more than a year. She was depressed, anxious, and obsessive. She had to drop out of her PhD program in clinical psychology because she couldn't focus or remember. Five antidepressants and three therapists later, she was giving up hope.

- Shawn, 35, broke his neck in four places in a surfing accident. After a remarkable physical recovery, he noticed his mood, memory, and cognition failing him. He was having suicidal thoughts when he first came to see us.

- Lew, 67, was a navy pilot and instructor for 40 years. He had to stop flying because he was not able to think through his flight plans. He and his wife were shocked when he made a mistake regarding some finances, causing a significant loss.

- David, 62, had become a recluse. His doctor had recently diagnosed him with Alzheimer's disease. After beginning a new medication, he seemed confused.

- Jesse, 42, had recently been diagnosed with multiple sclerosis. She struggled with her mood and memory. She had been put on immune-suppressing drugs, but the side effects made her feel terrible.

- Anita, 38, thrived for years in her roles as a teacher and mom of three. Then suddenly she began feeling exhausted, sad, and forgetful. She couldn't sleep well and had little energy. Nothing she tried seemed to boost her energy level or mood.

- Kyle, a 51-year-old CEO, was successful in leading his family's meat-packing business, but he was not doing well personally. He had diabetes and sleep apnea, and he wasn't following his doctor's treatment plan.

You will meet all these people in *Memory Rescue*. Over the past 30 years, people with stories like these, plus tens of thousands of others, have come to Amen Clinics for help. They all have had one thing in common: The physical functioning of their brains needed improvement. Through a series of events in my life, it has become my mission to help people have better brains and better lives.

At 18, I was trained as an infantry medic in the US Army, where my love of medicine was born. While still in the service, I became an X-ray technician and developed a passion for medical imaging. As our professors used to say, "How do you know unless you look?" Then, when I was a second-year medical student, someone I loved tried to kill herself. I arranged for her to meet with an outstanding psychiatrist and came to realize that if he helped her (which he did), he would ultimately help her children and grandchildren, too, because they would be influenced by someone who was happier and more stable. I was drawn to psychiatry because I realized its potential to change generations of people for the better.

Yet psychiatry then, and even now, remains the only medical specialty that virtually never looks at the organ it treats—the brain. Frustrated, I decided to learn more about brain imaging tools, which have revolutionized my life and the lives of my patients, coworkers, family members, and friends. I first learned about SPECT (single photon emission computed tomography) during a lecture conducted by the chief of medicine at our local hospital in 1991. Convinced that such imaging could provide invaluable information, my colleagues and I adopted the technique and began building a database of brain scans related to behavior. Today it is the world's largest database, totaling more than 135,000 scans on patients from 111 countries taken over the past 25-plus years.

Ultimately, the scans led me to five conclusions:

1. **Brain health is central to all health and success in life.** When your brain works right, you are happier, healthier (because you make better decisions), wealthier (again because you make better decisions), and more successful in everything you do.

2. **When your brain is troubled, for whatever reason, you are likely to be sadder, sicker, poorer, and less successful.**

3. **You are not stuck with the brain you have.** You can make it better, even if you have been bad to it—and I can prove it. This has been the most exciting lesson of my professional life, and it is one of the main topics in this book.

4. **To save your brain, you have to get your mind right.** Too many people give themselves excuses to stay sick. I call them the "little

lies" that keep them fat, depressed, and feeble-minded. Here are the most common justifications I've heard over the years, along with my responses to patients.

LITTLE LIES	RESPONSE
This will be hard.	Focusing on getting well is dramatically easier than being sick or losing your mind. Initially change is hard because the brain hates change and likes to do what it has always done. But with the right attitude and strategies, it can be very rewarding.
I don't want to deprive myself.	When you make poor health decisions, you are robbing yourself of what you really want—energy, memory, and good health. Getting well is about abundance, never deprivation. *Memory Rescue* will help you avoid hypertension, heart disease, cancer, diabetes, depression, and dementia.
It is too expensive.	Being sick is much more expensive than thoughtfully spending your resources to get and stay well. With a better-functioning brain, you will have more money because the quality of your decisions will be better.
I don't have time.	Spending time and energy to optimize your brain will help you live longer and be cognitively sharper, giving you much more time overall.
Everything in moderation. Just a little can't hurt.	This is the gateway thought to illness. It is generally an excuse to justify doing something unhealthy. "Just a little can't hurt" leads to just one more cigarette, one more piece of cake, etc.

5. **You are in a war for the health of your brain.** Just about every-where you go, you are offered toxic food that will kill you early. The real "weapons of mass destruction" are highly processed, pesticide-sprayed, high-glycemic, low-fiber food-like substances in plastic containers. Such fare is destroying the health of America: Two-thirds of us are overweight or obese; 50 percent are diabetic or prediabetic; and 60 percent are hypertensive or prehypertensive—all conditions that damage the brain. In addition, news channels repeatedly pour toxic images into our minds, stoking our fear that disaster is every-where and constantly exposing our brains to stress chemicals that

can damage our brains' memory centers. Technology companies continually produce addictive gadgets that steal our attention and distract us from our loved ones. According to a study from Microsoft, the human attention span is now eight seconds; a goldfish's is nine seconds.[1]

For three decades, my staff and I have been at war, too, seeking to restore the mental health and brain health of thousands of people who've come to Amen Clinics. Just a few years ago, my staff and I began referring to those patients who took up the fight themselves as brain warriors.

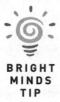

BRIGHT MINDS TIP

To rescue your memory, you must counteract the dangers to your health. You must become a *brain warrior.*

Throughout the book, I will tell you about brain warriors who've embraced a healthier mind-set and changed their lifestyle habits to save their own brains and those of the people they love. In this book, I'll tell you how to become a brain warrior and a memory rescuer, too.

That's because one of the most important symptoms of an unhealthy brain is memory problems. Once your memory starts to slip, everything in your life becomes harder, including your health, relationships, work, and finances. Such problems can even strip you of your independence. Let me be clear: I love my children very much, but I never want to live with them. I never want to be a burden to them, and I would prefer they not make decisions for me. I don't want them taking my driver's license from me or deciding what I'll wear and eat. If that is true for you, too, it means you need to think about your brain now, not 20 years from now. The truly exciting news is that you can start to change your brain and memory, beginning today.

Join me on a fascinating and important journey into improving your brain, memory, and life.

PART 1

MEMORY IS LIFE

CHAPTER 1

A BREAKTHROUGH APPROACH TO MEMORY ISSUES, AGING, AND ALZHEIMER'S

Memory is all we are. . . . Take a man's memories and you take all of him. Chip away a memory at a time and you destroy him as surely as if you hammered nail after nail through his skull.

MARK LAWRENCE, *KING OF THORNS*

Memory is the fabric of our souls. It enables us to integrate and make sense of the experiences of our bodies, minds, and spirits. It makes us who we are and allows us to keep our loved ones close, even when they are far away. Memory houses our joys, our hurts, and all of life's lessons. It reminds us who is trustworthy and who isn't, who has helped us and whom we need to help. Memory enables us to recall the important events in our lives and keeps us centered and growing. And because it contributes to our values and outlook, it also provides us with a sense of purpose that gives our lives meaning.

Our memories are such a part of us that we often take them for granted. Yet when our memory is damaged, the costs can be high. A diminished memory can rob us of our ability to make good decisions (because we forget important life lessons) and disconnect us from those we love. Memory problems limit our success at work, steal our independence, and ultimately make us vulnerable to anyone who might take advantage of us.

When someone's mental abilities, including memory, deteriorate enough to affect daily life, we say that person has dementia. Worldwide, a new person is diagnosed with dementia every seven seconds.[1] *Of the approximately 318 million Americans living today, 45 million—about 15 percent—will get*

Alzheimer's disease (AD) at some point in their lives. Tens of millions more will experience other forms of dementia, and 75 percent of older adults will suffer from memory problems.[2] Plus, more than 200 medication trials have failed to reverse Alzheimer's disease and other forms of dementia.[3] Given the complexity of the illness and how early it begins altering the brain, we are likely never going to have a medicine that cures it.

Yet new research suggests that a "memory rescue" program, like the one presented in this book, can dramatically improve memory and can prevent and sometimes even reverse some forms of dementia.[4] Given how most doctors approach this issue, however, you cannot count on traditional medicine to rescue your memory.

THE OLD APPROACH TO MEMORY COMPLAINTS

Here is a common scenario: You are having difficulty remembering conversations, forgetting where you put your reading glasses, or briefly getting lost driving in familiar areas. So you see your primary care physician or local neurologist, who asks you a few questions, gives you some short tests, orders an MRI (magnetic resonance imaging), and tells you, "Everyone has memory problems as they age. You're normal." It's also common for family members and friends to downplay forgetfulness.

A week or so later, you meet again with your doctor, who says that the report on your MRI came back as "mild, age-appropriate brain atrophy." He or she tells you that you have mild cognitive impairment (MCI). You're reassured that it's common and that you'll likely retain your personality and long-term memory until later in the illness. You're encouraged to get your affairs in order, given a prescription for Aricept (donepezil, a common memory medication that has short-term benefits but loses its effects after 18 months[5]), and told to schedule a follow-up appointment in six months. Typically, there is no discussion about eliminating risk factors through exercise, diet, supplementation, or memory training exercises.

That's literally the extent of the workup in 80 to 90 percent of the memory-related cases that come to us at Amen Clinics from the traditional medical system. *It's completely ineffective, heartbreaking . . . and unconscionable given what we know now.*

Until recently, health-care professionals assessing the presence of memory problems in patients classified their cognitive functioning as: (1) normal with no symptoms; (2) mild impairment observed by patients or their families;

or (3) Alzheimer's disease, in which dementia was becoming significant and getting worse.

The National Institute on Aging announced a significant change in 2011. Based on new brain imaging data, they added a new "preclinical" level. As a result, the current staging guidelines are

1. normal
2. preclinical: no obvious symptoms, but negative changes can be seen on biomarkers such as brain scans
3. mild cognitive impairment
4. Alzheimer's disease

Can you see the problem here? Long before symptoms develop, your brain may already be beginning to deteriorate, years or even decades before you realize it![6] A UCLA study found that 95 percent of people with Alzheimer's are not diagnosed until they are in the moderate to severe stages of the disorder. Yet the brain of a person diagnosed with Alzheimer's disease at age 59 likely started to show signs of deterioration by the time that person turned 30.

No matter your age, memory symptoms should be taken seriously. Developing brain fog or feeling as if your memory is slipping when you are in your forties, fifties, sixties, seventies, or even eighties is common, but it's not normal. It is a sign of impending doom. Ten years after you notice a problem (called subjective cognitive decline), there is an estimated 70 to 100 percent chance of your getting worse and slipping into dementia.[7]

But while it is true that memory issues are common with age, they are not inevitable. In the presymptomatic stage, when memory problems are minor, help is likely to be most effective. If you're struggling with your memory, even if it seems inconsequential, *now* is the time to get serious about your brain's health.

A BREAKTHROUGH CONCEPT: MEMORY RESCUE

Our decades-long experience at Amen Clinics of looking at the brain, together with the latest scientific research, has convinced me that the traditional approach to memory problems is misguided and leads to unnecessary disease and disability.

Just as many tributaries feed a river that is about to flood and destroy a community, we've discovered that there are many different causes of memory loss. It is no longer accurate to talk about mild cognitive impairment or AD as single entities with single causes, just as at Amen Clinics we no longer talk about a single type of depression, addiction, attention deficit hyperactivity disorder, or obesity. The ability to identify and address each of the potential causes of memory problems has enabled us to develop a plan to prevent or even reverse these devastating issues. Steve's story illustrates how effective our approach can be.

Steve: staring down Alzheimer's

Steve, a 60-year-old father and CEO, lost both his father and grandfather to AD. Steve was named after his grandfather, and they were very close. Steve found it heart-wrenching to watch him deteriorate to the point that his grandfather no longer recognized him. But watching it happen to his father was even worse. He worried about his dad every day for a decade. His father got lost, acted irrationally, and spent money in ways that jeopardized his life savings and family. In addition, Steve's mother always seemed sad and stressed.

Steve was terrified he'd get AD too. When his own memory began slipping, he went to see his family physician. His doctor did a cursory physical examination, ordered some blood work and a brain MRI, and saw him for follow-up a few weeks later. Steve's physician told him that his blood work was "mostly" within normal limits but didn't elaborate; his MRI was "normal for age with mild atrophy." He also told Steve it was "normal" for most people to struggle with memory problems as they aged. His doctor, who was Steve's age, said that he was having more senior moments too. Plus, he said, if Steve had early AD, there was nothing he could do for it, so why worry? The last thing the doctor said was "Make sure you have your affairs in order and let me see you in six months."

Deeply unsettled by the appointment, Steve came to see us at Amen Clinics. We have heard stories like Steve's over and over, and our approach is dramatically different. We know that the best way to prevent and even reverse significant memory problems is to identify them as early as possible and work to eliminate or treat all the risk factors that may be contributing to them. The mnemonic I developed to help us remember the risk factors is BRIGHT MINDS.

B – Blood Flow
R – Retirement/Aging
I – Inflammation
G – Genetics
H – Head Trauma
T – Toxins

M – Mental Health
I – Immunity/Infection Issues
N – Neurohormone Deficiencies
D – Diabesity (diabetes, prediabetes, and obesity)
S – Sleep Issues

When I reviewed Steve's records, I noticed that he had several important risk factors. He was prehypertensive (**blood flow**) and 60 years old (**retirement/aging**). His blood tests showed he had markers of **inflammation**. He also had a family history of severe memory problems (**genetics**) and was under chronic stress from watching his father's health decline and taking care of his mother (**mental health**). He was not eating organic or paying attention to the products he put on his body (**toxins**). His vitamin D (**immunity/infections**) and testosterone levels (**neurohormone deficiency**) were low, his fasting blood sugar and HbA1c levels were high, and he was overweight (**diabesity**). He had not been sleeping well for three years (**sleep**). Steve's risk factors and our recommended interventions (both of which will be explained in more detail in chapters 5 through 15) are summarized in the box below.

BRIGHT MINDS	STEVE'S RISK FACTORS	INTERVENTIONS
Blood Flow	Low blood flow on SPECT; prehypertension	Exercise, diet, ginkgo biloba
Retirement/Aging	60 years old	New learning exercises
Inflammation	High CRP and homocysteine	Diet; omega-3 fatty acids
Genetics	Strong family history of Alzheimer's	Serious focus on brain health
Head Trauma		
Toxins	Using multiple toxic products daily; not eating organic	Eliminate toxic products; eat organic
Mental Health	Chronic stress	Stress management tools
Immunity/Infections	Low vitamin D	Vitamin D3 supplements
Neurohormone Deficiencies	Low testosterone	Weight training, supplements, and no sugar
Diabesity	Prediabetes; overweight	Memory Rescue Diet
Sleep	Insomnia for three years	Sleep strategies

Steve's Memory Rescue risks and plan

As part of Steve's evaluation, I ordered much more extensive blood work and a SPECT (single photon emission computed tomography) scan, which measures blood flow and activity in the brain. SPECT is different from a CT (computed tomography) or MRI, which are anatomy scans that look at brain structure. SPECT looks at function. Functional problems almost always precede structural problems. SPECT tells us three things about the brain: Is there good blood flow? Too little activity? Or too much?

Steve's SPECT scan showed very low blood flow, the number one predictive sign of future trouble and Alzheimer's disease.[8]

Steve became serious about his self-care (he became a brain warrior), and within nine months of being on the Memory Rescue: BRIGHT MINDS program, Steve felt sharper, his memory was better, and he was hopeful that he could do something about his risk of Alzheimer's. A year later his scan showed remarkable improvement. Armed with this information, he taught his children about brain health.

STEVE'S "BEFORE" AND "AFTER" BRAIN SPECT SCANS

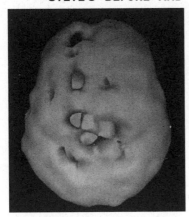 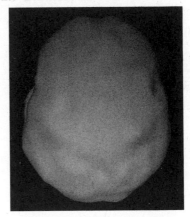

Low overall blood flow   Marked overall improvement

THE *MEMORY RESCUE* PROMISE

Memory Rescue will teach you the most common reasons for memory loss and help you identify the specific factors affecting your brain health. It will then provide you with a step-by-step approach to get your memory back, strengthen it, and keep it healthy for a lifetime.

You will learn:

- How to assess your brain on a regular basis to pick up issues early
- How to test for each of the risk factors
- Strategies to decrease or eliminate avoidable risks through exercises, nutritional supplementation, and diet
- How to follow the Memory Rescue Diet (one of the most powerful weapons for memory sustainability)
- Memory training and workouts to keep your brain sharp
- Innovative strategies to enhance brain function

Before we dive into those details, join me on a fascinating and important journey into your brain, the place where memories are truly made.

CHAPTER 2

HOW THE BRAIN WORKS
LEARN ABOUT THE MOST
IMPORTANT PART OF YOU

A woman's pastor saw her in the grocery store and asked her why she hadn't been to church lately. "Aren't you concerned about the hereafter?" he asked. "I'm concerned every day," she replied. "I go into the kitchen or the bedroom and am constantly asking myself what am I hereafter?"

ATTRIBUTED TO REVEREND CHARLES ARA

When we consider uncomfortable topics like death or dementia, human nature often leads us to joke about them, just as Reverend Ara did. Humor gives us a measure of control, particularly when we haven't been affected personally by something.

Yet if you have trouble remembering things, memory loss is no laughing matter. For the last decade, I've been a consultant to FranklinCovey, the business consulting giant founded by Dr. Stephen Covey. One of the first people I met at the company was Todd, their "chief people officer." He was recording a conversation with me for one of their productivity programs. Todd started the interview by telling me he was 53 and his memory was terrible.

"I often have no idea where I put my keys and sometimes find them in the refrigerator, next to the eggs." He quickly chalked it up to his age.

"It is definitely not normal," I told him, pointing out that though I was older than he was, my memory was as sharp as ever. "It is one of the little lies people tell themselves to justify their memory problems and bad habits. The denial prevents them from getting the help they need. Tell me about your diet and exercise."

Todd's face brightened as he explained that he worked out five times a week. "I run long distances and am in great shape," he added.

"And your diet?" I asked.

Todd looked uncomfortable. "It's not so great," he said. "I usually have a Diet Coke and Pop-Tarts on the way to work. The rest of the day doesn't get much better."

We'd hit on one key source of Todd's memory troubles. A luxury car running on cheap fuel doesn't perform well, regardless of how much time and money an owner spends on its frame. Likewise, no matter how much Todd exercised, his brain was suffering because of the cheap fuel he was putting into his body.

I told Todd, "It's time to begin treating yourself as someone special rather than abusing your body." During the rest of our interview, I pointed out several ways he could better care for his brain.

When we talked again three months later, Todd told me he had fallen in love with his brain and was taking much better care of it. His memory had also significantly improved.

Smiling, he said, "You now haunt me at every meal."

I hope I can convince you to love your brain too. Perhaps the best way to do that is to help you understand just how complex and powerful it is—and appreciate the many parts of your brain that are involved in creating and retaining memory.

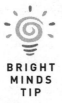

BRIGHT MINDS TIP

Fall in love with your brain.
It runs everything in your life.

Of course, your brain does far more than that. It runs your life and makes you who you are, producing your thoughts, feelings, plans, and behavior. It's the organ that enables you to learn, love, and work and it is at the center of every decision you make. A healthy brain leads to better decision making, which in turn leads to better relationships, job performance, finances, physical health, and overall happiness. Even though your brain makes up only about 2 percent of your body's weight (about three pounds), it uses 20 to 30 percent of the calories you take in, as well as 20 percent or more of the oxygen and blood flow in your body. The brain uses its approximately 86 billion neurons, which fire 18 trillion times a second,[1] to perceive and analyze incoming data; decide what, if anything, to do about it; and then execute your responses.

To understand how to strengthen your memory, it's important to understand how a healthy brain works and the role each of the four regions plays in the creation, storage, and retrieval of memories. Get ready for a fascinating insider's tour of the brain. My goal as your guide is that you come away from this chapter with a sense of wonder and awe and a better grasp of why it's so important to love and care for your brain. You get only one in life, and medical science sees no prospects for transplants for the foreseeable future. Taking care of your unique brain will contribute to your living a happier, healthier, more memorable life.

A GRAND TOUR OF THE BRAIN

The brain is divided into four main regions or lobes: frontal, temporal, parietal, and occipital. Generally speaking, the back half (the parietal and occipital lobes and the back part of the temporal lobe) perceives one's surroundings. The front half integrates what the body's senses take in and then analyzes that information before planning and carrying out decisions. The cerebellum lies behind the brain stem at the back and bottom of the brain.

The brain's CEO: frontal lobes and prefrontal cortex

The frontal lobes (the front half of the brain) are divided into three sections: the motor cortex, which controls the body's motor movements (such as jumping, chewing, and wiggling your fingers); the premotor area, which is involved in planning those movements; and the prefrontal cortex (PFC), which directs executive functions like forethought, judgment, and impulse control. Short-term and working memories are first processed in the PFC as well.

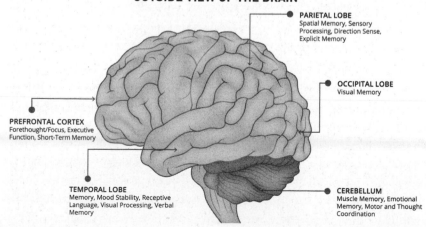

OUTSIDE VIEW OF THE BRAIN

PARIETAL LOBE
Spatial Memory, Sensory Processing, Direction Sense, Explicit Memory

OCCIPITAL LOBE
Visual Memory

PREFRONTAL CORTEX
Forethought/Focus, Executive Function, Short-Term Memory

TEMPORAL LOBE
Memory, Mood Stability, Receptive Language, Visual Processing, Verbal Memory

CEREBELLUM
Muscle Memory, Emotional Memory, Motor and Thought Coordination

The prefrontal cortex is responsible for the success of the human species. It enables us to learn from our mistakes and make plans. When the PFC is healthy, we behave consistently in ways that enable us to reach our goals. When it works as intended, we are organized, goal directed, thoughtful, empathetic, and able to express feelings appropriately. The PFC is often called the executive part of the brain and is closely associated with judgment, impulse control, attention span, self-monitoring, problem solving, and critical thinking. The prefrontal cortex is the brain's brake. It stops us from saying or doing stupid things.

I was once at a conference with a 42-year-old friend I'll call Joelle. She had been in a car accident that damaged her PFC a few years earlier. As we sat waiting for the next presentation, we overheard two women in the row in front of us talking about why they were heavy. One said to the other, "I don't know why I'm overweight; I just eat like a bird."

In a voice loud enough for everyone around us to hear, my friend said, "Yeah, like a condor."

Horrified, I gave Joelle a look that asked, *Why would you say that out loud?* Meanwhile the embarrassed and angry women moved away from us. Joelle put her hand over her mouth and said, "Oh no, did that get out?"

Not surprisingly, when the PFC isn't working as it should, problems such as impulsivity, distractibility, disorganization, faulty decision making, poor time management, and lack of empathy are evident. When such issues have been present someone's whole life, a developmental disorder such as attention deficit disorder (ADD), also known as attention deficit hyperactivity disorder (ADHD), might be to blame. Or if problems emerge early in life, they could be the result of a head injury, such as Joelle's. When developed later in life, they could be part of accelerated aging or a dementia-like process, such as frontotemporal lobe dementia or Alzheimer's disease in its later stages. If, say, Grandpa was a moral person his whole life but gradually began swearing more and doing unseemly things, such as making crude jokes or touching others inappropriately, it's likely a sign that his PFC is deteriorating.

Carl, 74, came to see us for depression, irritability, fatigue, and low motivation. His wife saw indications of short-term memory deficits, and he had more trouble making decisions. After grinding through a long series of failed therapies for years, his neurologist finally diagnosed him with Alzheimer's disease. Carl had nearly given up hope when he first considered seeing Brad Johnson, MD, at Amen Clinics outside of San Francisco. His insurance psychiatrist did not feel the need to do any imaging and discouraged him from coming to see us. When we scanned Carl's brain, we discovered a large benign tumor in his prefrontal cortex, crushing his brain. When it was removed, his depression and cognitive function dramatically improved.

CARL'S BRAIN SPECT SCAN

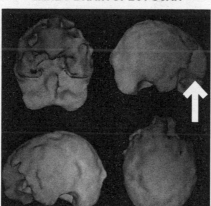

Severe deficit in prefrontal cortex

The social secretary: temporal lobes

The temporal lobes are located underneath your temples and behind your eyes. They are involved with encoding memories into long-term storage, as well as mood stability, receptive language (reading and hearing), the reading of social cues, and spiritual experience. The temporal lobes also house the "what pathway" in the brain, which helps you recognize objects by sight and name them. You can tell "what" they are.

A pair of thumb-sized structures on the inside of the temporal lobes are critical to our ability to learn and remember. Due to their shape, each is called the hippocampus, meaning "seahorse" in Greek. These are very special brain structures, because they house stem cells that can help produce new hippocampal cells under the right circumstances.[2] New research suggests we can produce up to 700 new cells a day if we provide them with a nourishing environment, which includes exercise (for better intake of oxygen and increased blood flow), proper nutrition, omega-3 fatty acids, and stimulation through mental exercise and social interactions.[3]

HIPPOCAMPUS COMPARED TO A SEAHORSE

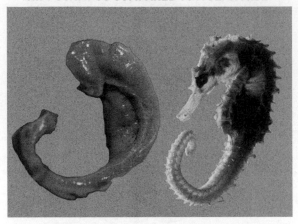

Our hippocampi (plural for *hippocampus*) encode new information and can store it for several weeks. If the information is reinforced, we keep it longer. In the movie *50 First Dates*, Lucy, Drew Barrymore's character, is in a severe car accident that damages her hippocampi. As a result, every evening when she falls asleep, memories of the prior day are wiped out. Although such a scenario is rare, it is possible. Each of the BRIGHT MINDS risk factors can also damage your hippocampi, making them smaller and weaker. *Memory Rescue* will give you many strategies to make them bigger and stronger.

BRIGHT MINDS TIP

The hippocampi are the star brain structures of your memory and this book. Without them you cannot store new information or experiences. Protect them at all costs.

UNDERSIDE OF THE BRAIN:
THE AMYGDALA AND HIPPOCAMPUS IN TEMPORAL LOBES

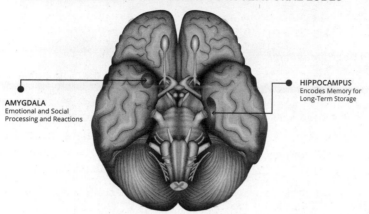

AMYGDALA
Emotional and Social
Processing and Reactions

HIPPOCAMPUS
Encodes Memory for
Long-Term Storage

In front of the hippocampus lies a critically important structure called the amygdala (derived from the Greek word for "almond" for its shape), which, as part of the brain's limbic system, coordinates emotional responses to what is happening around you. (Just as you have two hippocampi, you have a pair of amygdalae.) Strong emotions strengthen memory. Remember your first kiss? If you are older than 60, you likely remember where you were when President John F. Kennedy was shot in 1963 (I was in the third grade at Our Lady of Grace School, where I remember the nuns starting to cry at the news) or when the space shuttle *Challenger* exploded in 1986 (I was driving on the Likelike Highway on Oahu, where I was doing my child and adolescent psychiatry fellowship). And most Americans can recall what they were doing when the World Trade Center fell on 9/11 (I had just woken up at home in Newport Beach and turned on the television).

Emotional encoding of memories allows you to remember harrowing events, such as trauma, so that you can avoid them in the future, or awe-inspiring experiences, so that you can repeat them. In emphasizing the storage of certain experiences over others, the amygdala enables you to respond appropriately and rapidly in future situations; distancing yourself from someone lurking in a public stairway, for instance, could save your life. When the amygdala is operating correctly, your reactions to the world are logical. If your amygdala is overactive, you may overreact to events around you. If it is underactive, you may be unable to read situations accurately, and your response may be inappropriate. A good example: If you laugh when your boss tells you his mother died, your amygdala is underperforming.

Trouble in the temporal lobes can lead to both short- and long-term memory problems, along with reading difficulties, an inability to find the right words in conversation, trouble reading social cues, and mood instability. The temporal lobes, especially on the left side, have been associated with dark thoughts and temper problems.

The navigator: parietal lobes

The parietal lobes—the top, back part of the brain—are involved with important aspects of visual processing, such as seeing motion and tracking objects like a kite or a football in the air. They are involved with your sense of direction, as well as your ability to know right from left and to read and create maps in your mind. They are called the "where pathway" because they help us know where things are in space. Because they are involved in spatial awareness, when the parietal lobes are damaged, people tend to get lost, have trouble catching balls, or park cars at odd angles. The right parietal lobe perceives information from the left side of the body, while the left parietal lobe senses input from the right side. Additionally, these lobes help you understand what you read, perform basic symbolic operations involved in math (adding, subtracting, etc.), and rotate objects in your mind.

The parietal lobes are one of the first areas damaged in Alzheimer's disease. Because these lobes are heavily involved with directional sense, people with AD have trouble with navigation and driving, often getting lost. Because they may also have difficulty sensing their position or tracking objects visually, they may drop dishes, find parking a car difficult, or become confused when trying to put objects together (such as assembling an artificial Christmas tree). They also may experience trouble dressing, doing math, or writing; confuse their left and right; and have impaired copying, drawing, or cutting skills. Another symptom of impaired parietal lobes is denying these problems, so those affected may not even recognize the serious issues they may have with directions, driving, or communicating.

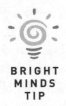

BRIGHT MINDS TIP

Be careful with your GPS. It may give you a false sense of "memory" security.

|||||||||||||||||||||||||||||||||||||||||||||||||||||||||||||||||||||||||||||||||||||||||

Why Is Alzheimer's Disease Being Diagnosed Later?

It's the smartphone in your pocket or purse. Twenty years ago, I would see patients with Alzheimer's disease soon after they had gotten lost driving to the home where they had lived for decades. They would end up on the other side of town in tears, and their family would bring them in the next week, anxious and upset. Now, because of the astonishingly accurate GPS devices built into most smartphones, when people get lost, they just ask the phone to take them home, which it does. This can delay the diagnosis and assistance, which is more likely to help when it is given early.

|||||||||||||||||||||||||||||||||||||||||||||||||||||||||||||||||||||||||||||||||||||||||

The seer: occipital lobes

The occipital lobes, located at the back of the brain, process visual information. Light enters the retinas, each of which sends signals to the occipital lobe on the opposite side. Light, shade, color, and basic shapes are sorted out in the occipital lobes. When these lobes are damaged, sight and perception are often affected. Visual hallucinations, illusions, or blindness sometimes occur. When one side of the occipital lobe isn't working, you can't see the opposite side of your environment. That means if the left lobe is malfunctioning, you can't see objects to your right. A type of dementia called Lewy body dementia (LBD), associated with Parkinson's disease, often begins with symptoms of occipital lobe damage, such as visual hallucinations.

The coordinator: cerebellum

The cerebellum, Latin for "little brain," is located behind the brain stem at the base of the brain and helps control physical coordination, as well as the precision of movement and timing. It also plays a role in the speed of thought, speech, and physical movement. Damage to the cerebellum can lead to slowed thinking, speaking, and moving.

New research shows that the cerebellum may also be involved with higher-level thinking, including attention, learning, working memory, language, judgment, and "thought" coordination, or our ability to integrate new information. The left side of the cerebellum plays a role with right-hemisphere tasks in the brain, such as seeing the big picture and reading social cues, while the right cerebellum assists with left-hemisphere tasks, such as language. Damage to one side of the frontal or temporal lobes tends to turn off the cerebellum on the opposite side, a condition called crossed cerebellar diaschisis. Coordination exercises, such as dance, tennis, table tennis, and tai chi, can strengthen this part of the brain.

BRAIN REGIONS: HOW THEY WORK, WHAT CAN GO HAYWIRE

BRAIN SYSTEM	FUNCTIONS	PROBLEMS
Prefrontal Cortex	Focus Forethought Judgment Impulse control Organization Planning Empathy Learning from mistakes	Short attention span Acting without thinking Poor judgment Impulse control problems Disorganization Lack of planning Lack of empathy Trouble learning from experience
Temporal Lobes	Hearing/listening Reading Interpreting social cues, including tone of voice Short- and long-term memory Recognizing objects by sight Mood stability Naming things	Mishears communication Dyslexia Socially inappropriate behavior Trouble reading social cues Memory problems Word-finding problems Poor visual recognition Mood instability Abnormal sensory perceptions Anger, irritability, dark thoughts
Parietal Lobes	Sense of direction Sensory perception Spatial processing Seeing motion Visual guidance, such as to grab objects Recognizing objects by touch Ability to know where you are in space Knowing right from left Reading and creating maps	Impaired sense of direction Trouble dressing or assembling objects Left-right confusion Denial of problems or illness Impaired position sense Difficulty with math or writing Neglect or unawareness of what one sees Problems copying, drawing, or cutting

Occipital Lobes	Vision Color perception Depth perception	Deficits in vision Deficits in perception Visual hallucination Visual illusions Functional blindness
Cerebellum	Motor coordination Thought coordination Impulse control Organization Speed of thought (like clock speed of computer)	Coordination problems Slowed walking Slowed thinking Slowed speech Disorganization Impulsiveness Poor learning

HOW THE BRAIN'S NEURONS TALK TO ONE ANOTHER

How does each region of the brain communicate with the others? Like every organ, the brain has its own set of specialized cells. Its primary working cell is the neuron, and there are roughly 86 billion of them in the brain. A neuron is similar in structure to other cells in the body, except it has two kinds of extensions (see "Healthy Brain Neuron" below). Dendrites, which look like bushes or tree branches, receive information from other brain cells, while the axon—a single, taillike extension—sends information to other neurons. Dendrites and axons can grow and be modified throughout life, depending on our experiences and the environment in which we live.

HEALTHY BRAIN NEURON

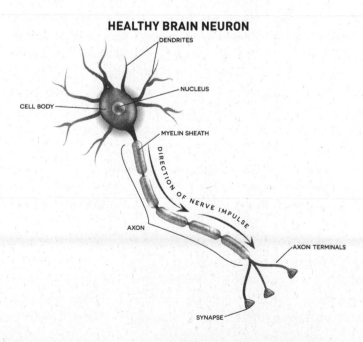

Neurons make up the brain's electrical information highway network. Their main job is to generate electrical signals to stimulate other neurons, like tiny lightning bolts traveling down axons at speeds as fast as 250 miles per hour. When an electrical signal reaches the end of the axon, it stimulates the release of neurotransmitters, or chemical messengers, into the synapse, or space between neurons, to excite or calm nearby neurons. Glutamate, the primary "excitatory" neurotransmitter, is released by 75 percent of all neurons in the brain. About 20 percent of neurons release GABA (gamma-aminobutyric acid), the primary "calming" neurotransmitter, which helps control anxiety. Other neurotransmitters include serotonin, which helps us feel happy and worry-free; dopamine, which improves motivation and focus; and acetylcholine, which helps us learn and remember. When enough neurons are stimulated, they create a network effect to perform specific brain functions, such as walking or thinking.

Each neuron is connected to as many as 1,000 other neurons. Scientists estimate that they exchange signals via about 100 trillion synaptic connections. Clearly the brain's storage capacity is vast, but it's nearly impossible to calculate exactly how many memories and pieces of information the human brain can hold.

HOW MEMORIES ARE MADE

Though the biology of memory is complex, the more you know about it, the better you'll understand how you can improve it. There are three main stages involved in memory: encoding, storage, and recall. Your senses—taste, sight, touch, smell, and hearing—linked with emotion are the raw ingredients for making memories. Your brain processes your experiences to form memories, whether it be through consciously focusing on something (like studying) or subconsciously creating associations (like attaching emotional significance to new information—think of your first day of school). With each new experience, your brain forms new connections and slightly rewires itself—an ability known as neuroplasticity.

Encoding is the first step to creating a memory. It occurs when your brain attaches meaning to experiences or determines why something happened. Studies show that we remember things better and retain them longer when we associate them with a purpose.

Storage is the next step in memory. Research suggests that the brain doesn't store memories in complete, exact recollections that it can simply retrieve. Rather, memories are stored in small bits scattered in different areas of the brain. The hippocampus is a critical gateway to long-term storage for memories. If the hippocampus is damaged, you may not be able to recall what happened yesterday.

Recall is how your brain retrieves a memory. During recall, your brain reconstructs the memory from the smaller stored pieces. When you remember something, it's not an exact "replay" of the experience. It's more like a creative reimagining, such as when you "remember" catching a 10-foot catfish last summer. That's why memories can change over time. When your brain recalls a memory, it stimulates nerve pathways that were created when the memory was formed. Repeatedly working your memory strengthens it over time.

Forming memories requires an intricate dance between cell membranes and the chemicals inside and outside of cells, especially glutamate and acetylcholine. As we age, glutamate tends to go up, which can overstimulate and be toxic for cells, while acetylcholine tends to go down, which is one reason memory suffers.

Variations of memory

The two tables below describe the different types of memory, how long they last, and the areas of the brain with which they are associated. Which ones are giving you trouble?

MEMORY DECODED

TYPE OF MEMORY	HOW LONG IT LASTS	ASSOCIATED BRAIN AREA
Sensory	< 1 second (most lost, since not encoded)	Visual-sensory cortex (parietal/occipital)
Short-term	< 60 seconds (such as a phone number)	Prefrontal cortex
Working	Seconds to hours (cramming for an exam)	Prefrontal cortex
Long-term	Hours to months	Hippocampus—the "gateway" brain structure. Long-term memories pass through the hippocampus and are then stored all over the brain: visual cues are stored in occipital lobes, sensory cues in parietal lobes, sounds in temporal lobes, etc.
Long-lasting	Months to a lifetime	Hippocampus, then all over the brain

LONG-TERM MEMORY

TYPES OF LONG-TERM OR LONG-LASTING MEMORIES	DESCRIPTION
Explicit	Conscious
Declarative	Facts and knowledge
Episodic	Life events and experiences
Semantic	Meaning of things (words, ideas, concepts)
Flashbulb	Emotionally charged
Implicit	Unconscious
Muscle	Automatic movements (riding a bike, swimming)
Emotional	Unconscious emotional reactions
Verbal	Words and abstractions of language
Spatial	Navigating space
Visual	How the world looks
Associative	Relationships between unrelated items, such as a person's name and the aroma of her perfume

BIRTH, AND DEATH, OF BRAIN CELLS

Neurogenesis is the word for the birth of new brain cells, but the birth cycle begins with death. Let's say someone goes to a New Year's Eve party and has a little too much champagne. He comes home and sleeps it off. By the time he wakes, several hundred thousand neurons may have died from alcohol toxicity. His brain will try to replenish its stores of neurons. The act of neurons dying triggers certain growth factors, such as the release of BDNF (brain-derived neurotrophic factor), to stimulate the growth of new neurons. But too many toxins over time can overpower neurogenesis. As a result, more cells die than are made, and the brain begins to shrink or atrophy.

Fortunately, you are not powerless to stop your brain from shrinking. In upcoming chapters, I will provide dozens of recommendations, from dietary changes to exercise options to beneficial supplements and more, designed to increase your brain's neurogenesis. If you love your brain, you can fight back to make it healthier and improve your memory.

MEMORY RESCUE: BRIGHT MINDS TAKEAWAYS

1. Fall in love with your brain. It's the most important part of you.

2. The prefrontal cortex is the brain's brake. It stops you from saying or doing stupid things. Protect it.

3. Your hippocampus is the gateway brain structure for memory.

4. Emotion anchors memory.

CHAPTER 3

WHAT TROUBLE LOOKS LIKE
HOW BRAIN IMAGING CHANGES EVERYTHING

Take away the brain, you take away the person.
MARIAN DIAMOND, PhD, UC BERKELEY

If you knew a train was going to hit you, would you get out of the way? A news story described the plight of two women trapped on an 80-foot-high railroad bridge in Indiana as a freight train barreled toward them. There was no way they could get out of its path! Ultimately, the women survived by lying down flat in the middle of the tracks, but what were they doing on an active railroad bridge with no escape route? I often include this story when I lecture because it reminds me of how blind most people are to the health of their brains. Like the women on the tracks, they are heading down a potentially deadly path. If you knew brain problems were coming for you, would you start making better decisions today to get out of the way?

All of us need a baseline brain health assessment to find out if our brains are in trouble. Unfortunately, this is rarely done. When I turned 50, my doctor wanted me to have a colonoscopy. I asked him why he didn't want to look at my brain. "Isn't the other end of my body just as important?" I asked. From colonoscopies and cardiac stress tests to mammograms and pap smears, baseline testing and preventive screening are done for most organs *except* the most important one—the organ that runs your life. That is just plain wrong when illnesses like Alzheimer's disease that rob people's very souls are expected to skyrocket in the coming decades.

This chapter will explore the early warning signs of trouble, a simple computerized test that can help you evaluate your cognitive abilities, and the brain imaging tests we use at Amen Clinics. Even if you never get a brain scan, the lessons they have taught us provide the foundation for *Memory Rescue*.

At Amen Clinics, the first thing we do when we meet a new patient is take a very detailed history. Understanding the story of a person's life is critical to getting the right diagnosis and developing an effective treatment plan. Since problems in the brain typically start years before people have any symptoms, it is essential to understand the early warning signs.

It's like the boiling frog analogy: If a frog is put suddenly into boiling water, it will jump out; but if the frog is put in cold water that is very gradually brought to a boil, it will not perceive the danger and will be cooked to death. We and our family members tend either to miss or discount the small, incremental changes that taken together can add up to significant problems.

A simple way to avoid making this mistake is to take a self-assessment regularly, beginning now and then every year hereafter. It highlights the most significant early warning signs of memory problems.

AMEN CLINICS' EARLY WARNING SIGNS QUESTIONNAIRE

Rate each question on a scale of 0–4, from Never (0) to Very Frequently (4).

0	1	2	3	4
Never	Rarely	Occasionally	Frequently	Very Frequently

Memory issues

1. ___ Tend to be forgetful?

2. ___ Notice that your memory, which has never been good, is getting worse?

3. ___ Misplace your keys or wallet?

4. ___ Wonder why you came into a room?

5. ___ Have trouble remembering names?

6. ___ Feel embarrassed by forgetting appointments?

7. ___ Read a book or an article, but don't remember much of it?

8. ___ Have trouble remembering things that happened recently?

9. ___ Struggle with brain fog?

10. ___ Have trouble remembering to consistently take medications or supplements?

11. ___ Rely more and more on memory aids or reminders on your phone?

12. ___ Know something one day but forget it the next?

13. ___ Forget what you're going to say right in the middle of saying it?

14. ___ Have trouble following directions that have more than one or two steps?

15. ___ Suspect that your memory is worse than it was 10 years ago?

16. ___ Lose track of the conversation?

17. ___ Find things in unusual places, like your keys in the refrigerator?

18. ___ Get mad at others, thinking they took your things, only to find out later you misplaced them?

Trouble planning and problem solving

19. ___ Have trouble making plans and sticking to them?

20. ___ Find it harder to follow a recipe or directions on how to put something together?

21. ___ Find it hard to focus on more complex tasks, especially those that involve math? For example, are you struggling with managing your bills or balancing your checkbook?

Confusion with times and places

22. ___ Have trouble driving to locations that had been familiar to you?

23. ___ Get easily confused or out of sorts?

24. ___ Get lost more easily or have to rely on GPS more than before?

Struggle with words

25. ___ Have more trouble finding the right word?

26. ___ Call things by the wrong name?

27. ___ Limit conversation with people, rather than join in?

28. ___ Have trouble following along in conversations?

29. ___ Keep repeating yourself?

Worsening judgment

30. ___ Struggle with making more bad decisions?

31. ___ Make mistakes with your finances?

Social withdrawal

32. ___ Feel more isolated from friends?

33. ___ Feel like cutting back at work because you just don't care as much?

34. ___ Feel less interested in activities you usually find fun?

35. ___ Take less care of your physical appearance?

Scoring:

Add up the number of questions that you answered 3 (Frequently) or 4 (Very Frequently).

    0   low risk of significant memory issues
    1–2 mild risk of significant memory issues
    3–5 moderate risk of significant memory issues
    6+ high risk of significant memory issues

Of course, everyone should take brain health and our BRIGHT MINDS approach seriously; the higher you score, the more serious you should be. If you are at moderate to high risk, it is important to get a thorough medical evaluation.

A RELIABLE COGNITIVE TEST

Several online cognitive tests can give you a sense of how well your brain is functioning compared to an age-matched group. At Amen Clinics, we use a comprehensive online test called Brain Fit WebNeuro that measures a wide range of cognitive and emotional functions. It takes about 35 minutes to complete and provides an objective assessment of how your brain works in 17 specific areas, scoring each one on a scale of 1 to 10. The test also generates an overall brain health score. Specifically, it measures:

1. Motor coordination
2. Processing speed (how quickly you process information)
3. Sustained attention (ability to maintain focus)

4. Controlled attention (ability to stop reactions when needed)
5. Flexibility (shifting attention)
6. Inhibition (self-control)
7. Working memory (ability to hold information for short periods)
8. Recall memory (ability to remember information)
9. Executive function (ability to plan and organize information)
10. Identifying emotions (reading faces)
11. Emotion bias (impact of emotions on decision making)
12. Stress level
13. Anxiety level
14. Depressed mood
15. Positivity-negativity bias (tendency to notice positive or negative emotions)
16. Resilience (coping during times of trial)
17. Social capacity (building and keeping relationships)

You can take this test through our online Brain Fit Life program (www.mybrainfitlife.com). It will provide you with a baseline score and, with retesting, a way to find out over time if your brain function is getting better or worse. Based on your scores, our program recommends targeted exercises in the form of fun brain games to strengthen vulnerable areas.

Determining the health of your brain with baseline testing is a critical strategy to keeping it strong over the long run. Studies have found that adding a brief objective assessment tool can improve early detection of trouble by more than nine times![1] New research shows that it is possible to detect the seeds of Alzheimer's disease in lower memory and thinking scores obtained up to 18 years in advance of a diagnosis,[2] when it is more likely that something can be done about it.

If you are at moderate or high risk for memory problems, consider taking the Brain Fit WebNeuro test every few months to chart your progress. I also recommend everyone 40 or older take this test annually to spot issues early. Baseline testing and regular checkups can also help you uncover problems when they first appear.

EXAMPLE OF WEBNEURO RESULTS

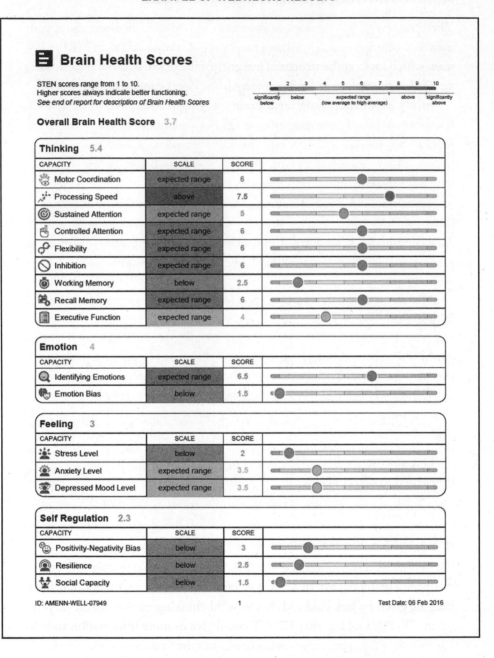

Be concerned about any individual scores below 5. In this example, there
are issues with working memory and executive function (judgment).
Emotion bias, stress, anxiety, depression, negativity, low resilience, and
social isolation also seem to be issues, which can weaken memory.

AMEN CLINICS' BRAIN IMAGING TOOLS

There are several ways to look at your brain if you are concerned about your memory. Most physicians will order an imaging study, such as an MRI or CT scan, which looks at the structural integrity of the brain. Most of these studies are read as normal, or as "mild atrophy (shrinkage) consistent with aging."

In my experience, functional brain imaging studies, like SPECT, PET (positron-emission tomography), or QEEG (quantitative electroencephalogram) are more useful, because *functional problems almost always precede structural ones.* These studies typically show problems before symptoms occur, which is when treatment is likely to be most helpful.

Functional studies are leading indicators of problems, meaning they show evidence of the disease process years before people show signs of it. Anatomical studies, such as CT and MRI, are lagging indicators. They show problems later in the course of the illness, when interventions tend to be less effective.

At Amen Clinics, we find two functional brain imaging studies particularly helpful.

1. Brain SPECT imaging: This scan looks at blood flow and activity patterns and shows us areas of the brain that are functionally healthy, underactive, or overactive.
2. QEEG testing: This scan shows the electrical activity in the brain.

Due to cost, PET scans are not commonly used, though they are sometimes used to detect plaques in the brain associated with Alzheimer's disease (see "What about Amyloid Imaging with PET Scans?" on page 38).

Brain SPECT imaging: seeing is believing

I became hooked on functional imaging, and SPECT in particular, because it made me a better doctor. In 1991, I went to my first lecture on brain SPECT imaging given by Jack Paldi, MD, a forward-thinking nuclear medicine physician. Dr. Paldi told us that SPECT could give us more information to help our patients. In fact, the scan results of eight of the first ten patients for which I ordered SPECT led me to change what I did for them. When it came to memory problems, the story of one woman remains deeply embedded in my own memory. In fact, I talk about her often because her case helped convince me of how invaluable SPECT can be.

||||||||||||||||||||||||||||||||||||||||||||||||||||||||||||||||||||||||||||||||||||||||||||

Dementia: Not Just Alzheimer's

Alzheimer's is the most common type of dementia—estimated to account for 60 to 80 percent of cases. Widespread damage occurs in the brain as neurons die after they stop functioning and connecting with other neurons. However, other forms of dementia also create serious problems. They include:

- *Vascular dementia*, the second most common type of dementia, typically occurs as a result of one or more strokes that have created blockages to the brain's blood vessels.
- *Lewy body dementia* refers to both Parkinson's disease and dementia with Lewy bodies, abnormal protein deposits that disrupt the brain's normal functioning.
- *Frontotemporal lobe dementia* is caused by progressive nerve cell loss in the frontal or temporal lobes, stemming from various uncommon disorders that cause the affected lobes to atrophy.

||||||||||||||||||||||||||||||||||||||||||||||||||||||||||||||||||||||||||||||||||||||||||||

Margaret: was it really Alzheimer's?

Margaret, 68, had been diagnosed with Alzheimer's disease by her family physician. She wanted to continue living independently, but her five daughters were afraid for her and wanted her to move into a supervised senior living facility. After Margaret left something burning on the stove—nearly burning down her home as a result—she was admitted to the hospital. Her family wanted her evaluated one more time before seeking a legal custody order to force her into supervised living.

When I first evaluated Margaret in the early 1990s, she appeared to have Alzheimer's disease. She was seriously forgetful, neglecting her appearance, and frequently getting lost driving. However, when I studied her SPECT scan, I realized that her brain did not look like one affected by Alzheimer's disease. The scientific literature in the late 1980s had described Alzheimer's as decreased blood flow in the parietal and temporal lobes. Those areas of Margaret's brain looked fine. But she had marked increases in blood flow in the emotional part of her brain.

Based on her scan, I suspected Margaret had something called pseudo-dementia, which is depression that results in dementia-like symptoms. I

MARGARET'S BRAIN SPECT SCAN

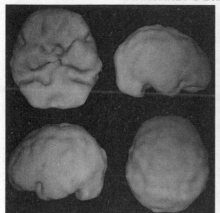

Full, even, symmetrical activity
not typical of Alzheimer's

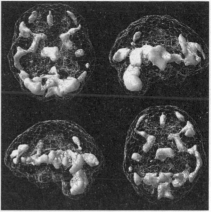

Increased activity in the emotional brain

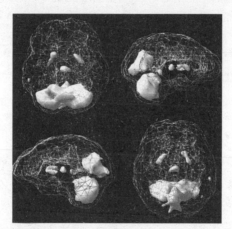

Normal active scan: In a healthy SPECT scan, the most active
areas are in the back part of the brain in the cerebellum.

prescribed the stimulating antidepressant Wellbutrin (bupropion), hoping
for the best. Within three weeks, Margaret had dramatically improved. She
was much more talkative, took better care of her appearance, and even led
cooking classes in the hospital. I have never forgotten her amazing transfor-
mation. She lived independently for another 15 years.

Brain SPECT imaging has taught me that there are many treatable causes
of memory problems. *But if you never look at how the brain functions, you will
never know how to address them.* Too many people diagnosed with Alzheimer's
disease or other forms of dementia have potentially treatable problems—and
may not even have a true form of dementia. A 2017 study from the University

of California at San Francisco using PET imaging drives this point home: When the researchers scanned 4,000 patients with mild cognitive impairment or dementia for the amyloid plaques that can be a sign of Alzheimer's, they discovered that just 54.3 percent of those with MCI and 70.5 percent of dementia patients had the plaques. Those who tested negative for the plaques—including some who'd been diagnosed with Alzheimer's—definitely did not have AD. Doctors altered the treatment for *two-thirds* of the enrolled patients as a result of the imaging.[3]

I learned early on that SPECT imaging can also be a useful tool when trying to distinguish Alzheimer's from other forms of dementia. That brings me to another case that was key to my understanding of SPECT imaging's potential.

Ed: the sign of the lobster

Ed, 72, came to Amen Clinics because his daughter Candace was concerned about his forgetfulness. His mood and judgment were poor, and when Candace looked at his finances, she discovered he had paid some bills twice and forgotten others. The local neurologist diagnosed Ed with Alzheimer's disease. Candace had read about SPECT imaging in my book *Change Your Brain, Change Your Life* and was unhappy that the doctor had made that diagnosis without ordering a scan. She then brought Ed to see us.

ED'S BRAIN SPECT SCAN

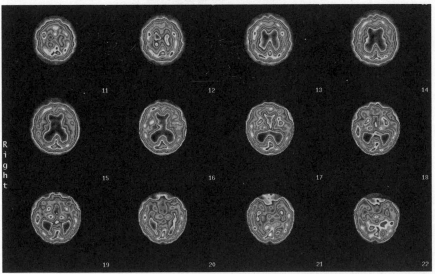

The image shows slices from the top to the bottom of the brain.
Slices 15 and 16 show the "lobster sign," which suggested that Ed
was suffering from a condition other than Alzheimer's.

Ed's SPECT scan revealed very large ventricles, or fluid-filled cavities, in his brain. I have labeled this pattern the "lobster sign" because it looks like an upside-down lobster in the brain slice images on page 36. The scan also revealed low activity in Ed's cerebellum (base of his brain). Ed definitely did not have the typical Alzheimer's pattern.

NORMAL BRAIN SPECT SCAN

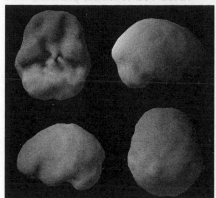

Full, even, symmetrical activity

ED'S BRAIN SPECT SCAN

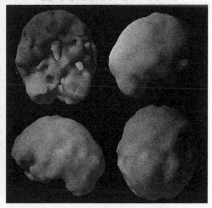

Not typical Alzheimer's pattern,
but large ventricles (middle hole)
and small cerebellum (bottom)

The reason finding the large ventricles was so important was that it is a classic sign of normal pressure hydrocephalus, or NPH. In this condition, the normal drainage of cerebrospinal fluid is gradually blocked. As a result, excessive fluid builds up slowly, over time. This disorder is often, but not always, accompanied by urinary incontinence and trouble walking. Because Ed did not have those other symptoms, his neurologist never suspected NPH. Subsequently, Ed's brain continued to deteriorate. Upon seeing his scan, I recommended Ed have an immediate neurosurgical consultation. The neurosurgeon agreed with me and placed a shunt in Ed's brain. Within three weeks, Ed's memory came back. *How do you know unless you look?*

Not one thing

As I have written about in several of my previous books, one of the biggest lessons from our brain imaging work at Amen Clinics is that *all* psychiatric illnesses, including ADHD, anxiety, depression, and addictions, are not single or simple disorders in the brain; they *all* have multiple types that need their own unique treatments.

SPECT has taught us that memory problems are similar. Just as there are many roads to depression, so, too, are there many roads to losing your memory. As we will see throughout the rest of the book, SPECT can help in the diagnosis of different types of memory problems. Not only can it help diagnose Alzheimer's disease and other forms of dementia, it can also suggest mild cognitive impairment stemming from such causes as head trauma, infections, toxins, and depression.

|||||||||||||||||||||||||||||||||||||||||||||||||||||||||||||||||||||||||||||||||||||||||||||||||||||||||||||||

What About Amyloid Imaging with PET Scans?

Many scientists believe that Alzheimer's disease is caused by the accumulation of toxic beta-amyloid plaques, sticky clumps of proteins that cause short circuits in the brain, as well as the formation of tangles inside neurons from inflamed tau proteins. The plaques and tau proteins begin forming before Alzheimer's symptoms become obvious.

AUTOPSY MICROSCOPIC BRAIN TISSUE

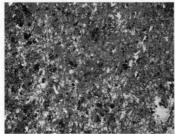 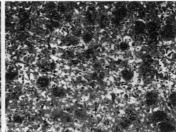

Healthy neurons:
no amyloid plaques

Unhealthy neurons:
loaded with amyloid plaques

Based on the assumption that early detection of these processes would lead to earlier detection—and possibly better outcomes—for Alzheimer's patients, several companies developed amyloid imaging agents for the brain, and they are currently working on tau imaging tools. Unfortunately, amyloid scans can tell only one thing: whether or not a person has classic Alzheimer's caused by amyloid. Plus, all the drugs that target the cleanup of these two toxic proteins have failed in clinical trials. Eliminating the amyloid plaques and tau proteins after they have caused damage has not been helpful. This suggests targeting Alzheimer's is more complicated than finding a one-size-fits-all solution.

SPECT imaging, on the other hand, potentially gives information on 10 different causes of memory loss, consistent with the BRIGHT MINDS risk factors. (See table below for a summary of the types of memory loss and dementia with the SPECT findings.) When evaluated with other presenting issues, it allows us to address the specific causes of memory loss.

||||||||||||||||||||||||||||||||||||||||||||||||||||||||||||||||||||||||||||||||||||||||||||||||||||

BRIGHT MINDS: CLINICAL ISSUES AND SPECT FINDINGS

RISK FACTOR	CLINICAL ISSUES	SPECT FINDINGS
Blood Flow	Memory loss tends to go down in a stepwise manner, rather than a consistently progressive decline	Overall low blood flow; larger strokes seen on SPECT
Retirement/Aging	Progressive memory loss with age	Overall low blood flow, especially in the parietal and temporal lobes
Inflammation	Progressive memory loss, also associated with depression and pain	Overall low blood flow, seen in all areas of the brain
Genetics	Progressive memory loss, direction sense, and thinking skills	Decreased blood flow in parietal and temporal lobes
Head Trauma	History of repetitive head trauma	Focal damage, especially affecting the frontal and temporal lobes
Toxins	History of toxic exposure or excessive alcohol intake	Overall decreased blood flow in a scalloped pattern
Mental Health	History of depression in self or family members	Increased limbic activity; less decreased activity than other types
Immunity/Infectious Issues	History of autoimmune or untreated infections, such as Lyme disease or syphilis	Overall decreased blood flow in a scalloped pattern
Neurohormone Deficiencies	Low thyroid, testosterone, estrogen, progesterone	Overall low blood flow

RISK FACTOR	CLINICAL ISSUES	SPECT FINDINGS
Diabesity	High BMI and blood glucose levels	Overall low blood flow
Sleep Issues	Sleep apnea, chronic insomnia	Decreased blood flow, especially in the parietal lobes

SPECT examples

HEALTHY

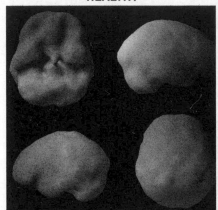

Overall full, even, symmetrical blood flow

CLASSIC ALZHEIMER'S DISEASE

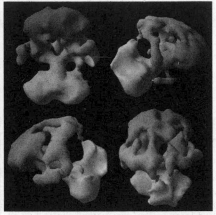

Parietal/temporal lobe decreases

FRONTOTEMPORAL LOBE DEMENTIA

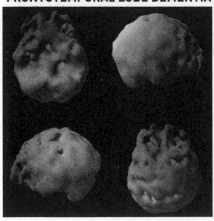

Frontotemporal lobe decreases

VASCULAR DEMENTIA

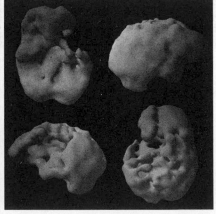

Due to blood vessel changes or one large stroke or multiple small strokes

LEWY BODY DEMENTIA, ASSOCIATED WITH PARKINSON'S

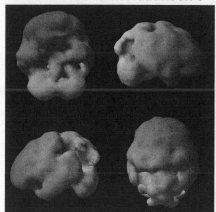

Occipital lobe decreases

NORMAL PRESSURE HYDROCEPHALUS

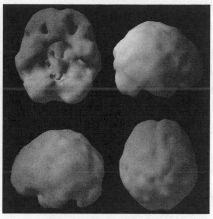

Large ventricles, with lobster pattern seen on brain slices

ALCOHOLISM

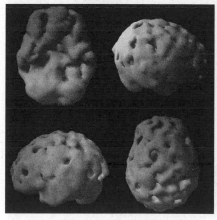

Overall decreased blood flow

INFECTION (LYME DISEASE)

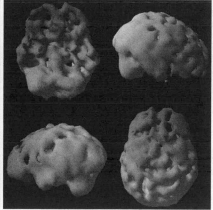

Overall decreased blood flow

TOXIN (MOLD EXPOSURE)

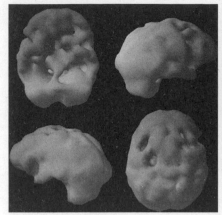

Overall decreased blood flow

TRAUMATIC BRAIN INJURY

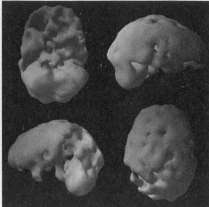

Decreases in areas hurt

DEPRESSION

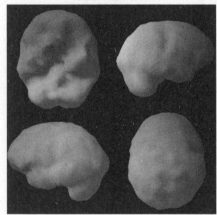

Outside surface often healthier

DEPRESSION

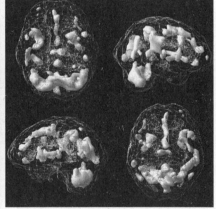

Increased activity in limbic structures

Quantitative electroencephalogram (QEEG)

QEEG is a tool we use for patients who are pregnant or are concerned about radiation exposure for any other reason. We may use it in combination with a SPECT scan if we need more information on the underlying cause of symptoms. With a QEEG, powerful computer programs take electrical signals from the brain and break them into five distinct brain wave patterns, showing how much of each is present compared to an age- and gender-matched healthy group. There are literally thousands of studies on QEEG for a wide variety of clinical indications, including memory problems, anxiety, depression, traumatic brain injury, and ADHD.

The five commonly discussed types of brain wave patterns, from the slowest to the fastest:

- *delta waves* (1–4 cycles per second): very slow brain waves, seen mostly during sleep
- *theta waves* (5–7 cycles per second): slow brain waves, seen during daydreaming and twilight states
- *alpha waves* (8–12 cycles per second): brain waves seen during relaxed states
- *beta waves* (13–20 cycles per second): fast brain waves seen during concentration or mental work states
- *high beta waves* (21–40 cycles per second): fast brain waves seen during intense concentration or anxiety

Memory issues typically show up as too much delta or theta activity, and QEEG helps us determine whether neurofeedback could be a helpful part of a patient's treatment plan.

QEEG EXAMPLES
No color represents normal limits. The deeper the gray color, the higher the activity in each band.

HEALTHY (ALL BANDS WITHIN NORMAL LIMITS)

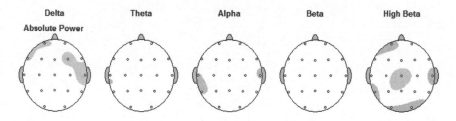

HIGH ALPHA IN EXPERIENCED MEDITATOR

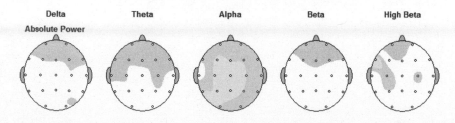

VERY HIGH THETA IN DEMENTIA PATIENT

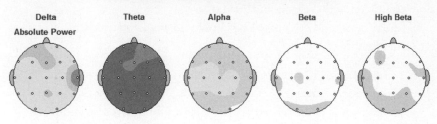

Delta   Theta   Alpha   Beta   High Beta
Absolute Power

   Throughout the course of my career I have often said, "A picture is worth a thousand words, but a map is worth a thousand pictures. A map tells you where you are and gives you directions on how to get to where you want to go."

   Without a map, you are lost. Not knowing the proper routes to get you back on track can cost you precious time in getting the help you need. At Amen Clinics we think of SPECT and QEEG as maps to help guide people to better brains and better lives.

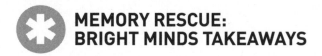 ## MEMORY RESCUE: BRIGHT MINDS TAKEAWAYS

Now that you know how to begin assessing the health of your brain, consider how you will use this information:

1. Do you have early warning symptoms? Which ones?

2. When will you test your brain?

3. Would you look at your brain, given the chance? I recommend people be screened at the age of 50, or as early as 40 if there is a history of dementia in their families.

PART 2

BRIGHT MINDS: THE ULTIMATE MEMORY FORMULA

CHAPTER 4

THE BRIGHT MINDS APPROACH TO RESCUING YOUR MEMORY

THE BEST WAY TO HELP PREVENT OR TREAT MEMORY DECLINE AND ALZHEIMER'S IS TO KNOW AND ADDRESS ALL YOUR RISK FACTORS

*If you are sitting on a tack, the treatment is not two Advil every three
to four hours. The treatment for "tack sitting" is "tack removal." Search
for the root and treat the cause rather than the symptoms.
If you are sitting on two tacks, removing one tack does not eliminate
50 percent of the symptoms. Complex conditions are "complex."
To be effective address all the underlying causes for resolution.*

SIDNEY BAKER, MD, INTEGRATIVE MEDICINE PIONEER

The reality is this: If you want a stellar memory, you need to know all the potential contributors that can destroy it and address each one. As Jesus told his followers, "You will know the truth, and the truth will make you free" (John 8:32, NCV). But first, at least when it comes to adopting a healthier lifestyle, the truth is likely to make you miserable!

We don't like to face the truth about ourselves—our weaknesses, bad habits, and vulnerabilities. However, until we own up to them and get serious about change, our attempts will likely be fleeting, and we'll be distracted by the next popular fad.

And change we must. I truly believe that *a single pill will never fix memory decline, aging, or Alzheimer's disease because there are too many ways trouble can occur.* This is a war that must be fought on multiple fronts.

I have organized the key risk factors on the following pages according to my BRIGHT MINDS model, with each component weighted in terms of just how damaging it can be to your brain and memory. In the following chapters, I'll go through all of the risk factors and provide strategies to turn each of them around. But first you need to know where you stand.

Mark the risks that apply to you. If you don't know whether you have a risk factor, refer to the specific chapter to learn more. When you get to the end of the assessment, add up your score. The number in parentheses next to each risk factor is the relative increase in risk for memory problems, accelerated aging, and AD compared to those without that risk factor. Here's how it translates: 1.3 = 30 percent increased risk; 1.5 = 50 percent increased risk; 2 = double the risk, 3 = triple the risk, and so on.

Blood Flow

1. History of a stroke (5)[1]
2. History of cardiovascular disease, including coronary artery disease, heart attacks, heart failure, and heart arrhythmias (2)[2]
3. Prehypertension or hypertension in midlife (2)[3]; low blood pressure in later life (1.3)[4]
4. Erectile dysfunction (1.7 for all ages; 6.1 between 50 and 64; and 27.2 for men over age 65)[5]
5. Limited exercise (less than twice a week) (2)[6]

Retirement/Aging

6. Age: 65 to 84 (2), 85 and older (38)[7]
7. Too much television viewing (more than two hours a day) (2)[8]
8. A job that does not require new learning (2)[9] or retirement without new learning endeavors
9. Loneliness or social isolation (2)[10]

Inflammation

10. Periodontal (gum) disease (2)[11]
11. Presence of inflammation in the body, indicated by high homocysteine or C-reactive protein (2)[12]
12. Low omega-3 fatty acids (see information on the Omega-3 Index test, page 102, chapter 7) (2)[13]

Genetics

13. One family member with Alzheimer's or dementia (3.5); more than one family member with Alzheimer's or dementia (7.5)[14]

14. One apolipoprotein E (*APOE*) e4 gene (2.5) or two *APOE* e4 genes (10)[15] (if known, based on genetic testing)

Head Trauma

15. A single head injury with loss of consciousness (2)[16]
16. Several head injuries without a loss of consciousness (2)[17]
17. Loss of one's sense of smell (2)[18]

Toxins

18. Smoking cigarettes for 10 years or longer (currently or in past) (2.3)[19]
19. Alcohol dependence or drug dependence (currently or in past) (4.4)[20]
20. History of radiation for head and neck cancers (3);[21] chemotherapy for breast cancer (1.5),[22] colorectal cancer (1.25),[23] and possibly other cancers
21. Chronic exposure to heavy metals, such as lead, cadmium, mercury, arsenic, or aluminum (1.5)[24]
22. Chronic mold exposure (1.5)[25]
23. Kidney dysfunction (2)[26]

Mental Health

24. Post-traumatic stress disorder (4),[27] bipolar disorder (2),[28] schizophrenia (2),[29] depression (3.5),[30] or chronic stress (2)[31]

Immunity/Infection Issues

25. Autoimmune issues, such as multiple sclerosis (1.5), rheumatoid arthritis (3),[32] systemic lupus erythematosus (2),[33] Crohn's disease (1.5),[34] severe psoriasis (3)[35]
26. Adult asthma (1.3)[36]
27. Chronic Lyme disease or other infectious process in brain/body not fully treated (2)[37]
28. Cold sores or genital herpes (2)[38]

Neurohormone Deficiencies

29. Low in thyroid,[39] estrogen (in females),[40] or testosterone[41] (males and females) (2 for each one)
30. Hysterectomy without estrogen replacement (2)[42]
31. History of prostate cancer with testosterone-lowering treatment (2)[43]

Diabesity

32. Prediabetes or diabetes (3)[44]
33. Being overweight or obese in middle age (3)[45]
34. Being underweight in older age (2)[46]

Sleep Issues

35. Chronic insomnia (2.3)[47]
36. Sleep apnea (2)[48]

Total Score: Add up the total number of risk factors you have plus the total of all the numbers in parentheses (relative risk factors).

____ Total number of risk factors

____ Relative risk factors (the total score from the parentheses)

Interpretation of Relative Risk Factors:

If the score is 0–6: You likely have a low risk of developing AD.

If the score is 7–14: You have a moderate risk; consider annual screening (lab tests, repeat of WebNeuro cognitive testing, and checkup with health-care provider) after age 50.

If the score is greater than 14: Consider annual screening (lab tests, repeat of WebNeuro cognitive testing, and checkup with health-care provider) after age 40.

Looking at memory loss risk, based on risk factors, has a precedence in a large study from Finland. Specifically, researchers looked at age, gender, education, blood pressure, weight, cholesterol, and physical activity in a large sample of middle-aged adults. They found a significant increase in dementia within 20 years among those with a higher number of risk factors.[49]

ADDRESS ALL RISK FACTORS TO KEEP YOUR BRAIN HEALTHY

The Amen Clinics Memory Rescue program eliminates or treats as many of the risk factors above as possible. If you follow the program, you will also improve your mood, weight, blood pressure, blood sugar, gum health, and sleep. If you want the best results and best health, read up on all the risk factors and try to incorporate as many of the recommendations from each as you can. But if you have fewer risk factors, focus on the recommendations provided in the BRIGHT MINDS chapters relevant to your issues. Those are the factors that are stealing your memory *now*. Chapters 5 through 15 will help you understand each of these risk factors, how to diagnose them, and what to do to properly treat, reduce, or eliminate them.

How to make positive changes—and make them stick

Whether you have many risk factors that are affecting your brain and memory or just a few, you will want to make sure the new habits you adopt from the BRIGHT MINDS Program will last. Thankfully, researchers have been looking into what can help you in this process. When you first start to make a big lifestyle change, you often feel positive and empowered. You want to feel healthier and get your memory back, and you are resolved to make the necessary lifestyle changes. But eventually you may get distracted or busy at work, leading you to skip your workout, grab fast food, or skimp on sleep.

Don't give up! It's natural to temporarily lapse into previous habits because your brain still recognizes those old behavior pathways. But your brain has tremendous plasticity and can learn new pathways to healthier behaviors if you keep repeating them. Here are several strategies to help you succeed.

Make a commitment. Research has shown that making a resolution or goal and then putting it on paper (or on your computer) can help you be more successful, especially when your initial gung ho spirit wanes. Even better, share your intention with a supportive friend and send a regular progress report to that person.

Make a note of it. Another way to stay on target is to write down the health-boosting actions you take. You might want to start a journal to track your progress.

Plan ahead. Some of the activities you begin will require time in your schedule. In order to be successful, you need to create space for these new behaviors and clue in your family and other people in your life so that they can support your program. If you are successful, they will benefit too! Look for ways to adapt your schedule: Mark off time to exercise or make healthier meals, for instance, and treat these activities as you would important appointments.

Celebrate your small victories. Instead of looking ahead to what you haven't yet done, take a few moments every few days or each week to look back at what you have achieved. This is known as the "horizon effect." This viewpoint helps to build enthusiasm and the drive to keep going. It's a way to continue inspiring yourself.

When you make mistakes, be curious and not furious at yourself, so you can learn from them. Everyone messes up at some point, and you will too. And not just once! Stop any negative thoughts by reminding yourself of what you have accomplished (enlist a supportive friend or family member if you have trouble with this part). The key to improving your memory and your brain is making little changes that accumulate over time and being as consistent as possible.

WHAT SHOULD EVERYONE DO, NO MATTER WHAT?

Everyone should take the following five steps to protect their memory and brain.

1. **Assess your brain regularly.** As mentioned in the last chapter, Amen Clinics use an online test called Brain Fit WebNeuro, which is available at www.mybrainfitlife.com. You don't have to use our test, but it is important to assess yourself on a yearly basis.

2. **Know your important health numbers.** Many business leaders operate by the old adage that "you cannot change what you do not measure." That is true of your health as well, so it is critical that you know your important numbers, which will be explained throughout this book. If, for example, your body mass index is too high, you can get serious about your weight, or if your Omega-3 Index is too low, you can eat more fish or take an omega-3 fatty acid supplement. If blood tests are needed to assess your risk, you can ask your healthcare provider to order them, or you can visit one of our clinics.

General Numbers to Know
- Body mass index (BMI)
- Waist-to-height ratio (see page 233)
- Blood pressure

Blood Tests

- Complete blood count (CBC)
- General metabolic panel (kidney and liver function)
- Lipid panel
- Fasting blood sugar
- Hemoglobin A1c (HbA1c)
- Fasting insulin
- Homocysteine
- C-reactive protein (CRP)
- Ferritin level (measure of iron store)
- Thyroid panel
- Testosterone level
- DHEA level
- Vitamin D
- Folate
- Vitamin B12 level
- Plasma zinc
- Serum copper
- Magnesium
- Omega-3 Index
- *APOE* gene type

3. **Know, treat, and eliminate your specific risk factors (see chapters 5–15).**

4. **Follow the Memory Rescue Diet (see chapter 16).** This is one of the most important strategies for lasting health.

5. **Take basic supplements daily, including a 100 percent multivitamin/mineral complex with extra vitamin B6, B12, folate, and vitamin D, plus omega-3 fatty acids EPA and DHA.** Then use targeted nutraceuticals (which I define as supplements with medicinal properties) based on your specific BRIGHT MINDS needs (explained in the next 11 chapters).

THE SCIENCE BEHIND NUTRACEUTICALS

Many doctors will say that you don't need supplements or that they are a waste of money, but I agree with my friend Mark Hyman, MD, director of Cleveland Clinic's Center for Functional Medicine. He wrote that people who "eat wild, fresh, whole, organic, local, nongenetically modified food grown in virgin mineral- and nutrient-rich soils" that has not been "transported across vast distances and stored for months before being eaten" may not need supplements if they "work and live outside, breathe only fresh unpolluted air, drink only pure, clean water, sleep nine hours a night, move their bodies every day, and are free from chronic stressors and exposure to environmental toxins."[50] But because we live in a fast-paced society that makes it convenient to run to the drive-through, skip meals, buy chemically treated and processed foods, and indulge in sugary treats, we could all use a little help from a multivitamin/mineral supplement.

Over the last 25 years I have been excited to see the research showing that high-quality, targeted supplements can have a positive impact on the brain. Here's a powerful example: In 2009, Amen Clinics performed the world's first and largest brain imaging study on active and retired NFL players. Many of them complained of memory problems and scored very poorly on the cognitive tests we gave them. As a group, their brain SPECT scans looked awful. For the treatment arm of the study, we used brain health education and targeted nutraceuticals. Our protocol demonstrated increased blood flow to multiple brain areas, including the prefrontal cortex and hippocampus, and improvements in memory, attention, and processing speed.[51]

My interest in nutraceuticals started after I began using brain SPECT imaging to help understand and treat my patients. One of the early lessons SPECT taught me was that some medications, especially those for anxiety and pain, had a negative effect on the scans, revealing areas of low blood flow (see next page). Later I learned some studies show that these medications increase the risk of dementia and strokes.[52] In medical school, I was taught, "First do no harm. Use the least toxic, most effective treatments."

As I looked for alternatives to these medications to help the children and adults I was serving, I discovered that many natural supplements had strong scientific evidence with fewer side effects than prescription medications. For this reason, I give specific nutraceutical recommendations in each of the BRIGHT MINDS chapters.

MEDICATIONS THAT ARE TOXIC ON SPECT SCANS

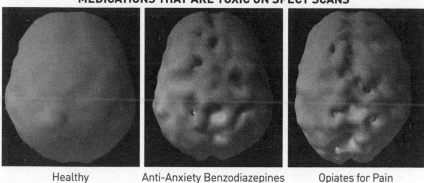

Healthy   Anti-Anxiety Benzodiazepines   Opiates for Pain

Pros and cons of nutraceuticals

In considering nutraceuticals, it is important to understand their pros and cons. First, many have been studied extensively and have a significant scientific body of research pointing to their effectiveness. Nutraceuticals generally have far fewer side effects than most prescription medications and are much less expensive. Also, because prescriptions for medications become part of your medical records and can affect your insurability (people are often denied or forced to pay higher rates for health, life, disability, and long-term care insurance because they have taken certain medications), natural alternatives that work are sometimes a better option.

Yet nutraceuticals have some drawbacks. These supplements can also have side effects, so they need to be used carefully. (Just because something is natural doesn't mean it can't be harmful. After all, arsenic and cyanide are natural!) Also, though nutraceuticals are generally less expensive than medications, they may prove costlier because they are usually not covered by insurance.

A major concern about nutraceuticals is the lack of quality control in their production. Studies have shown that supplements don't always contain what their labels claim, which means they might be ineffective or even harmful. Many people get their advice about these products from the clerk at the health food store, who may not have the best information. You may need to do some work on your own to find brands you can trust. The best approach to finding quality supplements is to develop a relationship with the brand and communicate your questions and issues to their technical and quality control staff.

Even considering these issues, the benefits of nutraceuticals (and their relatively low risks compared to medications) make them worth considering, especially if you can get thoughtful, research-based information. Every day I

personally take targeted nutraceuticals because I believe they make a significant difference in my life.

||||||||||||||||||||||||||||||||||||||||||||||||||||||||||||||||||||||||||||||||||||||||

Are Your Medications Making You Sick?

Many medications deplete important nutrients that help keep us
well. Here is a list of some of the most common troublemakers.

- Antacids: decrease stomach acid (which helps you digest your
  food), calcium, phosphorus, folate, and vitamin K
- Female hormones: decrease folate, magnesium, B vitamins,
  vitamin C, zinc, selenium, and CoQ10
- Antidiabetics: decrease CoQ10 and vitamin B12
- Antihypertensives: decrease vitamins B6 and K, CoQ10, magnesium, and zinc
- Anti-inflammatories, such as ibuprofen: decrease calcium,
  zinc, iron, folate, and vitamins B6, C, D, and K
- Cholesterol-lowering: decrease CoQ10, omega-3 fatty acids,
  carnitine
- Antibiotics: decrease vitamins B and K
- Oral contraceptives: decrease B vitamins, folate, magnesium,
  zinc, selenium, tyrosine (building block for dopamine), and
  serotonin (critical for mood). Being on oral contraceptives
  increases the risk for depression by 40 percent.

Be sure to consult with your physician before stopping any
medication.

||||||||||||||||||||||||||||||||||||||||||||||||||||||||||||||||||||||||||||||||||||||||

MEMORY RESCUE: BRIGHT MINDS TAKEAWAYS

The following to-do list will help you customize and begin your own Memory Rescue program:

1. Know your specific risk factors.

2. Learn the steps to make lasting positive changes.

3. Assess your important health numbers on a yearly basis.

4. Adopt easy strategies for each of the BRIGHT MINDS risk factors.

5. Start simple with supplements: a multivitamin/mineral complex and omega-3 fatty acids EPA and DHA. Know and optimize your vitamin D level.

CHAPTER 5

<u>B</u> IS FOR BLOOD FLOW
UNLOCKING THE KEY TO LIFE

Yes, exercise is the catalyst. That's what makes everything happen: your digestion, your elimination, your sex life, your skin, hair, everything about you depends on circulation.

JACK LALANNE

JIM: MARKERS OF MEMORY PROBLEMS

Jim, 61, was a successful businessman whose life started unraveling because of memory loss and erratic behavior several years before he came to our clinic just outside Washington, DC. Throughout his life, Jim had struggled with a short attention span, distractibility, and restlessness. He said he was unable to sit still and was "always on the go."

Family and friends told Jim he likely had ADD (attention deficit disorder). He was dyslexic and didn't learn to read until the sixth grade. Jim excelled at football and played for 10 years (middle school, high school, and college) as a linebacker, one of the worst brain-damaging positions. As a young adult, he drank heavily and smoked cigarettes and marijuana. Despite his many challenges, Jim was an outstanding businessman who owned seven automobile dealerships.

Two years before Jim came to see us, he was involved in a serious car accident in which he lost consciousness and stopped breathing three times. First responders used a defibrillator to restart his heart. During his hospital stay, he told us, he was not evaluated for a concussion. However, his memory deteriorated even more afterward, and his behavior became uncharacteristically erratic. He withdrew from his family and started having an affair, which led to a legal separation from his wife. He also described forgetting things he had asked his employees to complete, and so he ended up asking them more than once. He started drinking vodka martinis and said he "was probably drinking more than he should." He became more anxious and had trouble sleeping, so his doctor prescribed Xanax and Ambien. Jim's father had developed severe memory problems in his early seventies, which progressed to a diagnosis of Alzheimer's disease. Given his family history, Jim worried that he could be exhibiting early signs of dementia.

When we first saw Jim, he was overweight and had high blood pressure and high cholesterol. His sugar intake was "higher than it should be," and his fasting blood sugar, HbA1c, ferritin, homocysteine, and C-reactive protein were all high. His vitamin D level was low. His cognitive testing showed significant memory problems, and his brain SPECT scan showed marked overall decreased blood flow, the number one predictor of serious memory problems in the future.

JIM'S BRIGHT MINDS RISK FACTORS AND INTERVENTIONS

BRIGHT MINDS	JIM'S RISK FACTORS	INTERVENTIONS
Blood Flow	Severe low blood flow on SPECT, hypertension, three episodes where Jim stopped breathing after being knocked unconscious	Exercise, diet, ginkgo biloba, and other supplements
Retirement/Aging	High ferritin (iron) level	New learning exercises
Inflammation	High CRP and homocysteine	Diet, omega-3 fatty acids EPA and DHA, vitamins B6 and B12, and folate
Genetics	Father with Alzheimer's	
Head Trauma	Ten years playing football; motor vehicle accident with loss of consciousness	
Toxins	History of significant alcohol and marijuana use	Stopped drinking alcohol

BRIGHT MINDS	JIM'S RISK FACTORS	INTERVENTIONS
Mental Health	ADD; Xanax for anxiety	Medication for ADD; discontinued Xanax
Immunity/Infection Issues	Low vitamin D	Vitamin D3 supplements
Neurohormone Deficiencies	Low testosterone	Testosterone, weight training, supplements, and no sugar
Diabesity	High HbA1c and fasting blood sugar; obesity	Weight loss and improved blood sugar control with the Memory Rescue Diet
Sleep Issues	Sleep issues since motor vehicle accident; Ambien for insomnia	Sleep strategies to replace Ambien

JIM'S "BEFORE" BRAIN SPECT SCAN

SPECT SCAN AFTER NINE MONTHS

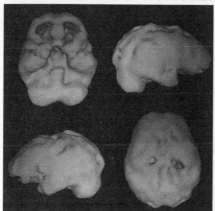
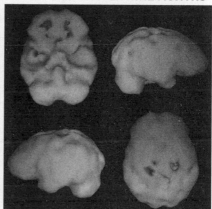

Overall low blood flow

Overall improvement

The cognitive testing and scan really got Jim's attention. He did everything his psychiatrist, Lantie Jorandby, MD, asked him to do. He stopped drinking, changed his diet, started to exercise, and took medication for ADD as well as and targeted supplements to support his brain. These changes, along with strategies to improve Jim's sleep, made it possible for Dr. Jorandby to take Jim off Xanax and Ambien. Nine months later he felt much better and his cognitive test scores and brain SPECT scan were markedly improved. Jim's wife wrote to Dr. Jorandby, "Thank you for all of your help. I believe you and the Amen Clinics saved Jim's life, our marriage, and our family. We are extremely grateful."

*Low blood flow in the brain is the number one predictor
of future memory problems and Alzheimer's disease
and how quickly your brain will deteriorate.*[1]

Blood is the channel that supplies cells with nutrients and clears toxins. To keep our brains sharp and healthy for as long as possible, it is critical to protect our blood vessels. In fact, brain cells don't age as quickly as once believed; research shows it is the blood vessels supporting our neurons that age.[2]

Noting that 20 percent of the body's blood flow is used by the brain, I often tell patients, "Whatever is good for your heart is good for your brain, and whatever is bad for your heart is also bad for your brain." Not only that, but *if you have blood flow problems anywhere, you probably have them everywhere.*

Case in point: Commercials for drugs that treat erectile dysfunction, such as Viagra, Levitra, and Cialis, are now commonplace on television. Just as this condition is rapidly increasing in men, so are brain problems. When I wrote *The Brain in Love* in 2007, I realized I had overlooked the connection between the two. Now I say, "Whatever is good for your heart is good for your brain is good for your genitals. And whatever is bad for your heart is bad for your brain and bad for your genitals. It's all about blood flow." Circulation goes down in both organs, not one or the other. Sexual dysfunction and low blood flow are also increasingly problems in women.

Forty percent of 40-year-old men have erectile dysfunction, according to the Massachusetts Male Aging Study, which likely means that 40 percent of 40-year-old men also have brain dysfunction. The rate rises to an alarming level in older men: The same study reported that 70 percent of 70-year-old men had erectile dysfunction, which likely means that 70 percent of 70-year-old men likely also have brain dysfunction.[3]

Besides erectile dysfunction and a loss-of-oxygen experience (like a near drowning or heart stoppages, as in Jim's case), there are several other vascular or blood flow risk factors:

- Cardiovascular disease, including:
    a. atherosclerosis (hardening and narrowing of the arteries)
    b. high LDL or total cholesterol
    c. heart attack
    d. atrial fibrillation
    e. hypertension or prehypertension
- A stroke or transient ischemic attack (TIA)
- Exercising less than twice a week and/or a slow walking speed

The Blood Brain Barrier: Don't Let Yours Leak

No discussion of blood flow to the brain is complete without mentioning the blood brain barrier (BBB), the protective membrane between blood vessels and brain tissue. The BBB acts as a gatekeeper, allowing nutrients like water, oxygen, glucose, vitamins, and hormones to cross into brain tissue and ushering out waste products like carbon dioxide. The BBB also protects the brain from toxins, infections, and allergens.

Although this protective layer is only a single cell thick, the cells forming it are tightly connected into a strong barrier. However, age, high blood pressure, trauma, inflammation, lack of oxygen, and other assaults can fray or damage the cell connections. When that happens—when the connections become "leaky"—disease is much more likely to occur because unwanted substances, like toxins, can cross into the brain.

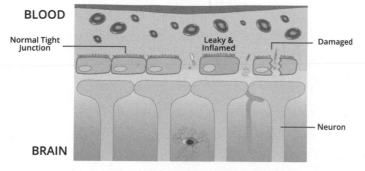

BLOOD BRAIN BARRIER

BLOOD

Normal Tight Junction

Leaky & Inflamed

Damaged

Neuron

BRAIN

Likewise, certain infections, such as syphilis and Lyme disease, can cross the BBB, which may be why they often are associated with cognitive and emotional problems. Some researchers suggest that gluten and milk proteins can also disrupt this barrier.[4] As we age, the BBB first becomes leaky in the area of the hippocampus,[5] which may be a big reason memory issues are much more common as we grow older. See page 71 ("Prescription to Reduce Your Brain Blood Flow Risk") for ways to help strengthen the BBB.

BLOOD FLOW RISK FACTORS EXPLAINED

Cardiovascular diseases

Given how important blood flow is to the brain, heart and blood vessel disease is a major risk factor for memory decline. Let's look at each potential contributor.

Atherosclerosis, the main culprit behind cardiovascular diseases, is caused by a buildup of fatty deposits called plaques on the inside walls of arteries. As plaques get larger, arteries gradually narrow and can become clogged, restricting blood flow to areas that need it. Blood vessels also become less elastic (so-called "hardening of the arteries"), which raises blood pressure and makes the vessels brittle, more likely to break (causing strokes). People with the *APOE* e4 gene have an increased risk of coronary artery disease (in the arteries that feed the heart) and Alzheimer's disease.[6] The most common risks for developing atherosclerosis are high blood LDL cholesterol levels (see below), advancing age, being male (women are more often affected after menopause), high blood pressure, diabetes, smoking, obesity, and physical inactivity. The risk is also greater in people with close relatives who had heart disease or a stroke at a relatively young age.

High levels of LDL cholesterol increase dementia risk, while high levels of HDL seem to lower it. In a four-year study of 1,037 women under 80 who had coronary artery disease, those who had elevated levels of LDL cholesterol had almost double the risk of memory loss, cognitive impairment, or dementia. But lowering LDL cholesterol into the normal range eliminated this increase in risk. One caveat: Lowering *total cholesterol* below 160 milligrams per deciliter (mg/dL) can increase the risk of depression and aggression. Maintaining proper cholesterol levels is particularly important for people with an *APOE* e4 gene.

Having a *heart attack* significantly increases the risk for future memory problems. That's because damage to the heart decreases its ability to pump blood and keep blood flowing effectively.

Atrial fibrillation is a type of heart rhythm abnormality (arrhythmia) that reduces the amount of blood the heart can pump. This fluttering rhythm also allows blood clots to form, which are then pumped into the bloodstream. A-fib, as it's commonly known, is a recognized risk factor for stroke and dementia.

Hypertension, or high blood pressure, increases the risk of memory problems. Optimal blood pressure is critical for brain health. High blood pressure and even blood pressure at the higher end of the normal range (prehypertension) is associated with lower overall brain function and blood flow to the brain.[7] According to the CDC about one-third of Americans have hypertension; another one-third are prehypertensive.[8] Being hypertensive is the second leading preventable cause of death and is associated with heart disease and stroke, other risks for memory problems. Chronically elevated pressure causes the blood vessel walls to enlarge and stiffen, making them more narrow and likely to break, much like atherosclerosis. Common causes of hypertension include genetics, being overweight, sleep apnea, and kidney disease. Hypertension can also be a side effect of oral contraceptive use.

Stroke or transient ischemic attacks

A stroke occurs when a blood vessel breaks or a clot chokes off blood supply to the brain, killing cells. The risk of developing dementia is six to ten times greater in a person who has had a stroke than in the general population.[9] Even a stroke that is caused by a clot smaller than a pencil eraser increases the risk for dementia. Having one or more strokes means blood vessels are significantly more vulnerable. However, risk factors such as high blood pressure, smoking, heart disease, and diabetes develop over a long time, meaning people generally have time to address these risk factors before it's too late. And the benefits to the brain can be substantial. Recently, Canadian researchers reported that a stroke-prevention program in Ontario had a very positive side effect: a 15.4 percent reduction in dementia over a decade in those ages 80 and over. The program included following a healthy diet, exercising, staying tobacco-free, and taking blood pressure medication, if needed.[10]

BE-FAST is a mnemonic (memory device) to help people remember the early warning signs and problem areas associated with a stroke:

Balance: sudden loss of balance or coordination
Eyes: sudden loss of vision in one or both eyes

Face: drooping on one side
Arms: weakness; inability to raise both arms without one arm drooping
Speech: slurred or jumbled
Time: prompt medical help is critical; call 911

Sometimes the warning signs of a stroke last for only a few minutes before disappearing, but that does not mean the problem is resolved. Ministrokes, also called transient ischemic attacks (TIA), don't last long or cause permanent damage, but they are a major warning sign of a greatly increased risk for more serious strokes and progressive memory problems.

RIGHT-SIDE FRONTAL, TEMPORAL LOBE STROKE—

BEFORE TREATMENT   AFTER TREATMENT

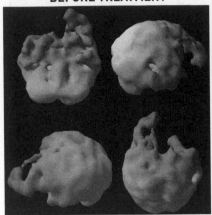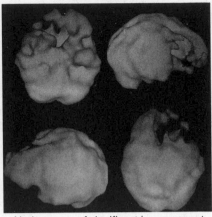

Overall severe decreased activity   Notice areas of significant improvement

If you've had a stroke or a TIA and want to rescue your memory, you must be very serious about your health. I've seen significant improvement in people who have had a stroke when they put their brains in a healing environment—specifically, when they followed all the BRIGHT MINDS strategies and used hyperbaric oxygen therapy (HBOT), which helps boost blood flow in the area surrounding the stroke.[11] (See chapter 19 for more on HBOT.)

Loss of oxygen

Your brain is oxygen hungry, and when it is deprived, it prematurely ages and is damaged. Sleep apnea can cut off oxygen (see chapter 15), as can near-drowning episodes, cardiac arrest, or voluntary asphyxiation, which is more common than most people know. I've treated a number of patients who would hold their breath as long as they could underwater, and others who would knowingly engage in autoerotic asphyxiation without realizing the damage they were doing to their brains.

Limited or no exercise

Not exercising is a major risk factor for memory loss, in large part because physical activity keeps blood vessels healthy. Exercise helps to boost a chemical called nitric oxide, which is produced in the walls of blood vessels and helps to control their shape. If blood vessel walls do not receive pulses of blood flow regularly from exercise, they begin to distort, flatten out, and limit blood flow overall. As a result, the body's tissues, including the brain, do not receive the nutrients they need or have a good mechanism to rid themselves of the toxins that build up in the body. If the deep areas of the brain are starved of oxygen and glucose, a person will have problems coordinating his or her limbs and processing complex thoughts, as during deep conversations. Regular physical exercise is a major preventive strategy for memory loss,[12] no matter the age someone begins.

Yalla imshi. As a child, I heard those two Lebanese words a lot from my father. They mean "Let's go" or "Hurry up." I am the third of seven children, and we were often in a hurry to get to school, pick someone up from baseball, or go to the store. I still hear this phrase in my head and have used it once or twice with my own children. Little did my dad know how important those two words are. The faster we walk as we age, the longer we live and the sharper we think. An 80-year-old person who walks one mile per hour has only a 10 percent chance of living until 90. But if that same 80-year-old moves faster, say at 3.5 mph, he or she has an 84 percent chance of reaching 90.[13] As walking speed goes down, so do executive function and decision-making skills.[14] If you haven't walked at a fast pace for a long time, start slowly and work your way up safely. Falls are also a major cause of memory loss.

IIIIIIIIIIIIIIIIIIIIIIIIIIIIIIIIIIIIIIIIIIIIIIIIIIIIIIIIIIIIIIIIIIIIIIIIIIIIIIIIIIIIIIIIIIIIIIIIIIII

The Miracle of Exercise

Physical exercise needs to be part of your everyday life for many reasons. For instance, it stimulates neurogenesis, the ability of the brain to generate new neurons. Research shows that, when laboratory rats are engaged in physical activity, new neurons are generated in the frontal lobe and hippocampus, which survive for about four weeks and then die off unless they are stimulated.[15] If you stimulate these new neurons through mental or social interaction, they connect to other neurons and become integrated into brain circuits that help maintain their functions throughout your life. This is why people who go to the library or take music lessons after a workout are smarter than those who work out and then veg out.

Exercise also protects the hippocampus from stress-related hormones, like cortisol,[16] which normally shrink it. Even leisurely walking has been shown to increase the size of the hippocampus in women.[17]

Many other health benefits stem from physical activity; for example, it

- helps increase the size of the hippocampus,[18] the holy grail of any memory enhancement program;
- stimulates the production of growth factors, such as BDNF (brain-derived neurotrophic factors), that nurture stem cell production;
- decreases beta-amyloid plaque formation;[19]
- improves cognitive flexibility and function;[20]
- elevates mood and focus;
- enhances the heart's ability to pump blood throughout the body and brain, which increases oxygen and nutrient delivery;
- boosts nitric oxide production and the flexibility of blood vessels, which decreases the risk for high blood pressure, stroke, and heart disease;
- enhances insulin's ability to lower high blood sugar levels, reducing the risk of diabetes;
- helps you maintain coordination, agility, and speed;
- increases levels of the hormone DHEA, which is critical to brain health;
- improves blood pressure;
- increases flexibility and agility;
- allows for greater detoxification through sweat;
- enhances the quality of sleep; and
- boosts immunity.

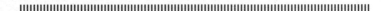

 ## CHECKUP FOR BLOOD FLOW ISSUES

Blood pressure

Here are the numbers you should know:

Optimal
Systolic 90–120
Diastolic 60–80

Prehypertensive
Systolic 120–139
Diastolic 80–89

Hypertensive
Systolic > or = 140
Diastolic > or = 90

If you have diabetes or chronic kidney disease, you should have a target blood pressure below 130/80.[21] However, blood pressure that is too low can also be a problem.

Hypotensive
Systolic < 90
Diastolic < 60

Lab tests

- **Complete Blood Count (CBC):** This blood test checks the health of your blood, including red and white blood cell counts. Low red blood cell count (anemia) can make you feel anxious and tired and can lead to memory problems. It may indicate internal bleeding or a vitamin or iron deficiency, among other causes. Enlarged red blood cells may mean you are drinking too much alcohol. A high level of white blood cells may indicate infection. Check with your health-care provider for treatment suggestions.

- **Lipid Panel:** Cholesterol and triglyceride (fat) levels in the blood are also important, especially because they can negatively affect blood delivery to the brain. Cholesterol that is either too high or too low is bad for the brain. Higher cholesterol later in life has been associated with better cognitive performance[22] and a decreased risk of dementia.[23] Normal levels are:

  - Total Cholesterol (135–200 milligrams per deciliter [mg/dL], yet a level below 160 has been associated with depression, suicide, homicide, and death from all causes, so the optimal level is 160–200 mg/dL)
  - HDL (>/= 60 mg/dL)
  - LDL (<100 mg/dL)
  - Triglycerides (<150 mg/dL)

Knowing the particle size of your LDL cholesterol (your health-care professional can order this test) is important because large particles are less toxic than smaller particles. If cholesterol is a concern for you, I recommend two books: *The Great Cholesterol Myth* by Stephen Sinatra, MD, and Jonny Bowden, PhD, and *What Your Doctor May Not Tell You about Heart Disease* by Mark Houston, MD.

FROM THE BRAIN WARRIOR'S WAY LIVE CLASS

"I finally got myself to the lab to get my lipid test done, and my doctor actually messaged me and told me she was really happy with my numbers, all my numbers. She said, 'Whatever you are doing, keep doing it!' I'm proud of myself. And thank you, Dr. Amen and Tana [Amen]; I couldn't have done it without you too! These numbers were much worse before I started your program."

Balance test: how long can you stand on one foot?

Throughout life, your eyes, ears, muscles, brain (especially your cerebellum), and nerves work together to keep you upright, balanced, and steady on your feet. But as you age, your balance tends to become less dependable, especially if you don't engage in regular coordination exercises. Unsteady footing makes it difficult to engage in any habitual physical activity, putting you at greater risk for cardiovascular disease. Poor balance and an unsteady gait are also associated with a higher incidence of falls and memory problems.[24]

A simple way to check your balance is called the static-balance test. How long can you stand on one leg with your eyes closed before you lose your balance? Follow these simple instructions to find out.

1. Enlist the help of someone who has a watch or timer.

2. Stand barefoot on a flat, hard surface. Stand close to something to grab on to, or ask your partner to stand close to steady you in case you start to fall.

3. Close your eyes.

4. Lift one foot off the ground about six inches, bending your knee at a 45-degree angle. (Use your left foot if you're right-handed; your right foot if you're left-handed).

5. Ask your partner to start timing.

6. Keep still for as long as you can without jiggling, teetering, falling, or opening your eyes.

7. Repeat the test three times, add up the results, and divide by three to get the average. Then check your time against the chart below.

Balance Time: Balance-Based Age

4 seconds: 70 years
5 seconds: 65 years
7 seconds: 60 years
8 seconds: 55 years
9 seconds: 50 years
12 seconds: 45 years
16 seconds: 40 years
22 seconds: 30–35 years
28 seconds: 25–30 years

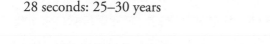

PRESCRIPTION TO REDUCE YOUR BRAIN BLOOD FLOW RISK

The Strategies

The strategies below can help support your overall blood flow and improve your cholesterol levels and blood pressure.

1. **Avoid anything that hurts vascular health.** Examples include a sedentary lifestyle, caffeine and nicotine (which both constrict blood flow to the brain and other organs), and dehydration.[25]

2. **Seek treatment for anything that damages your blood flow.** Be serious about addressing coronary artery disease, heart arrhythmias, prediabetes and diabetes, prehypertension and hypertension, insomnia, sleep apnea, and drug and alcohol abuse.

3. **Lose weight if your BMI is over 25.** BMI, an abbreviation for Body Mass Index, is a measure of body fat that is based on a person's height and weight. To determine your BMI, check any online BMI calculator. (The National Institutes of Health provide one at https://www

.nhlbi.nih.gov/health/educational/lose_wt/BMI/bmicalc.htm.) See also chapter 14.

4. **Spend 10 to 20 minutes a day in deep prayer or meditation.**[26] Both prayer and meditation have been shown to improve blood flow to the brain, particularly in areas involved in memory and thinking skills.

BRIGHT MINDS TIP

Not only do prayer and meditation boost blood flow to the brain, these spiritual practices are also wonderful stress management tools.

---

5. **Strengthen your blood brain barrier (BBB).** Eliminate gluten, dairy, and toxins (see chapter 16), and treat any infections (see chapter 12). Many of the supplements I recommend in the Memory Rescue program also seem to help with the integrity of the BBB, such as folate, vitamins B6, B12,[27] and D,[28] acetyl-L-carnitine,[29] alpha-lipoic acid,[30] alpha GPC,[31] curcumin,[32] resveratrol,[33] and omega-3 EPA and DHA.[34]

6. **Adopt natural strategies to keep your blood pressure healthy.**

    • Eat more plant-based foods.
    • Limit dairy.
    • Limit salt intake (about 1,500 mg a day is recommended; no more than 2,300 mg).
    • Eat more foods high in magnesium (e.g., pumpkin seeds) and potassium (e.g., bamboo shoots, cabbage).
    • Eat more foods with blood pressure–lowering effects, such as broccoli, celery, garlic, chickpeas, spinach, and mushrooms.
    • Eliminate alcohol, caffeine, fruit juices, and sodas (including diet sodas).[35]
    • Drink water! People who drink at least five glasses of water a day have half the risk of hypertension as those who drink fewer than two a day.

- Focus on getting seven to eight hours of sleep a night, and if you have sleep apnea, get it assessed and treated.
- Take supplements that research-based evidence has shown to lower blood pressure:[36] These include magnesium, potassium, CoQ10, vitamins C and D, aged garlic, and omega-3 EPA and DHA.

7. **Take medication if you need it.** At Amen Clinics we prefer to take a natural approach to health problems, but hypertension or excessively high cholesterol levels can become a crisis if not managed properly. The thoughtful use of medicine can be very helpful.

8. **Exercise!** Regular exercise helps to boost nitric oxide and keep blood vessels open and flexible. (See "The Miracle of Exercise" on page 67 for additional benefits.) The following four types of exercise are great for your brain. Of course, you should check with your physician before starting any new exercise routines.

   - *Burst training.* This workout involves several surges of intense activity lasting 30 to 60 seconds, each followed by a few minutes of lower-intensity exertion for recovery. An easy way to incorporate this into your routine is to take a 30- to 45-minute walk every day. Include four or five one-minute periods to "burst" (walk or run as fast as you can), and walk at a normal pace for two to three minutes between bursts. A 2006 study at Canada's University of Guelph found that burst training burns fat faster than continuous, moderately intensive activities. Short burst training also raises endorphins, lifts your mood, and energizes you. It also may improve the health and number of your mitochondria, the energy storehouses inside your cells.[37] Whenever you walk during ordinary activities, walk as if you are late. Seniors who walk faster live longer and have better executive function.[38] *Yalla imshi!*

   - *Strength training.* Aim to complete two 30- to 45-minute weight-lifting sessions a week, a day or two apart. One session should focus on the lower body (abs, lower back, and legs); the other on the upper body (arms, upper back, and chest). The stronger you are as you age, the less likely you are to get Alzheimer's disease. Canadian researchers found that resistance training helps prevent cognitive decline[39] and benefits people with mild cognitive impairment.[40]

- *Coordination activities.* Exercises such as dancing, tennis, and table tennis (the world's best brain sport) increase activity in the cerebellum, which is involved with both physical and thought coordination. Although the cerebellum makes up only 10 percent of the brain's volume, it contains 50 percent of its neurons.

- *Mindful exercise.* Yoga, tai chi, and other mindful exercises have been found to reduce anxiety and depression and increase focus and energy. So although they don't offer the same BDNF-generating benefits as aerobic activity, these types of exercise can still improve your brain health.

||||||||||||||||||||||||||||||||||||||||||||||||||||||||||||||||||||||||||||||||||||||||||||||||||||

Table Tennis, Tennis, and Other Sports That Boost Longevity

To get the biggest benefit from exercise, pick up a table tennis or tennis racquet and get moving. A 2016 study published in the *British Journal of Sports Medicine*[41] that tracked more than 80,000 adults for nearly a decade found that those who played racquet sports, such as tennis, table tennis, badminton, or squash, had the lowest risk of dying during the study compared to other exercisers. In fact, they had a 47 percent lower chance of dying from all causes compared to those who didn't play racquet sports and were 56 percent less likely to die as a result of cardiovascular disease (blood flow problems).

Table tennis is my favorite sport for the brain, because it is one of the fastest racquet sports, with balls flying close to you at speeds of up to 60 miles per hour. Table tennis's demanding visual and spatial requirements, together with strategy and aerobic exercise, offer powerful brain benefits. A study of 164 Korean women age 60 and older showed that table tennis improved cognitive function more than dancing, walking, gymnastics, or resistance training.[42] Other research suggests table tennis may help with ADHD.[43]

If racquet sports are not your thing, get in the water:

Swimmers were 28 percent less likely to die for any reason and 41 percent less likely to die of cardiovascular disease than other exercisers in the British study. Or try Zumba or aerobics—those who did were 27 percent less likely to die of any cause and 36 percent less likely to die of cardiovascular disease.

||||||||||||||||||||||||||||||||||||||||||||||||||||||||||||||||||||||||||||||||||||||||||

The Nutraceuticals

- *Ginkgo biloba extract*[44] has been shown to help cerebral blood flow and memory. In fact, the prettiest brain SPECT scans I see often belong to people who are taking this Chinese herb concentrate. The typical adult dose is 60 to 120 mg twice a day. I recommend starting at the lower dose for several weeks and then increasing to the higher amount to determine at which dosage your focus, energy, and memory are sharpest.

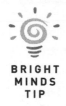

BRIGHT MINDS TIP

For better blood flow, consider taking 60 mg of ginkgo biloba twice a day.

- *Cocoa flavanols*[45] have been shown to boost blood flow to the brain, promote healthy blood pressure,[46] and improve some cognitive functions,[47] even in those who are sleep deprived.[48] I recommend one piece of sugar-free, dairy-free dark chocolate every day. Being the grandson of a candy maker, I was so excited about this finding that I made our own sugar-free, dairy-free, gluten-free, non-GMO chocolate bar called Brain in Love, which tastes amazing and has nine grams of fiber (www.brainmdhealth.com/brain-in-love-chocolate-bar-case).

- *Omega-3 fatty acids* can increase blood flow;[49] decrease brain atrophy;[50] increase working memory,[51] executive function,[52] and mood;[53] and decrease inflammation.[54] The active omega-3s are EPA (eicosapentaenoic acid) and DHA (docosahexaenoic acid). The reliably effective daily dose seems to be well above 1,000 mg (1 gram) per day of EPA and DHA. I recommend that most adults take 1.4 grams or more in about a 60/40 EPA/DHA ratio. (Check out more detailed information on the Omega-3 Index on page 102.)

- *Green tea catechins* (GTC—especially epigallocatechin gallate, or EGCG) have been shown to increase blood flow,[55] improve blood vessel tone, and help manage blood pressure.[56] An analysis of a group of studies indicates taking GTC daily lowers the risk of stroke.[57] GTC has also been shown to help improve cholesterol management[58] and blood sugar regulation.[59] Daily consumption of GTC may improve depression[60] and significantly lowers the risk of cognitive decline, especially for females and those at genetic risk for Alzheimer's.[61] A note of caution: I recommend not taking more than 600 mg a day.

- *Pycnogenol*, a standardized extract of flavonoids from the bark of the maritime pine (*Pinus pinaster*), is a powerful antioxidant and anti-inflammatory that protects the circulation and also the brain—especially the endothelium, a delicate single layer of cells that line the blood vessels and regulate their functioning.[62] The most intensively researched of all the nutraceuticals, Pycnogenol has shown benefits for memory, attention, and other cognitive functions in both students and the elderly. An effective dose ranges from 30 to 150 mg per day and occasionally much higher since Pycnogenol is very safe to take.[63]

- *Resveratrol* at 75 mg a day can increase blood flow to the brain.[64]

- *Probiotics* may lower LDL cholesterol, blood pressure, inflammatory markers, blood sugar levels, and BMI,[65] according to researchers who have found accumulating evidence of probiotics' benefits. For more information, see page 106 in chapter 7.

The Foods
AVOID (OR LIMIT):

Caffeine, which has been shown to constrict blood flow to the brain

Sugary and diet sodas, which are harmful to both your health and your brain. Sugar-sweetened sodas can raise blood pressure and cause other heart problems,[66] and diet sodas have now been linked to a higher risk of dementia, Alzheimer's disease, and stroke.[67]

Baked goods, which can lead to clogged arteries, hypertension, and heart failure

French fries and other foods fried in vegetable oils

Trans fats, found not only in some processed snacks but in many
   margarines and powdered coffee creamers

Low-fiber "fast" foods

Alcohol (I recommend no more than two to four servings a week.)

CONSIDER ADDING:

Spices: cayenne pepper,[68] ginger, garlic,[69] turmeric,[70] coriander and
   cardamom,[71] cinnamon,[72] rosemary, and bergamot (which has
   cholesterol-lowering properties)

Arginine-rich foods to boost nitric oxide and blood flow: beets, pork,
   turkey, chicken, beef, salmon, halibut, trout, steel-cut oats, clams,
   pistachios, walnuts, seeds, kale, spinach, celery, cabbage, and
   radishes. Drinking nitrate-rich beet juice has been found to lower
   blood pressure, increase stamina during exercise and in older people,
   and boost blood flow to the brain.[73]

Vitamin B6, Vitamin B12, and folate-rich foods: leafy greens, cabbage,
   bok choy, bell peppers, cauliflower, lentils, asparagus, garbanzo
   beans, spinach, broccoli, parsley, salmon, sardines, lamb, tuna,
   beef, and eggs

Vitamin E–rich foods, which widen blood vessels and decrease clotting:
   green leafy vegetables, almonds, hazelnuts, and sunflower seeds

Magnesium-rich foods, which relax blood vessels: pumpkin and
   sunflower seeds, almonds, spinach, Swiss chard, sesame seeds, beet
   greens, summer squash, quinoa, black beans, and cashews

Potassium-rich foods to help control blood pressure: beet greens, Swiss
   chard, spinach, bok choy, beets, brussels sprouts, broccoli, celery,
   cantaloupe, tomatoes, salmon, bananas, onions, green peas, sweet
   potatoes, avocadoes, and lentils

Fiber-rich foods, which have been shown to lower blood pressure[74] and
   improve cholesterol levels[75]

Vitamin C–rich foods: See more in chapter 12, page 200.

Polyphenol-rich foods: See page 118 in chapter 8.

Garlic-rich foods to lower cholesterol

Omega-3-rich foods: See page 107 in chapter 7.

Maca, a root vegetable/medicinal plant native to Peru, to reduce blood pressure[76]

 ## PICK ONE HEALTHY BRIGHT MINDS HABIT TO START TODAY

1. Focus on drinking more water—blood is mostly water.

2. Avoid caffeine and nicotine.

3. **Take up a racquet sport.***

4. Have a small piece of sugar-free dark chocolate.

5. **Take ginkgo biloba.**

6. Spice up your food: Add cayenne pepper.

7. Add arginine-rich foods, including beets.

8. Add vitamin E foods, including green leafy vegetables.

9. Add magnesium-rich foods, including pumpkin seeds.

10. Drink green tea.

---

*Note: Items in bold may be the most effective way to begin addressing a particular risk factor.

CHAPTER 6

R IS FOR RETIREMENT AND AGING
WHEN YOU STOP LEARNING, YOU START DYING

Although Moses was one hundred and twenty years old when
he died, his eye was not dim, nor his vigor abated.

DEUTERONOMY 34:7, NASB

SHERMAN: SCARED STRAIGHT

One of my best friends was deeply concerned about her husband, Sherman, an accomplished artist. At 71, he had begun to struggle with decision making, memory, and worry, waking up in the middle of the night infested with what I call ANTs (automatic negative thoughts). He wrestled with sadness and lack of enjoyment in life. He felt he was simply "going through the motions" without truly connecting to his work, other people, or even himself. Sherman's sense of estrangement from himself was foreign, and it scared him. He feared that the decline in his mood and outlook was his "new reality," and he felt increasingly hopeless about his future.

When I scanned Sherman's brain, it looked awful, in a pattern similar to Alzheimer's disease. I was horrified for him and wondered why it looked so bad. When I took his history, I learned he had high cholesterol and low thyroid and testosterone, which were all being treated. For anxiety, he took a benzodiazepine (Klonopin), which lowers blood flow to the brain and, in some studies, increases the risk of dementia. As a teenager, he had been struck by a car while riding his bike and had lost consciousness. His lab work showed high blood glucose, ferritin, and homocysteine levels; low vitamin D; and a low Omega-3 Index. He was also 20 pounds overweight and drank three glasses of Scotch whiskey in the evening to calm himself down, his standard practice for years.

SHERMAN'S BRIGHT MINDS RISK FACTORS AND INTERVENTIONS

BRIGHT MINDS	SHERMAN'S RISK FACTORS	INTERVENTIONS
Blood Flow	Low blood flow on SPECT, high cholesterol	Exercise, diet, ginkgo biloba
Retirement/Aging	71 years old, high ferritin level	Blood donations, new learning exercises
Inflammation	High homocysteine, low Omega-3 Index	Diet; omega-3 fatty acids EPA and DHA; vitamins B6 and B12; and folate
Genetics	Mother with dementia	
Head Trauma	Knocked unconscious as a teenager	
Toxins	Three glasses of Scotch whiskey a day, benzodiazepines	Stopped drinking alcohol and taking Klonopin
Mental health	Depression, chronic work stress	Stress management tools, learned to kill the "ANTs"
Immunity/Infection Issues	Low vitamin D	Vitamin D3 supplements
Neurohormone Deficiencies	Low thyroid and testosterone	Thyroid medicine, weight training, no sugar
Diabesity	Prediabetes and overweight	Weight loss and improved blood sugar control with the Memory Rescue Diet
Sleep Issues	Erratic sleep	Sleep strategies

SHERMAN'S "BEFORE" SPECT SCAN

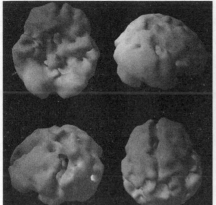

AFTER 6½ MONTHS

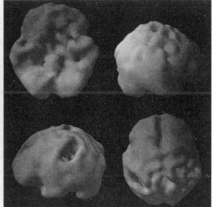

Overall low blood flow, similar
to Alzheimer's disease

Marked improvement

From the moment Sherman saw his scan during our first clinical meet-ing, he was scared straight into doing everything he could to make his brain better. Some people will just try to make one small change at a time, whining and complaining all the while, but Sherman recognized how serious his situation was and went all in with what I recommended. He stopped drinking and taking Klonopin, closely adhered to the Memory Rescue Diet, donated blood to lower his ferritin level, and was faithful in taking targeted supplements and exercising. After three months, he had lost 22 pounds and was excited to be at his college weight. He also noticed that his memory and mood were better. He felt less anxious and was positive about his progress. After six and a half months, he felt he was healthier than before he had started to slip. His follow-up scan showed remarkable improvement, which called for a day of celebration—but without the Scotch whiskey.

Mental decline is normal with age, but it's not inevitable. Increasing age is the most significant clinical risk factor for memory loss and Alzheimer's disease. Our research shows that most people's brains become less and less active with age. Blood flow drops, and people become much more vulnerable to memory problems, brain fog, and depression.

To the right is the SPECT scan of a typical 55-year-old man with mild memory problems.

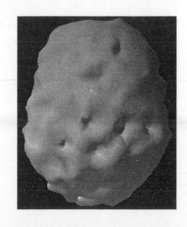

And below is a brain SPECT scan of a typical 82-year-old woman who suffers from memory problems, low energy, and depression. Over her lifetime, she gave virtually no thought to taking care of her brain . . . and it shows.

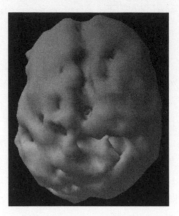

Now compare these scans to this one of Doris Rapp, MD, a world-famous allergist, taken when she was 80 years old. She has taken care of her brain all her life and still practices medicine and plays tennis.

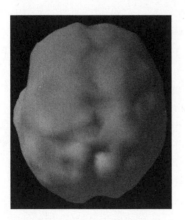 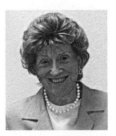

One of the most exciting lessons I've learned from looking at all these scans is that your brain does not have to deteriorate. With a little fore-thought, you can slow or even reverse the aging process in the brain.

I recently met a woman who told me now that she was 60 years old, she didn't want to have to worry anymore about what she ate or whether she exercised. She said she was done with that part of her life. If that describes you, I have a question: Are you okay with the consequences of having an older-functioning brain—less energy, brain fog, depression, and bad decisions? As we age, we have less room for error if we want to stay vibrant and healthy. To be at our best and rescue our memory, we have to be vigilant with our health.

Since the 2008 recession, many people who thought they could retire have had to continue working. The average retirement age rose from 60 to 62. But there can be a silver lining to working longer. A study of nearly 500,000 people found that for each additional year of work, the risk of getting dementia is reduced by 3.2 percent.[1] Working keeps us physically active, socially connected, and mentally stimulated, all of which help prevent cognitive decline. But if your brain is not healthy, you'll have trouble competing against younger talent. Don't let that be you.

My father, who is 88, still goes to work five days a week. He owns a chain of grocery stores and is active on the board of Unified Grocers, a four-billion-dollar company, where he was the long-term chairman. He told me he goes to work because all of his friends who retire either die or lose their minds. It seems there may be something to his thinking. Of course, if you actively engage your brain in retirement, it can be one of the best times of your life. But never forget that your brain is like a muscle: You have to use it, or it will get smaller and smaller. When you stop learning, your brain starts dying.

Beware of "old person's speech"

Before my father turned his health around at age 86 (after a health crisis that my wife, Tana, and I wrote about in *The Brain Warrior's Way*), he had what I call "old person's speech," which goes something like this:

> "I am too old."
> "I am too tired."
> "Leave me alone."
> "I know I'll die soon."
> "Why should I care anymore?"
> "I've done it this way my whole life; I cannot change now."
> "I'd rather get Alzheimer's disease than give up sugar, wine, chips . . . you name it."

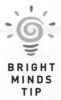

BRIGHT MINDS TIP

Keep your self-talk positive. Remember: The words you tell yourself are the movie script your brain plays out.

Your brain is very powerful and brings to life what you verbalize and project. If you think you are old and slow, you will act and feel old and slow.

MECHANISMS OF AGING

There are several recognized mechanisms that lead to faster aging, including lowered blood flow, inflammation, higher blood sugar levels, excessive caloric intake, and overproduction of molecules known as free radicals that can wreak havoc throughout the body. Blood flow, inflammation, and blood sugar are covered elsewhere in this book and the BRIGHT MINDS program, so let's focus in this chapter on how to care for our mitochondria (cell energy producers) and address other risk factors of aging, including:

- free radicals and oxidative stress
- too much (or too little) iron
- telomere length
- AGEs (advanced glycation end products)
- loss of neurotransmitters (serotonin, dopamine, and acetylcholine)
- social isolation

Mitochondria: your body's (and brain's) powerhouses

Inside your cells are tiny power plants called mitochondria, which convert oxygen into energy in the form of ATP (adenosine triphosphate). Different types of human cells have varying numbers of mitochondria. Red blood cells don't have any, liver cells can have up to 2,000, and cells that require the most energy (heart, retina, and brain) can have up to 10,000 mitochondria per cell.[2] The prefrontal cortex (which is involved with focus, forethought, judgment, and impulse control) is the area of the brain most densely populated with mitochondria. When these engines are healthy, they crank out ATP and you feel energized; when they are inefficient or damaged, you feel tired, foggy headed, and old.

Aging is the most common reason that mitochondria stop working productively.[3] Their efficiency drops an estimated 50 percent from your thirties to your seventies, which could help explain why diseases such as Alzheimer's or Parkinson's tend to occur later in life.

Free radicals and oxidative stress

A natural by-product of mitochondrial energy production is highly reactive molecules called free radicals. Normally, our bodies have defenses against these unstable molecules, but when free radicals are produced in excessive amounts or our ability to mop them up is impaired, they can damage our cells and accelerate aging. This is known as oxidative stress, and its effects are similar to that of rust on metal. Many things can generate free radicals and promote oxidative stress, including cigarette smoking, excessive sun exposure, the consumption of charred meats, exposure to pesticides and mercury, liver dysfunction, and high iron.

Too much—or too little—iron

Iron loves to make oxygen into free radicals; having excessive iron in your body promotes oxidative stress and internal "rusting." High levels are associated with inflammation, insulin resistance, and neurodegenerative illnesses such as Alzheimer's and Parkinson's diseases.[4] Low levels are associated with anemia, restless legs, ADHD, low motivation, and fatigue. Balance is important. Premenopausal women often have lower iron stores than men, due to monthly blood loss from menstruation. Some scientists theorize that this is one reason women tend to live longer than men.

Telomere length

When it comes to your brain, size matters! You never want to do anything to cause your brain to shrink or atrophy. Size also matters when it comes to your telomeres (the casings at the ends of chromosomes, which are similar to the plastic caps at the ends of shoelaces). The job of telomeres is to prevent "fraying" when a cell replicates. As a cell ages, its telomeres become shorter and shorter. Eventually, the telomeres become too short for accurate replication, and the cell dies. In 2003, Richard Cawthon, MD, PhD, from the University of Utah discovered that people with longer telomeres live longer than those with shorter telomeres.[5] Anything that increases oxidative stress and chronic inflammation (such as smoking, sodas, trans fats, processed foods, infections, heavy metal exposure) can shorten telomeres, while a diet high in antioxidants that reduce oxidative stress can slow telomere shortening.[6]

TELOMERES: THE END CAPS ON CHROMOSOMES

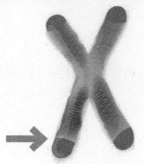

Akin to the ends of shoelaces

AGEs (advanced glycation end products)

I've always been amused by this acronym because it so clearly teaches us that sugar is associated with accelerated aging. Think of what happens when a cook caramelizes onions in a frying pan; it makes a delicious but sticky and gooey mess. That process is known as glycation, the result of sugar reacting with proteins and fats to form sticky molecules called AGEs. When AGEs circulate in the bloodstream, they gum up your biological system and fast-track aging by increasing free radicals and inflammation. AGEs help produce wrinkles in your skin and damage all your cells. They are also implicated in heart, eye, liver, and pancreatic disease, as well as in memory loss. Limiting or eliminating your sugar intake will help decrease your biological age, wrinkles, and AGEs!

Loss of neurotransmitters—
especially serotonin, dopamine, and acetylcholine

As we age, we lose brain cells that produce important neurotransmitters, chemicals that help our neurons to communicate effectively. These include

- serotonin (increasing the risk of depression)[7]
- dopamine (increasing the risk of Parkinson's disease and loss of motivation and pleasure)[8]
- GABA (increasing the risk of anxiety)[9]
- acetylcholine (affecting learning and memory)[10]

Protecting your brain will help support your neurotransmitter producers and decrease your risk of "normal" age-related memory decline. When it comes to memory, both dopamine and acetylcholine are particularly important.

Social isolation

We are all social animals. It is hardwired into our brains, and when we are lonely and disconnected from others, it can have negative physical and neurological effects.[11] Being socially isolated, which is more common as we age, is associated with an increased rate of cognitive decline.[12] In a recent study, more than one in eight people reported having no close friends.[13] As part of the US Health and Retirement Study, more than 8,300 adults ages 65 and older were assessed every two years from 1998 to 2010; researchers reported that the loneliest among them experienced cognitive decline approximately 20 percent faster than people who were not lonely, regardless of any other factors.

 ## CHECKUP FOR <u>R</u>ETIREMENT/AGING ISSUES

Your age!

As we age, we must be more careful about our health, because our natural healing mechanisms are usually much less effective.

Lab tests

The following tests measure the blood markers of aging[14] and should be part of an annual checkup.

- **C-reactive protein** (CRP) is a measure of inflammation. A healthy range is 0.0 to 1.0 mg/L. (See page 101 in chapter 7 for more on CRP.)

- **Fasting blood sugar and hemoglobin A1c** are two blood tests that screen for prediabetes and diabetes; age is one of the primary risk factors for both. (See pages 233–234 in chapter 14 for the specific numbers you should be aiming for on these tests.)

- **DHEA (dehydroepiandrosterone)** and **testosterone** are two neurohormones essential to check. DHEA drops with age; higher levels are associated with longevity. Too little testosterone—in both men and women—is associated with depression, poor memory, and low sex drive. (See chapter 13 for more on these and other hormones.)

- **Ferritin** blood test measures iron stores. Levels between 50 and 100 ng/mL (nanogram per milliliter) are ideal. Low levels can cause issues, but generally a high number is more problematic. The higher it goes over 100, the worse the iron overload, and levels over 300 are particularly toxic. They may eventually cause serious brain damage in people who sustain those levels long-term.[15]

- **Telomere length** is measured by a number of companies, which will test your blood and then compare your score to a "healthy" or "average" population.[16] However, some researchers[17] believe that telomere length is really a measure of other aging issues, such as inflammation and blood sugar control. For that reason, testing your C-reactive protein (inflammation) and HbA1c (long-term blood sugar biomarker) is likely a cheaper way to measure something similar.

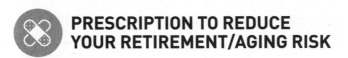

PRESCRIPTION TO REDUCE YOUR RETIREMENT/AGING RISK

The Strategies

1. **Be serious.** After looking at thousands of seniors' brains, I know I'm in a battle for the health of mine now that I'm in my sixties. But I have also seen many healthy 92-year-old brains, and I'm planning for mine to be one of them. When I don't feel like exercising or eating right, I ask myself, *Which brain do you want? An old or a young one? Which do you want?*

2. **Focus on new learning.** If you want to keep your brain sharp, you must engage in lifelong learning (see chapter 17).

3. **Keep your iron on target.** A common cause of too much iron is regular alcohol consumption, which increases the absorption of iron from your diet. If you drink wine with your steak, you will likely absorb more iron than you need. Cooking in iron pans, eating processed foods like iron-fortified cereals, drinking well water that's high in iron, or taking vitamin or mineral supplements with extra iron can also raise its level. In addition, some people have a genetic predisposition to absorbing too much iron from food.

    If your iron level is low, consider taking an iron supplement. If it is too high, you can lower it by donating blood, which benefits you as well as someone else.[18] An alternative? Being bled by leeches. Really! A few years ago, while visiting a spice market in Istanbul, I actually saw leeches for sale. I prefer donating blood.

Green tea and rosemary are rich in beneficial substances called polyphenols, which can reduce iron absorption.[19] Curcumin also may help to eliminate iron.[20]

4. **Intermittent fasting.** As discussed, memory loss is associated with the brain producing too much of certain toxic proteins that damage cells. One way your brain gets rid of these proteins is through a process called autophagy (from the Greek word for "self-devouring"). Think of tiny trash collectors cleaning up the toxins and pieces of dead and diseased cells that gunk up your brain. This cleaning process lowers inflammation and helps to slow down the aging process.

   Nightly 12-to-16-hour fasts (aka "intermittent fasting") have been shown to turn on autophagy. Experiment: If you eat dinner at 7 p.m., for example, try not eating again until 7 a.m. (or 11 a.m. for a longer fast). Fasts of 24 hours can also be helpful. Mark Mattson, PhD chief of the laboratory of neurosciences at the National Institute on Aging and a leading researcher in this field, reportedly limits his diet to no more than 2,000 calories a day and skips breakfast and lunch on Mondays, Wednesdays, and Fridays.[21]

5. **Strengthen your telomeres.** Avoid things that may shorten them, such as:

   - smoking[22]
   - alcohol[23]
   - inflammation and high C-reactive protein[24]
   - high homocysteine[25]
   - oxidative stress[26]
   - lower dietary intake of beta carotene, vitamin C, or vitamin E[27]
   - poor quality sleep[28]
   - chronic emotional stress and high cortisol levels[29]
   - type 2 diabetes[30]
   - high body mass index[31]

   Protect your telomeres using the following strategies:

   - exercise[32]
   - stress reduction[33]

- continuing education[34]
- mindfulness meditation[35]
- omega-3 fatty acids EPA and DHA[36]
- astragalus herb supplement[37]
- vitamin D[38]
- lowering LDL cholesterol[39]
- daily multivitamins (lengthens telomeres by 5 percent)[40]

6. **Get social.** To reduce the risk of loneliness and isolation, get involved with your family, church, or other groups. Take a class, form new friendships, share experiences, get physically active, and stay connected with others. New research shows that people who help care for others live longer.[41] Grandparents who care for their grandchildren, for example, live longer on average than grandparents who do not.

7. **Make love regularly.** New research suggests that sex not only protects your telomeres, it also improves cognitive function in older adults, especially when they engage in weekly lovemaking.[42]

The Nutraceuticals

- *Alpha GPC (alpha-glycerylphosphorylcholine).* Occurring naturally in our cells, this phospho-lipid has been shown to improve memory and other cognitive functions in Alzheimer's. GPC provides choline, an essential nutrient for gene regulation as well as acetylcholine production in the brain. In a double-blind two-year Alzheimer's trial, when taken along with the Alzheimer's drug Aricept (donezepil), GPC improved cognition and other clinical measures better than donezepil alone. GPC has been used in Europe for decades to treat Alzheimer's, stroke, comas, and even autism in children. GPC also elevates growth hormone (GH), a major hormone for tissue maintenance and renewal. GPC is found in mother's milk in high concentrations and is a major source of choline for growing babies. It is known to be a powerful brain protectant, and recent research suggests it protects mitochondria and improves their efficiency.[43] The typical starting dose for adults is 600 mg a day, which can be increased to 600 mg twice a day if needed.

- *Phosphatidylserine (PS).* An essential phospho-lipid component of cell membranes and critically important to their functions, PS powers all our cells and especially our neurons. It is concentrated in brain tissue, especially at the synapses that pass signals between the neurons.[44] PS helps maintain neuronal integrity, receptor density, neurotransmitter actions, and neuronal network efficiency, so the brain can continue to form and retain memories. As we age, brain cell membranes begin to lose their receptors for neurotransmitters and growth factors, which results in decreased cellular communication and interferes with storing memories. The upshot is that age-related memory declines. Clinical trials demonstrate that PS improves attention, learning, memory, and verbal skills in aging people with cognitive decline and may help "turn back the clock" on brain aging.[45] The best food sources of PS are egg yolks, muscle meats, and organ meats, but these amounts are low so it's best to get it from supplements. The typical therapeutic dose: 200 to 300 mg a day.

- *Acetyl-L-carnitine (ALCAR).* ALCAR is naturally produced in our cells and is essential for our mitochondria to work. Its levels have been shown to decrease as memory problems progress to Alzheimer's disease.[46] Its many benefits include supporting the mitochondria's ability to burn fat; reducing fatigue; improving insulin sensitivity and blood vessel health; decreasing inflammation; protecting neurons; and helping repair nerve-cell damage caused by diabetes and diabetic neuropathy. It has also been shown to have a beneficial effect on mild cognitive impairment.[47] ALCAR is often used to support brain function and increase energy and alertness. The typical dose is 500 to 2,000 mg a day. I usually start patients at the smaller dose and work up over time.

- *NAC (N-acetylcysteine)* is an oral source of cysteine, which cells use to make glutathione (GSH), a powerful antioxidant (cysteine itself is too unstable to use as a nutraceutical). Cysteine is the most abundant antioxidant in the blood and, together with GSH, helps eliminate heavy metals[48] and excrete environmental pollutants.[49] NAC can also decrease inflammation[50] and delay brain atrophy in Alzheimer's disease.[51] The typical adult dose is 600 to 2,400 mg daily, but doses above 1,800 mg can cause stomach upset. I usually start patients at 600 mg twice a day.

- *Huperzine A.* This remarkable compound, studied in China for nearly twenty years, works by blocking the enzyme that breaks down acetylcholine, thereby leaving more of the neurotransmitter to do its work in facilitating learning and memory.[52] It has been shown to be effective in patients who suffered cognitive impairment from several types of dementia, including Alzheimer's disease and vascular dementia.[53] Researchers have also found that it protects against oxidative stress.[54] Possible adverse side effects include gastrointestinal issues, headaches, dizziness, and increased urination. Caution: Taking huperzine A with medications that increase acetylcholine, such as Aricept or Exelon, may produce additive adverse effects and should be used only under a doctor's supervision. The typical adult dose is 50 to 100 micrograms (mcg) twice a day.

- *Saffron.* For more than 3,000 years, saffron has been an expensive and coveted spice throughout the world. It is extensively used in Persian, Indian, European, Turkish, and Arab cuisines to add flavor and color and is used as a traditional medicine to treat more than 90 illnesses.[55] Saffron contains more than 150 potentially active compounds. Recent studies have found that saffron helps with depression,[56] premenstrual syndrome (PMS),[57] and sexual function.[58] It has also been shown to be a potent antioxidant,[59] a neuroprotectant,[60] and a memory enhancer, even in people with mild cognitive impairment[61] and Alzheimer's disease,[62] comparing favorably with dementia medications such as Namenda.[63] It appears to aid memory by protecting the hippocampus and improving blood flow,[64] boosting acetylcholine,[65] and protecting neurons against beta-amyloid toxicity[66] and abnormal tau proteins.[67] The typical dose of saffron is 30 mg per day of a concentrate produced from the flower. The dose of the patented preparation of saffron called Satiereal (often used as a natural weight-loss aid) is 176.5 mg a day.

- *Bacopa (Bacopa monnieri).* This icon among Indian traditional herbs has been used since antiquity to improve memory, learning, and other brain functions. It contains a variety of bacosides and other substances that can improve the brain's intrinsic neurotransmitter and growth factor actions, which are vital for making, consolidating, and recalling memories. In controlled clinical trials, Synapsa, a highly concentrated, standardized Bacopa extract, has been shown to improve memory in aging brains, whether healthy or at risk for Alzheimer's. The effective dose of Synapsa for adults is 250 to 500 mg per day.[68]

- *Sage.* Herbalists have touted the benefits of this herb for hundreds of years. One of the most notable was Nicholas Culpeper, a seventeenth-century botanist who spent much of his life cataloging descriptions of medicinal herbs. Sage, he observed, "is of excellent use to help the memory, warming and quickening the senses." Scientists now believe they know why sage helps improve memory. Like huperzine A, it increases acetylcholine, which is typically deficient in older people with memory issues. Several studies show the cognition-enhancing effects of sage extracts.[69]

The typical dose for improved mood, alertness, and cognitive performance is 300 to 600 mg of dried sage leaf in capsules per day. Sage essential oil can also be used in doses of 25 to 50 microliters (mcL). *Caution:* Those who have hypertension or seizure disorders should use it only under the supervision of their health-care providers.

The Foods
AVOID:

If retirement or aging is one of your risk factors, begin by avoiding certain foods, especially sugar and foods that turn to sugar, as they increase AGEs. Limit your consumption of charred meats because when cooked at a high temperature, meat forms polycyclic aromatic hydrocarbons (PAHs), which are associated with cancer. (Cigarette smoke and car exhaust are also high in PAHs.) Steer clear of trans fats, and if your ferritin level is high, avoid foods with high dietary iron, including red meat, soybeans, collard greens, leeks, beans, sprouts, kelp, and olives.

CONSIDER ADDING:

Antioxidant-rich spices:[70] cloves, oregano, rosemary, thyme, cinnamon, turmeric, sage, garlic, ginger, fennel

Antioxidant-rich foods: acai fruit, parsley, cocoa powder, raspberries, walnuts, blueberries, artichokes, cranberries, kidney beans, blackberries, pomegranates, chocolate, olive and hemp oil (though don't use either one for cooking at high temperatures), dandelion greens, green tea

Choline-rich foods: to support acetylcholine and memory:[71] shrimp, eggs, scallops, chicken, turkey, beef, cod, salmon, shiitake mushrooms, chickpeas, lentils, collard greens

Allicin-rich foods: See page 200 in chapter 12.

Polyphenol-rich foods: See page 118 in chapter 8.

Vitamin B12 and folate-rich foods: See page 77 in chapter 5.

PICK ONE HEALTHY BRIGHT MINDS HABIT TO START TODAY

1. Limit charred meats.

2. **Get your ferritin level checked.**

3. Donate blood.

4. Try a daily 12-to-16-hour fast.

5. Season food with cloves, a potent antioxidant.

6. Take an acetyl-L-carnitine (ALCAR) supplement.

7. Add acetylcholine-rich foods, such as shrimp.

8. Stay connected; volunteer.

9. Begin or continue musical training.[72]

10. **Start a daily practice of learning something new.**

CHAPTER 7

I IS FOR INFLAMMATION
MANAGE THE INTERNAL FIRE THAT DESTROYS YOUR ORGANS

Inflammation is the cornerstone of Alzheimer's disease and Parkinson's, multiple sclerosis—all of the neurodegenerative diseases are really predicated on inflammation.

DAVID PERLMUTTER, MD

SARAH: FAITH IN WHAT MATTERS MOST

Sarah, a 62-year-old grandmother with six grandchildren, worried that her memory was starting to fail. Several months before she first saw me, she'd had a ministroke that temporarily paralyzed her right side before subsiding 30 minutes later. Her doctor called it a transient ischemic attack (TIA). Sarah's faith was critically important to her, and she wanted to pass it on to her grandchildren and great-grandchildren, but she feared that if she lost her mind, she would be unable to share with them what she had learned in life. Because faith adds a great deal of richness and meaning to my own life, I understood why it mattered so much to her.

Sarah also complained of chronic intestinal problems, joint pain, and mental fogginess. She was a "sugaraholic" and couldn't imagine giving it up, especially since she loved baking cookies with her granddaughters. Sarah's SPECT scan showed very low activity overall. Her inflammation markers (CRP and homocysteine) were high, as were her weight, blood sugar, and LDL cholesterol levels. In addition, she had low levels of omega-3 fatty acids and vitamins B12 and D. She told me she never ate fish because she could not stand the taste. She also had an abnormal gene for folate. Her cognitive testing showed significant weakness in her memory and executive function.

Sarah's test results—the seriously low activity on her SPECT scan, her poor memory scores, and her abnormal lab tests—got her attention. She realized that if she didn't get serious about her health, she would become a burden to her children and grandchildren. She told me that sugar wasn't worth losing her mind over, and she changed her diet, took targeted supplements (including omega-3 fatty acids EPA and DHA and probiotics), and started to exercise. Over the next year, she dropped 40 pounds, and all her important health numbers improved. In follow-up testing, her scan and memory scores were dramatically better.

SARAH'S BRIGHT MINDS RISK FACTORS AND INTERVENTIONS

BRIGHT MINDS	SARAH'S RISK FACTORS	INTERVENTIONS
Blood Flow	Low blood flow on SPECT, high LDL cholesterol, history of vascular disease (TIA)	Exercise, ginkgo biloba
Retirement/Aging	Age 62	
Inflammation	High CRP and homocysteine, low Omega-3 Index, low vitamin B12, abnormal gene for folate	Diet, omega-3 fatty acids EPA and DHA, probiotics, vitamin B12 and methyl folate, curcumin
Genetics		
Head Trauma		
Toxins		
Mental Health		
Immunity/Infection Issues	Low vitamin D	Vitamin D3 supplements
Neurohormone Deficiencies		
Diabesity	Prediabetes and obesity	Weight loss and blood sugar stabilization
Sleep Issues		

SARAH'S "BEFORE" SPECT SCAN

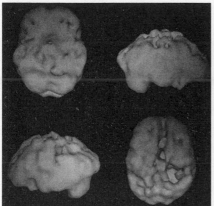

**SARAH'S SPECT SCAN
ONE YEAR LATER**

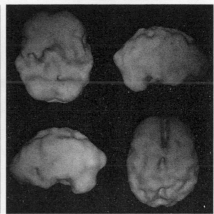

The word *inflammation* comes from the Latin *inflammare*, meaning "to set on fire." Chronic inflammation acts like an ongoing, low-level fire that destroys organs. Just as poor blood flow and oxidative stress can devastate your brain, so can chronic inflammation.

Inflammation is your body's natural way of coping with an injury or insult. It's a vitally important response that must be elicited at the right time and in the right balance. You would never want to completely eliminate inflammation because your body would not be able to deal with foreign invaders or heal from injuries.

When you are injured or develop an infection, your body's natural defenses against foreign invaders jump into action: Blood vessels dilate, blood flow increases to the troubled area, and your immune system's white blood cells (plus substances they produce) rush to the scene to deal with the trouble, much like firefighters hurrying to a fire. Nearby areas become swollen, warm, and red as your immune system fights to destroy bacteria and clear the way for healing to begin.

Injury and infection aren't the only things that trigger or promote inflammation; others include the following:

- environmental toxins
- smoking
- low levels of vitamin D or omega-3 fatty acids
- hormone imbalances
- gum disease
- gastrointestinal problems ("leaky gut")

- emotional stress
- excess body fat—especially belly fat
- high blood sugar levels
- pro-inflammatory foods: sugar and foods that quickly turn to sugar; trans fats; excessive omega-6 fatty acids from vegetable oils

Inflammation that constantly remains on, rather than arising occasionally to heal an injury or infection, is called chronic inflammation. Even though it may operate at a low level, over time chronic inflammation can damage organs and contribute to a wide range of illnesses, including heart disease, arthritis, gastrointestinal disorders, cancer, Alzheimer's, Parkinson's disease, depression, and chronic pain.

This chapter will focus on two major causes of chronic inflammation that damage your memory: (1) leaky gut and (2) low omega-3 fatty acid levels.

LEAKY GUT: TROUBLE IN THE GASTROINTESTINAL TRACT

Here's a pop quiz:

1. Where are three-quarters of your neurotransmitters made?
2. What organ system contains two-thirds of your body's immune tissue?
3. What system contains 10 times more cells than the rest of your body combined?
4. What system hosts a foreign legion that protects you?
5. What do 70 percent of people have problems with?

Answer: the gut!

The gut—your gastrointestinal (GI) tract—is often called the second brain because it is loaded with nerve tissue. It is in direct communication with your brain, which is why you get butterflies when you're excited or have loose bowels when you're upset. Anxiety, depression, stress, and grief all express themselves as emotional pain and, quite often, GI distress. The gut lining is a single cell layer thick and connects your internal organs with substances from the outside world. It is one of your body's initial defenses against invaders. Big trouble happens when the lining becomes excessively permeable, a condition known as leaky gut.

Besides chronic inflammation, a long list of health problems is associated with a leaky gut, from autoimmune diseases (such as lupus, rheumatoid arthritis, Hashimoto's thyroiditis, and multiple sclerosis) and digestive issues (gas, bloating, constipation, and diarrhea) to seasonal allergies and skin problems (acne, rosacea). Not surprisingly, leaky gut is also linked to brain problems, including mood and anxiety disorders, ADHD, Parkinson's, and Alzheimer's.

Make friends with good bugs

Your gut plays an important role in the health of your brain. About 100 trillion microorganisms (bacteria, yeast, and others) live in your GI tract. This community of "bugs" is collectively known as the microbiome. For you to be healthy, your microbiome should contain about 85 percent good bugs and only about 15 percent troublemakers. When that ratio is reversed, you can develop a leaky gut, along with corresponding physical and mental problems. *Keeping your gut microbiome in proper balance is essential to your mental health.*[1]

The microbiome functions to protect your gut lining, digestion, and nutrient absorption. It synthesizes vitamins (K, B12) and neurotransmitters, such as serotonin. It is involved in detoxification and helps manage inflammation, immunity, appetite, and blood sugar levels. New evidence indicates that friendly gut bacteria deter invading troublemakers, such as *E. coli* bacteria, and help us withstand stress. If the good bugs are deficient—either from a poor diet that feeds yeast overgrowth (such as from sugar) or excessive use of antibiotics (even as far back as childhood), which kills good bacteria—you are more likely to feel anxious, stressed, depressed, and tired.

‖‖‖

What Decreases Healthy Gut Bacteria?

The level of healthy bacteria in your gut can be compromised by a number of factors, including:

- medications (antibiotics, oral contraceptives, proton pump inhibitors, steroids, NSAIDS)
- stress
- sugar and high fructose corn syrup
- artificial sweeteners
- gluten

- allergies to the environment or food
- insomnia (especially among soldiers and those involved in shift work)
- toxins (antimicrobial chemicals in soaps; pesticides; heavy metals)
- intestinal infections (H. pylori, parasites)
- low levels of omega-3 fatty acids
- low levels of vitamin D
- radiation/chemotherapy
- high intensity exercise
- excessive alcohol[2]

||||||||||||||||||||||||||||||||||||||||||||||||||||||||||||||||||||||||||||||||||||||||||||

Actually, most of your exposure to antibiotics comes, not from those prescribed by your doctor, but from your food. An estimated 80 percent of the antibiotics used in the United States are given to livestock, and the prevalence of these drugs in conventionally raised meats and dairy may disturb the balance of good to bad bacteria in the gut. This is why it is critical to eat antibiotic- and hormone-free meats whenever possible.

In a 2016 study, mice given antibiotics showed decreased gut bacteria, which lowered the number of white blood cells that communicated among the gut, brain, and immune system.[3] Surprisingly, *the antibiotics stopped the growth of new cells in the hippocampus and impaired memory.* Probiotics and exercise reversed the trouble in the hippocampus. In short, you need to take care of your gut or your brain could be in big trouble.

LOW OMEGA-3 FATTY ACIDS: WHY EATING FISH BOOSTS BRAIN HEALTH

One of the leading preventable causes of death is having a low level of the omega-3 fatty acids EPA and DHA in your bloodstream, according to researchers at the Harvard School of Public Health.[4] Low levels of EPA and DHA are associated with

- inflammation[5]
- heart disease[6]
- depression and bipolar disorder[7]
- suicidal behavior[8]
- ADHD[9]
- cognitive impairment and dementia[10]
- obesity[11]

Unfortunately, most people are low in the omega-3 fatty acids EPA and DHA unless they focus on eating fish (which can be high in mercury and other toxins) or take an omega-3 fatty acid EPA plus DHA supplement. In 2016, Amen Clinics tested the omega-3 fatty acid levels of 50 consecutive patients who were not taking fish oil (the most commonly used source of EPA and DHA) and found that 49 had suboptimal levels. In another study, our research team correlated the SPECT scans of 130 patients with their EPA and DHA levels and found that those with the lowest levels had lower blood flow—the number one predictor of future brain problems—in the right hippocampus and posterior cingulate (one of the first areas to die in Alzheimer's disease). On cognitive testing, we also found low omega-3s correlated with decreased scores in mood.

Increasing scientific evidence points to a connection between cognitive function and the consumption of fish rich in omega-3 fatty acids EPA and DHA. For example, a team of Danish researchers compared the diets of 5,386 healthy older individuals and found that the more fish in the diet, the longer people were able to maintain their memory and avoid dementia.

These beneficial fatty acids are not to be confused with omega-6 fatty acids, which are plentiful in the American diet. Unfortunately, eating too much omega-6 fatty acids can erase the benefits of omega-3s. (For more on the distinction between these fatty acids, see chapter 16.)

 ## CHECKUP FOR INFLAMMATION ISSUES

Lab tests

Testing amounts of the following substances in your blood will help you and your doctor determine the level of inflammation in your body and provide direction on what to do about it.

- **C-reactive protein (CRP)** measures inflammation. The most common cause of elevated C-reactive protein is metabolic syndrome or insulin resistance. The second most common cause is sensitivity to food, such as gluten. High CRP levels can also indicate hidden infections. A healthy range is between 0.0 and 1.0 mg/L.

- **Interleukin 6 (IL-6)** is another measure of inflammation. IL-6 is a cytokine, a protein produced by immune cells that acts on other cells to help regulate and/or promote an immune response. Normally, IL-6 is not detected in the blood or is present in very low quantities. An elevated amount of IL-6 may mean an inflammatory condition is present, such as an infection or an autoimmune disorder. It is also associated with a worsening prognosis for memory issues.

- **Homocysteine** is an amino acid that, when elevated, is associated with inflammation, atherosclerosis (hardening and narrowing of the arteries), and an increased risk of heart attack, stroke, blood clots, and possibly Alzheimer's disease. Homocysteine is also a sensitive marker for folate deficiency. The level should be lower than 8 micromoles/liter.

- **Folate** aids in the production of DNA and other genetic material. It is required for the healthy regulation of our genes and is especially important when cells and tissues are growing rapidly, such as in infancy, adolescence, and pregnancy. Folate works together with vitamins B6 and B12 and other nutrients to control blood levels of homocysteine. It is common to have low levels of folate as a result of alcoholism, inflammatory bowel disease (IBD), celiac disease, and taking certain medications. A normal level is 2 to 20 ng/mL; the optimal level is thought to be greater than 3 ng/mL.

- **Vitamin B12** is critically important for healthy brain function. A vitamin B12 deficiency can potentially cause severe and irreversible damage, especially to the brain and nervous system. Symptoms such as fatigue, depression, and poor memory can occur at levels only slightly lower than normal. Vitamin B12 also can be depleted by medications, particularly those that impair stomach and intestinal function, such as proton pump inhibitors for acid reflux. Its deficiency can cause symptoms of mania and psychosis and can even masquerade as dementia. A normal range is 211 to 946 picograms per milliliter (pg/mL); an optimal level is greater than 600.

- **The Omega-3 Index** measures the total amount of omega-3 fatty acids EPA and DHA in red blood cells, which, as it turns out, directly reflects their levels in the brain. This test, requiring just a drop of blood, has been validated by more than 100 peer-reviewed research studies and is a helpful, clinically validated biomarker of your brain's health. A low Omega-3 Index increases the risk of cognitive decline by as much as 77 percent.[12] You can talk to knowledgeable integrative medicine health-care providers about this test. You should aim for an Omega-3 Index level above 8 percent.

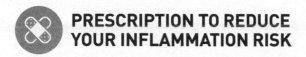

PRESCRIPTION TO REDUCE YOUR INFLAMMATION RISK

The Strategies

1. **Address the health of your gut with four strategies:**

   - Avoid anything that hurts your gut (see list on page 99).
   - Increase prebiotics (the food for probiotics): apples, beans, cabbage, psyllium, artichokes, onions, leeks, asparagus, and root veggies (sweet potatoes, yams, squash, jicama, beets, carrots, and turnips).
   - Increase probiotics to strengthen your microbiome. You can do this with probiotic supplements (see page 106) or fermented foods that contain live bacteria: kefir, kombucha, unsweetened yogurt (goat or coconut), kimchi, pickled fruits and vegetables, and sauerkraut.
   - Be careful with antibiotics. If you have had a lot of them in the past, taking probiotics and eating a healthy diet become even more important to maintaining brain health.

2. **Reduce homocysteine.** B vitamins, especially B6, B12, and folate, help lower high levels of homocysteine, and they also support brain health. A 2010 Oxford University study[13] tested the presumption that by controlling levels of homocysteine, the amount of brain shrinkage (which tends to precipitate Alzheimer's disease) could be reduced. Study participants received relatively high doses of B vitamins, including 800 mcg of methyl folate, 500 mcg of B12 (cyanocobalamin), and 20 mg of B6 (pyridoxine hydrochloride). Two years later, those who had received the vitamin B regimen suffered significantly less brain shrinkage than those who had received a placebo. After taking the vitamins, even the brains of those who had the highest levels of homocysteine at the start of the study shrank at half the rate of the brains of those taking a placebo. In another

study, participants taking high doses of folate and vitamins B12 and B6 lowered homocysteine and the associated brain shrinkage by 90 percent.[14]

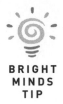

BRIGHT MINDS TIP

Load up on omega-3s. Getting more of the fatty acids EPA and DHA will improve your blood flow, mood, and weight, and they'll give your brain a boost.

---

3. **Boost your omega-3s.** The omega-3 fatty acids EPA and DHA can increase blood flow;[15] slow brain atrophy;[16] increase working memory,[17] executive function,[18] fluid intelligence (problem solving) and mood;[19] and decrease inflammation[20] and anxiety.[21] Before we started offering the Omega-3 Index to our patients, I tested our employees, several family members, and myself. When my test results came back, I was very happy: An Omega-3 Index score above 8 is good, and mine was nearly 11. But the results for nearly all of our employees and family members were not so good. In fact, I was horrified at how low their levels were, which put them at greater risk for both physical and emotional problems. It was an easy fix: They just needed to eat more clean, cold-water fish or take fish oil supplements.

EPA and DHA are practically vitamins because the body has very limited capacity to make them, and we have to obtain most of our supply from foods or supplements. Most Americans have low levels as measured by the Omega-3 Index. Plants don't make them, but cold-water fish are a good dietary source. You do have to be careful that the fish you eat don't poison you with mercury, PCBs, and dioxins. Check where they were caught and be sure they are free of such toxic contamination. The safest way to increase your Omega-3 Index is to take highly concentrated fish oil supplements that provide at least 1,000 mg of EPA plus DHA per day.

Increasing your intake of omega-3 fatty acids EPA and DHA is one of the best ways to improve your brain power, mood, and weight. EPA is important for controlling inflammation and maintaining a positive mood, and it works with DHA to help brain stem cells mature into functioning neurons. DHA is an important contributor to the lipids in your brain that build cell membranes, which play a vital role in how your cells function. DHA actually makes up a large portion of the gray matter of the brain. It is also a main component of the brain's trillions of synapses (where neurons come together to form connections). DHA and EPA work together to improve blood flow, which boosts overall brain function.

Researchers have discovered that a diet rich in omega-3 EPA and DHA helps maintain emotional health and positive mood as people age. Taking fish oil high in EPA and DHA helps ease symptoms of depression. In fact, a 20-year study of 3,317 men and women found that people with the highest consumption of EPA and DHA were less likely to have signs of depression.

Omega-3 EPA and DHA can benefit cognitive performance at every age. In 2010, scientists at the University of Pittsburgh reported that middle-aged people with higher DHA levels performed better on a variety of tests, including nonverbal reasoning, mental flexibility, working memory, and vocabulary. Swedish researchers surveyed nearly 5,000 15-year-old boys and found that those who ate fish more than once a week scored higher on standard intelligence tests given three years later than those teens who ate no fish. A follow-up study found that teens eating fish more than once a week also had better grades in school than students with lower fish consumption. Additional benefits of omega-3 EPA and DHA include increased attention in people with ADD, reduced stress, and a lower risk for psychosis. And when we put a group of retired football players on highly concentrated fish oil supplements, many of them were able to decrease or completely eliminate their pain medications.

4. **Take care of your gums.** This is an easy one. To decrease inflammation, it is critical to avoid periodontal (gum) disease, which is a risk factor for dementia.[22] Be sure to brush your teeth twice a day after meals and floss daily. *Flossing your teeth is a brain exercise!* And see a dentist regularly for checkups and cleanings.

The Nutraceuticals

Folate, vitamin B12, and vitamin B6: I recommend that my patients with high homocysteine levels take the following:

- *Folate:* Take 800 mcg a day of methyl folate (the body's naturally most active form), not folic acid (which is a synthetic).
- *Vitamin B12:* Take 500 mcg a day of methyl cobalamin; hydroxocobalamin is also safe. Both are preferable to cyanocobalamin, a widely sold form that contains potentially toxic cyanide.
- *Vitamin B6:* Take 20 mg a day of pyridoxine hydrochloride or as pyridoxal-5-phosphate. (Both are well absorbed and utilized.)
- *Betaine (trimethylglycine):* Take 1,000 to 3,000 mg a day of this substance, which is present naturally in our cells and is very useful as a methyl backup.

Omega-3s: My recommendation for most adults is 1,400 to 2,800 mg a day of EPA and DHA omega-3 fatty acids. Other omega-3s such as alpha-linolenic acid are not likely to be beneficial because they are so poorly converted to the larger active EPA and DHA molecules.

Curcumin: This is the collective name for the three active curcuminoids from turmeric root (used in making curries), which have potent anti-inflammatory effects. More than 7,000 published articles have revealed the benefits of curcumin, including its powerful antioxidant properties, its ability to help regulate blood sugar, and its anti-inflammatory and anti-cancer activities.[23] But the curcuminoids are poorly absorbed when taken by themselves. I recommend 500 to 2,000 mg a day of a highly bioavailable curcumin supplement. (Longvida is an excellent brand, proven to have high absorption.)

Probiotics: Clinical studies show that probiotics decrease homocysteine and inflammation.[24] They are even more effective when given with prebiotics,[25] which support and promote the growth of probiotics. Look for products that contain both *Lactobacillus* and *Bifidobacterium* strains. The number of probiotics in a supplement is less important than the quality of the strains. The probiotic I often recommend is effective at 3 billion live organisms a day.

The Foods
AVOID (OR LIMIT):

High omega-6 vegetables: corn and soybeans

High omega-6 vegetable oils: corn, safflower, sunflower, soybean, canola, cottonseed

Sugar and foods that turn to sugar, such as refined grains

Wheat flour

Trans fats: products containing vegetable shortening or "partially hydrogenated" oils in the list of ingredients

Processed meats: Sodium nitrites can combine with amines to form nitrosamines, which are carcinogenic.

Grain-fed meats: Because these are a source of excessive omega-6s, choose grass-fed meat whenever possible.

Food additives: MSG, aspartame, etc.

Foods that disrupt the gut lining, such as gluten

CONSIDER ADDING:

Anti-inflammatory spices: turmeric,[26] cayenne, ginger,[27] cloves, cinnamon,[28] oregano, pumpkin pie spice, rosemary, sage, fennel[29]

Folate-rich foods: spinach, dark leafy greens, asparagus, turnips, beets, mustard greens, brussels sprouts, lima beans, beef liver, root vegetables, kidney beans, white beans, salmon, avocado

Omega-3-rich foods: A number of studies show that flaxseeds, walnuts, salmon, sardines, beef, shrimp, walnut oil, chia seeds, and avocado oil lower cardiovascular risk and inflammation. The animal sources provide EPA and DHA directly, but the plant sources have to be converted, and some people's enzyme systems are poor at making this conversion. Track your Omega-3 Index!

Prebiotic-rich foods: dandelion greens, asparagus, chia seeds, beans, cabbage, psyllium, artichokes, raw garlic, onions, leeks, root vegetables (sweet potatoes, yams, squash, jicama, beets, carrots, turnips)

Probiotic-rich foods: brined vegetables (not vinegar), kimchi, sauerkraut, kefir, miso soup, pickles, spirulina, chlorella, blue-green algae, kombucha

Tart cherry juice decreases levels of inflammatory CRP.[30]

Magnesium-rich foods: See page 77 in chapter 5.

Polyphenol-rich foods: See page 118 in chapter 8.

Allicin-rich foods: See page 200 in chapter 12.

Fiber-rich foods: See page 239 in chapter 14.

 ## PICK ONE HEALTHY BRIGHT MINDS HABIT TO START TODAY

1. Floss your teeth daily and care for your gums.

2. Eat more green leafy vegetables.

3. Test your CRP and homocysteine levels.

4. **Test your Omega-3 Index; aim to get above 8.**

5. Eliminate trans fats.

6. Limit omega-6-rich foods (corn, soy, processed foods).

7. Increase omega-3-rich foods (fish, avocados, walnuts).

8. Take vitamin B6, vitamin B12, and methylfolate.

9. Add prebiotic foods to your diet.

10. **Add probiotic foods and/or supplements.**

CHAPTER 8

G IS FOR GENETICS
GENES ONLY LOAD THE GUN; YOUR BEHAVIOR PULLS THE TRIGGER

I lavish unfailing love to a thousand generations. I forgive iniquity, rebellion, and sin. But I do not excuse the guilty. I lay the sins of the parents upon their children and grandchildren; the entire family is affected—even children in the third and fourth generations.

EXODUS 34:7

BUD: LEARNING TO MITIGATE THE GENETIC FACTOR

Bud, 52, came to see me because he was concerned about his memory, focus, and energy. His mother had died of Alzheimer's disease, and he had a wife 20 years his junior and two young children, ages five and seven. From his history, I learned he had untreated ADHD and bouts of depression that were becoming more frequent as stress piled up at work. He also had one copy of the *APOE* e4 gene variant; mild hypertension; prediabetes; high CRP, ferritin, and LDL cholesterol; low vitamin D, DHEA, and testosterone levels; untreated sleep apnea; and erectile dysfunction. In addition, Bud carried an extra 30 pounds, putting him in the obese category. His BrainFit WebNeuro showed significant memory, attention, and executive problems. His SPECT scan showed decreased activity in the frontal and temporal lobes. Bud was clearly headed for serious trouble. He had multiple risk factors that were damaging his brain, his fortune, and his family.

BUD'S "BEFORE" BRAIN SPECT SCAN

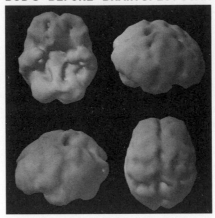

BUD'S BRIGHT MINDS RISK FACTORS AND INTERVENTIONS

BRIGHT MINDS	BUD'S RISK FACTORS	INTERVENTIONS
Blood Flow	Low blood flow on SPECT, hypertension, high LDL cholesterol, erectile dysfunction	Exercise, ginkgo biloba
Retirement/Aging	Age 52, high ferritin (iron)	Blood donation to lower ferritin, antioxidant-rich diet
Inflammation	High CRP	Diet, omega-3 fatty acids EPA and DHA
Genetics	Family history of Alzheimer's, *APOE* e4 positive	
Head Trauma		
Toxins		
Mental Health	Chronic stress, ADHD, mild depression	Stress management tools, ADHD treatment
Immunity/Infection Issues	Low vitamin D	Vitamin D3 supplements
Neurohormone Deficiencies	Low DHEA and testosterone	Exercise, weight lifting, limited sugar, DHEA supplements
Diabesity	Prediabetes and obesity	Memory Rescue Diet
Sleep Issues	Sleep apnea	CPAP machine

After seeing his scan and test results, Bud was determined to become an active participant in his health. He radically changed his diet by cutting out his usual six daily sodas, severely restricting his sugar intake, increasing the protein and healthy fat in his diet, and reducing grains and processed carbohydrates. He started weight lifting twice a week and replaced his typical once-or-twice-weekly slow walks (30 minutes apiece) with burst training three times a week (see page 73 for more on this type of exercise). He started wearing his CPAP machine to treat his sleep apnea and was faithful with his supplement regimen.

Over the next year, Bud lost 30 pounds, and his blood sugar and blood pressure dropped to normal levels without any medication. He reported that his memory, focus, and energy were better than they had been in 30 years. Plus, his sexual function improved—a common outcome of the treatment. As I've said before, when blood flow gets better anywhere in the body, it typically gets better everywhere.

YOUR GENES DON'T HAVE TO BE YOUR DESTINY

About 20 years ago, I was on a committee of a professional medical society, advocating for the use of neuroimaging tools like SPECT for the diagnosis of Alzheimer's disease and other memory disorders. I argued that people should have access to more information about their own health and that SPECT was one of the best tools to evaluate brain function. One of my colleagues from a major Midwestern university disagreed. He suggested that since there was nothing people could do about the risk, there was no point in worrying them. It turned into a heated discussion because I believed then, and know now, that you can take a number of steps to decrease your risk.

In the BRIGHT MINDS mnemonic, *G* is for genetic risk factors. Humans receive 23 pairs of chromosomes—one set from each parent—that are found in the DNA in the nucleus of cells. Each chromosome contains the genes that provide instruction, or coding, for producing the different kinds of proteins that make up our cells. A healthy person has just the right number of chromosomes and the right number of genes. When the number of chromosomes is wrong, or there are extra or defective genes, health problems occur.

People who have family members with severe memory problems, Alzheimer's disease, or another form of dementia, or those who have one or two copies of the *APOE* e4 gene or several other genes, have a higher risk for memory problems. This is especially true for those with a first-degree relative (mother, father, brother, or sister) with memory issues. They are 3.5 times more likely to develop symptoms. A family history of Parkinson's disease also makes it more likely that people will develop memory issues. A recent study revealed that people with first-degree relatives with Parkinson's disease were six times more likely to develop dementia than those in the general population.[1]

I think of the brain as a magnificent, complex series of spiderwebs (nerve cell fields) suspended in water, with neurons communicating at speeds of up to 268 miles per hour. Two of the prevailing theories about what causes severe memory loss include (1) the abnormal accumulation of beta-amyloid plaques—think of beta amyloid as a sticky, gooey substance that gets dropped into nerve cell fields, causing short circuits; and (2) twisted tangles of tau proteins within brain cells, called neurofibrillary tangles, that disrupt brain cell function.

For years, researchers have debated whether beta-amyloid plaques or tau proteins lead to severe memory loss. At times the hostility between the two camps has grown as bitter as a religious war, with some calling it a battle between the "baptists" (beta-amyloid believers) and the "tauists." It now seems that both mechanisms are important, but cleaning up beta amyloid and toxic tau proteins after a person develops memory issues has not helped in human studies.[2] They must be purged as early as possible, before they short-circuit brain cell networks.

At least four genes are known to increase beta-amyloid production:

1. the e4 version of the apolipoprotein E (*APOE*) gene on chromosome 19, which is associated with late-onset Alzheimer's disease[3]

2. the amyloid precursor protein (*APP*) on chromosome 21, which is overproduced in people with Down syndrome, sometimes causing memory problems between the ages of 35 and 65

3. the presenilin 1 gene on chromosome 14 (*PSEN1*), which often causes Alzheimer's disease

4. the presenilin 2 gene on chromosome 1 (*PSEN2*), which also often causes Alzheimer's

Tau proteins are found inside neurons and provide the structure, like train tracks, to help cells expel unwanted and toxic proteins. When tau proteins function properly, they clear the cells of toxic proteins such as beta amyloid. When they act abnormally, the tracks fail, trash accumulates, and damage occurs,[4] sort of like a car wreck. Tangled and abnormal tau deposits can result from repeated head trauma, which is found in football players with dementia (also called chronic traumatic encephalopathy, or CTE).[5] Besides trauma, errant genes on chromosome 17 can cause tau protein problems, as can excessive iron stores.[6]

The APOE *gene: do you have an e4?*

Everyone has two *APOE* genes. These genes alone are not dangerous; we need them to function. They help in the development, maturation, and repair of cell membranes. They also help regulate the amount of cholesterol and triglycerides in nerve cell membranes.

There are three versions of the *APOE* gene: e2, e3, and e4. As with all genes, we inherit one copy from each parent, which means everyone has one of the following combinations:

e2/e2	e3/e3
e2/e3	e3/e4
e2/e4	e4/e4

A person with one *APOE* e4 gene inherited it from one parent. Someone with two *APOE* e4 genes received one from each parent. A person with one *APOE* e4—or worse, two genes—has a high chance of experiencing memory problems. This gene increases the beta-amyloid deposition and plaque formation that are found in the brains of people with Alzheimer's disease, so it increases the chance of developing late-onset Alzheimer's disease—by 2.5 times if you have one e4, or 5 to 15 times if you have two e4s.[7] For people who carry the *APOE* e4 gene but whose Alzheimer's is due to other causes, symptoms appear two to five years earlier than in people without the gene.

About 15 percent of the population has at least one *APOE* e4 gene. With just one *APOE* gene, the odds of developing Alzheimer's after age 65 are 25 percent, versus a 5 to 10 percent risk for people with no *APOE* e4 gene. That's quite a difference. But there is good news: Not everyone with the gene will develop Alzheimer's disease; in fact, 75 percent will not. Even if someone with one *APOE* e4 gene develops dementia, the cause may be something other than Alzheimer's disease. However, if someone with two *APOE* e4 genes develops dementia, the odds are high that Alzheimer's disease is the culprit. In fact, having two e4 copies may increase the risk of developing Alzheimer's by 12 times. Having one or two copies of the *APOE* e4 gene also increases the risk of vascular problems.[8] The *APOE* e4 gene is associated with overall lower blood flow to the brain,[9] which means it is absolutely essential that people with this gene take good care of their blood vessels.

The presenilin genes (PSEN1 and PSEN2): another route to Alzheimer's disease

Two other genes, presenilin 1 and 2 (*PSEN1* and *PSEN2*), have been found in families where a number of members have Alzheimer's disease. *PSEN1* is on chromosome 14, while *PSEN2* is on chromosome 1. Both of these gene mutations greatly accelerate beta-amyloid production. *PSEN1* causes symptoms to appear early, when people are between the ages of 35 and 55. The *PSEN2* gene is rarer, and dementia symptoms may appear early or late, between ages 40 and 85.[10]

EPIGENETICS MAY BE JUST AS IMPORTANT

For the past few decades, scientists have been exploring the new field of epigenetics, or the way behaviors, emotions, and environment can turn certain genes on or off. As a result, some illnesses become more or less likely, in us as well as in our children, grandchildren, and even great-grandchildren. Geneticists now know that our habits, feelings, and environment affect our biology so deeply that they cause changes in the genes that are transmitted to future generations. These epigenetic "etches" tell your genes to switch on or off or to express themselves more loudly or softly.

In other words, environmental factors like diet, stress, toxins, and prenatal nutrition can affect the activity of the genes that are passed on to your offspring and beyond. A 2006 study demonstrated that prepubescent boys (age 11 or 12) who started smoking cigarettes increased the risk of obesity in their children.[11] Unwise decisions at such a young age could affect future generations. And obesity[12] is just the beginning. Some researchers believe that epigenetics could also help us better understand certain cancers, forms of dementia, schizophrenia, autism, and diabetes.[13]

CHECKUP FOR GENETICS ISSUES

Know your family history

Not everyone has taken the time to find out what happened to Aunt May or Great-Uncle Willie. Reach out to family members so that you can be aware of any branches of your family tree in which memory troubles have appeared—and address those issues, if necessary.

Lab test

- **Apolipoprotein E gene (APOE) status:** Get tested to know your risk; any doctor can order this test for you. Many people tell me they do not want to know whether they carry an APOE e4 gene, but if you find out that your genetics put you at increased risk, you have an opportunity to make a more concerted effort to decrease all the other risk factors.

   Some studies show that the APOE e4 gene also increases the risk of memory problems and Alzheimer's in the presence of cancer chemotherapy and head injuries.[14] I believe children and teens who want to play contact sports should be screened for the APOE e4 gene. If they have it, they should play less risky sports. Presenilin and other more sophisticated genetic testing may be worthwhile if people in your family have early-onset memory issues. Consult with your family doctor about this.

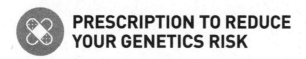 ## PRESCRIPTION TO REDUCE YOUR GENETICS RISK

The Strategies

1. **Go for screening early.** For those who have genetic risk factors (a family history of memory problems, dementia, or Alzheimer's), early screening—around age 40—that includes questionnaires, cognitive testing, and possibly brain SPECT imaging is important. New research shows that having the APOE e4 gene is not necessarily a dementia death sentence.[15] Early screening gives you a window in which to address the other risk factors.

2. **Take your brain health seriously.** If you suspect you have a genetic predisposition to memory issues, caring for your brain is critical. Studies have shown that the risk of dementia was significantly lower in people with one or two of the e4 variants of the *APOE* gene if they had higher education levels and engaged in leisure activities like sports or hobbies that involved new learning. They also did better if they took care of their blood vessels and had fewer vascular risk factors, such as hypertension, smoking, or heart problems.

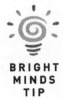

BRIGHT MINDS TIP

Being hypervigilant about keeping your brain healthy could make all the difference, particularly if you've watched family members struggle with dementia.

---

3. **Hop on the exercise bandwagon.** Research has found that physical exercise can decrease beta-amyloid buildup in the brain in *APOE* e4 carriers.[16] Research teams in Finland and Sweden found that exercising at least twice a week in middle age lowered the chance of getting dementia more than 20 years later, and this protective effect was stronger in people with the *APOE* e4 gene. All of us should exercise, engage in new learning, and take care of our blood vessels, but it is even more imperative if you have one or two *APOE* e4 genes.

4. **Avoid head trauma.** To protect your head from injuries and concussions (which can increase abnormal tau proteins), avoid contact sports and falls, which are much more common as you age. Practice balance exercises and strengthen your muscles to keep them in shape.

The Nutraceuticals

The following nutrients have been shown to decrease beta-amyloid plaque formation and tau protein deposits in animal studies:

- *Blueberry extract*[17]

- *Resveratrol*[18]

- *Green tea catechins (GTC)*, including EGCG[19]

- *Acetyl-L-carnitine (ALCAR)*[20]

- *Curcumin:*[21] In a 12-month study of 96 older adults with cognitive decline, those who took 1,500 mg a day derived significant benefits compared to those who took a placebo.[22]

- *Ashwagandha*[23]

- *Ginseng*[24]

- *NAC (N-acetylcysteine):*[25] NAC improved cognition in Alzheimer's patients compared to a placebo.[26]

- *Coenzyme Q10* (CoQ10)[27]

- *Magnesium*[28]

- *Vitamins B6 and B12*[29]

- *Vitamin D:*[30] People with the lowest levels of vitamin D have as much as a 25-fold higher risk of having mild cognitive impairment, the predecessor to Alzheimer's, when compared to those with the highest vitamin D levels.[31]

- *DHA*, one of the omega-3 fatty acids[32]

The Foods
AVOID (OR LIMIT):

Meals with high-glycemic foods and lots of saturated fat: These foods (think fast-food pizza, ribeye steak and mashed potatoes, pancakes with syrup and bacon) raise the levels of blood sugar, insulin, and cholesterol in our bodies, which can contribute to diabesity.

Processed cheeses and microwave popcorn: They contain diacetyl, a flavoring chemical that increases beta amyloid.

CONSIDER ADDING:

Spices to help decrease beta amyloid: sage, turmeric, cardamom, ginger, saffron, cinnamon (which decreases tau aggregation)

Foods to decrease beta amyloid: salmon, blueberries, curry

Polyphenol-rich foods: chocolate, green tea, blueberries, kale, red wine, onions, apples, cherries, cabbage. These foods contain quercetin and other ingredients that increase circulation, prevent LDL oxidation, and decrease inflammation and beta-amyloid plaques.

Vitamin B6, vitamin B12, and folate-rich foods: See page 77 in chapter 5.

Magnesium-rich foods: See page 77 in chapter 5.

Vitamin D–rich foods: See page 200 in chapter 12.

A ketogenic (very low carbohydrate) diet: This eating plan has been shown to decrease beta amyloid in animal models.[33]

PICK ONE HEALTHY BRIGHT MINDS HABIT TO START TODAY

1. **If you have dementia in your family, be serious about brain health starting now and get early screening for memory problems.**

2. Test your *APOE* gene type.

3. If you have the *APOE* e4 gene, avoid contact sports or other head trauma risks.

4. Limit high-glycemic, saturated-fat foods, such as pizza.

5. Limit processed cheeses and microwave popcorn.

6. **Take a curcumin supplement to decrease beta-amyloid plaques before they damage your brain.**

7. Eat organic blueberries to decrease beta-amyloid plaques.

8. Cook with sage to decrease beta-amyloid plaques.

9. Take a ginseng supplement.

10. Take a coenzyme Q10 (CoQ10) supplement.

CHAPTER 9

H IS FOR HEAD TRAUMA
THE SILENT EPIDEMIC

*I wouldn't let my six-year-old son near any football field. And if any coach
asks my son to play football, I'll sue that coach, and I'll sue the school.*

**BENNET OMALU, MD, NEUROPATHOLOGIST
WHO DISCOVERED CTE (FOOTBALL DEMENTIA)**

SHAWN DOLLAR:
THE SURVIVAL STORY OF A BIG WAVE SURFER

When I first met with Shawn Dollar at our clinic, I was transfixed by this professional surfer's story. On September 7, 2015, 35-year-old Shawn was surfing in a remote area off the coast of Big Sur. As a 25-foot wave approached, Dollar stood up on his surfboard and dove headfirst under the wave. Unfortunately, the sharp edge of a boulder sat just below the surface, and his skull slammed into it. On impact, he heard his neck shatter. In fact, it had broken in four places, and he'd suffered a concussion. Although he was dazed, Shawn knew people weren't supposed to move after breaking their spine.

As Shawn floated in the ocean, trying to remain conscious but without moving, he realized

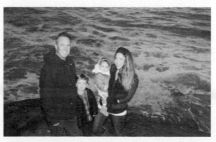

Shawn Dollar with his wife, Jenn; son, Kai, 5; and daughter, Kaylee, 1; in 2016 at the beach in Pleasure Point, California

he had three choices. He could drown, allow himself to be pounded against the rocks, or begin paddling toward shore and risk paralyzing himself. None sounded ideal, but as Shawn thought of his wife and kids, he was determined to try paddling the 30 to 40 feet to shore.

"I had to muster up all the strength I could to survive," he said. "It was terrifying." He had little strength to move or even mount his board. The waves relentlessly knocked him off his surfboard. Yet not only did Shawn make it to shore, he hiked up the beach and walked a mile through ravines and up switchback trails to get to his car at the top of a cliff.

As it turns out, surviving and then making it to the hospital were the easy part. The recovery ahead was far more brutal than Shawn could have imagined.

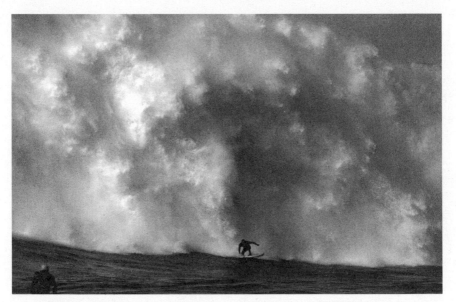

During a break between the semifinal and final heats of the 2010 Mavericks surfing contest, Shawn Dollar—though not a competitor—paddled into and then rode this 55-foot wave, setting a Guinness World Record. *Photo by Phil Gibbs. Used with permission.*

But one thing Shawn Dollar had going for him was tenacity. He isn't your average surfer. He's an internationally recognized professional who has broken the Guinness World Record twice for the largest wave ever paddled into—once during the legendary Mavericks competition near Half Moon Bay, California, and again off the coast of Cortes Bank, southwest of Los Angeles, where he rode a 61-foot-high wave.

After his injury, Shawn, a gifted athlete accustomed to training, did everything the doctors and physical therapists asked of him. He was deter-mined to make a complete recovery, and by November, his neck had healed.

"As soon as the neck brace came off, everybody thought I was back," Shawn told me. "But I could feel my life falling apart."

Shawn had severe migraines every day that made him throw up and kept him from sleeping. His mood swings were intense, accompanied by feelings of depression, anxiety, confusion, and even suicidal thoughts. His memory had also deteriorated: He couldn't focus, do simple math, or match his socks.

"He had trouble with recall," Shawn's wife, Jenn, said. "There were mem-ories that had gone missing, experiences that had fallen through the cracks."

After months with no improvement, Shawn explained his concerns to two neurosurgeons. Their advice? Relax. The standard medical protocol for concussions is rest, wait, and monitor, and that's what they urged Shawn to do.

But things did not get better; they got worse. One doctor gave Shawn the impression that, although his neck had healed, his mental condition might remain unchanged for the rest of his life. "The brain doesn't really heal," he told Shawn. "Once you have brain damage, that's it. That's what you've got."

Greatly concerned over his poor memory and mental state, Shawn began looking for other sources of help. He researched new doctors and therapists and experimented with various treatments. "A lot of the places I went to have one medium of care and that's what they focus on. It's frustrating because, you know, care needs to come in multiple ways," he said.

Then Shawn's wife, who loves health and fitness, told him about our work at Amen Clinics. She had seen my public television specials and during Shawn's recovery started showing him some of my online videos. A mutual acquaintance connected us. Of course, after we took his history, we had to see his brain.

"From my MRI to CT scans," Shawn said, "*everything* in my brain looked fine. The SPECT scan showed a totally different picture. . . . It put things into perspective. *This is when things started to get better.*"

After treating thousands of patients with traumatic brain injuries, coupled with my work with 200 active and retired NFL players, I had seen this type of brain before. The overall decreased blood flow, evidenced by what appear to be holes of inactivity, was consistent with the pattern of a severe traumatic brain injury (TBI). Like the football players we've seen, Shawn had been knocked around while surfing.

"I'd taken some bad wipeouts at Mavericks and come up feeling dizzy, but I always got better," he said. "Now I understand why I was not getting better this time. The scan gave me hope. It gave me the diagnosis to start to heal and to get everyone around me on the same page. My wife started to have more empathy for me as well, which helped our relationship."

SHAWN DOLLAR'S "BEFORE" BRAIN SPECT SCAN

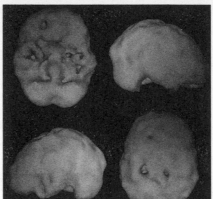

Shows damage to both of his temporal lobes and overall decreased blood flow

SHAWN'S BRIGHT MINDS RISK FACTORS AND INTERVENTIONS

BRIGHT MINDS	SHAWN'S RISK FACTORS	INTERVENTIONS
Blood Flow	Low blood flow on SPECT	Exercise, diet, ginkgo biloba
Retirement/Aging		
Inflammation		
Genetics		
Head Trauma	Serious	HBOT, neurofeedback, supplements
Toxins		
Mental Health	Depression, stress at home	SAMe, betaine supplement, stress management tools
Immunity/Infection Issues	Low vitamin D	Vitamin D3 supplements
Neurohormone Deficiencies		
Diabesity		
Sleep Issues	Insomnia after accident	Sleep strategies

We immediately began treatment, and Shawn attacked his recovery like he attacked the big waves. He did everything we asked of him, which included changing his diet, taking nutraceuticals, and undergoing neurofeedback and hyperbaric oxygen therapy (HBOT). HBOT is a noninvasive, safe, and well-established treatment for decompression sickness, a hazard of scuba diving. It delivers pure oxygen at greater-than-atmospheric pressure to improve poor circulation and increase the amount of oxygen your blood can carry. We recommended it as part of Shawn's treatment plan because an increase in blood oxygen helps stimulate the release of substances called growth factors and stem cells to help in the healing process (see more on neurofeedback and HBOT in chapter 19). Shawn said, "I felt significantly better after the first HBOT treatment."

Today, Shawn is happier and closer with his family than he has ever been. His focus and memory have improved as well. He is starting to surf and have fun again, but he has wisely decided not to surf big waves anymore. He and his wife, Jenn, are two of my favorite brain warriors and memory rescuers.

SOFT BRAIN, HARD SKULL

In multiple studies, having one or more head injuries has been associated with an increased risk of lasting memory issues.[1] If the injury occurred before the age of 25, a person has 2.5 times the risk of memory problems; if it occurred after 55, a person has almost 4 times the risk. And the risk is even higher if that person has the *APOE* e4 gene.[2]

Many people think of the brain as firm, fixed, and rubbery, but it's not. It only becomes that way after someone dies and the brain is fixed in form-aldehyde. During life, the brain has the consistency of soft butter, tofu, or custard—something between egg whites and Jell-O.[3]

Your very soft brain is housed in a really hard skull that has multiple sharp, bony ridges, which means that the brain is easily damaged. Whiplash, jarring motions (think shaken baby syndrome), blast injuries, and blows to the head can cause the brain to slam into the hard interior ridges of the skull. Here are several mechanisms of brain trauma:

- bruising
- broken blood vessels and bleeding
- increased pressure
- lack of oxygen
- damage to nerve cell connections

- brain cells ripped open, spilling out proteins like tau that cause inflammatory reactions

In addition, because your pituitary gland (the master hormone regulator) sits in a vulnerable part of your skull, it is often damaged in head injuries, causing significant hormonal imbalances.

Soft brain + hard skull with sharp ridges = big trouble
when head injuries occur

A LOOK INSIDE THE SKULL

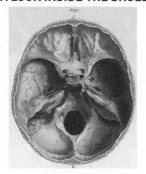

Notice the sharp, bony ridges. Looking down from the top, you
can see the protective bony ridges along the interior of the skull,
which can damage your soft brain in an accident or injury.

Each year about two million new traumatic brain injuries occur. At the time of this writing, more than 350,000 military veterans have sustained a TBI since 2000.[4] This means the Iraq and Afghanistan wars will likely have a 70-year tail, as these veterans will have an increased risk of psychiatric issues and dementia. They need our BRIGHT MINDS approach more than ever.

|||||||||||||||||||||||||||||||||||||||||||||||||||||||||||||||||||||||||||||||||||||||||||||||

Common Causes of Head Trauma

- Falls: falling out of bed, slipping in the bath or shower, tripping down steps, falling off ladders
- Motor vehicle–related collisions: involving cars, motorcycles, ATVs, or bicycles; also pedestrians involved in accidents
- Violence: caused by gunshot wounds, assaults, domestic violence, or child abuse

- Sports injuries: common, not only in football, but in soccer, boxing, baseball, lacrosse, skateboarding, hockey, cycling, basketball, and other high-impact or extreme sports
- Explosive blasts and other combat injuries

||||||||||||||||||||||||||||||||||||||||||||||||||||||||||||||||||||||||||||||||||||||||||||

PROTECT YOUR HEAD—IT COULD SAVE YOUR LIFE

This is worth repeating over and over: Protect your head. It contains your brain, which runs everything in your life. Seems obvious, right? Yet until very recently, this simple concept escaped the consciousness of many people in our society, me included. We let little children hit soccer balls with their heads and do dangerous gymnastic routines. People cheer at high school football games when the opposing quarterback is knocked out of the action after a vicious hit to his head. Many fans love the fights in hockey so much that the National Hockey League has not yet considered eliminating them from the game.[5]

I was once a crazy football fan. I played football in high school and for fun on weekends, and I was a passionate Los Angeles Rams and Washington Redskins fan. Football had been part of my life since I was young, and nothing in my medical training caused me to question my devotion to it.

That all began to change in 1991 when I started looking at the brain. One of the first big lessons I learned from our brain SPECT imaging work was that traumatic brain injuries (TBIs)—even those considered mild without a loss of consciousness and that occurred decades earlier—cause lasting damage that we could clearly see on scans. Those injured areas were wreaking havoc on people's lives, causing depression, suicidal thoughts, panic attacks, temper problems, addictions, and memory and learning issues. What's more, very few professionals knew it because most psychiatrists who see patients who struggle with these issues never look at their brains.

I also found (and still find) that I usually have to ask my patients multiple times whether they ever had a brain injury because many have forgotten even major events. The typical scenario goes like this: A person comes into one of our clinics complaining of a mood, anxiety, learning, memory, or relationship problem.

While taking the patient's history, we ask if he or she ever had a traumatic brain injury.

Usually the patient says no.

Then we examine the SPECT scan, which shows clear evidence of a TBI. We see damage to either one side of the brain or to both the front and back parts of the brain. (This pattern is the result of a coup-contrecoup injury, in which the force of a blow causes the brain to move in the opposite direction, hitting the other side of the skull and damaging that side of the brain as well.) Once we see evidence of a TBI, we ask again, this time with more persistence and specificity. We'll ask:

- Did you ever fall out of a tree or off a fence, or dive into a shallow pool and hit your head?
- Did you ever fall off a horse, ladder, or roof?
- Did you ever play contact sports and have a concussion?
- Did you ever repeatedly hit your head, such as when heading soccer balls or playing tackle football?
- Were you ever in a bicycle, car, or motorcycle accident where you hit your head?

At first, I was amazed at the number of people who answered no five, six, maybe even ten times, and then, all of a sudden, remembered falling out of a second-story window, being thrown from a vehicle moving at 30 miles per hour, or falling off a cliff 150 feet into a riverbed below. One man said his mother told him he had fallen down a flight of stairs at the age of three and was unconscious for days, but he had no recollection of it.

It became clear to me that traumatic brain injuries are a major cause of lasting psychiatric illness and memory problems.

Of course, I was not the first person to make this discovery. Researchers who study and understand this issue have linked TBI to drug and alcohol abuse, anxiety and panic attacks, depression, ADD/ADHD, learning problems, school failure, murder and violent crime, suicide, job failure, incarceration, and homelessness.[6] In a study of homeless people in Toronto, researchers discovered that 58 percent of the men and 42 percent of the women had a significant brain injury before they were homeless.[7] This problem was much bigger than I ever imagined.

Sadie: overcoming a kick in the head

I met 42-year-old Sadie after she had failed her sixth alcohol treatment program. She desperately wanted to stop drinking but couldn't follow through with any of the program recommendations because she was so impulsive and her memory was poor. Whenever alcohol was around, she just couldn't say no or remember the sobriety strategies she'd been taught. Her brain scan, below, showed severe damage to her prefrontal cortex (impacting focus, forethought, judgment, and impulse control) and temporal lobes (affecting learning and memory).

After about the tenth question on the topic of brain injury, Sadie told me that she had been kicked in the head by a horse and lost consciousness when she was 10. Once we focused on the injury and its aftermath, she remembered that her grades at school had started to slip and she became more rebellious at home. People treated her as though she was just a bad person, which made her feel sad and hopeless. In addition to the alcohol and brain injury, Sadie had a family history of dementia, was not sleeping, rarely exercised, had mild hypertension, was often depressed, and wasn't engaged in any type of new learning. Rehabilitating her brain with the BRIGHT MINDS strategies helped her to stay sober and rescue her life.

SADIE'S "BEFORE" BRAIN SPECT SCAN

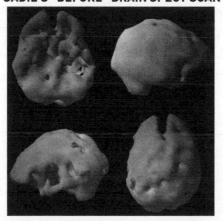

Brain injuries after a kick to the head by a horse

SADIE'S BRIGHT MINDS RISK FACTORS AND INTERVENTIONS

BRIGHT MINDS	SADIE'S RISK FACTORS	INTERVENTIONS
Blood Flow	Low blood flow on SPECT, low exercise, mild hypertension	Exercise, ginkgo biloba, omega-3s EPA and DHA, diet
Retirement/Aging	No new learning activities	New learning
Inflammation		
Genetics	Family history of dementia	

BRIGHT MINDS	SADIE'S RISK FACTORS	INTERVENTIONS
Head Trauma	Serious	HBOT, supplements
Toxins	Chronic alcohol abuse	Eliminate alcohol
Mental Health	Depression, stress of addiction	Supplements, exercise, and eliminating the ANTs (automatic negative thoughts)
Immunity/Infection Issues	Low vitamin D	Vitamin D3 supplements
Neurohormone Deficiencies		
Diabesity		
Sleep Issues	Chronic insomnia	Sleep strategies

Football and brain trauma

Although many of our patients, like Sadie, have forgotten long-ago head injuries that contribute to memory problems, I've spent decades working with a group of people who regularly take hits to the head: football players. When I first started looking at their brain scans, I noticed that many Pop Warner and high school players showed clear evidence of traumatic brain injuries. These young players were between the ages of 8 and 18, and I was horrified by what I saw. Then I saw college players whose brains showed damage that was even worse. One college player was referred to me after a domestic violence incident. The left side of his brain was clearly damaged (see below).

A COLLEGE FOOTBALL PLAYER'S "BEFORE" BRAIN SPECT SCAN

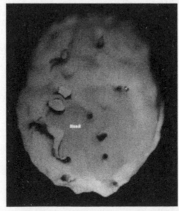

Note the damage to the left side of his brain scan.

In 1999, retired Minnesota Viking offensive guard Brent Boyd came to see me, complaining of headaches, depression, fatigue, dizziness, and cognitive dysfunction. He had suffered multiple concussions in his football career; in fact, his teammate Joe Senser told me that he heard one of the hits against Brent all the way across the field. Brent spent many years dealing with post-concussive syndrome.

Yet when Brent applied for disability through the NFL, the league denied his claim and said his injuries were not football related. It was disturbing. "It was hell," he said, "to experience decades of being called 'lazy and crazy' by friends and loved ones, not to mention employers—and then internalizing it and believing it myself." Prior to the concussions, Brent had been a highly motivated self-starter, graduating with honors at UCLA while playing football.

Brent's SPECT scans showed clear evidence of brain damage. Being able to see the damage changed the way he thought about himself. He later wrote to me, "I am eternally grateful to you for finally correctly diagnosing my problem and putting an end to the self-talk and put-downs by others. I had been so embarrassed by my condition that for over a decade I had cut myself off from friends, family, [and] ex-teammates and crawled under my blanket to die."

In 2007, Brent was the first NFL player to testify in front of Congress about brain injuries in football, especially about the ramifications for younger players.

BRENT'S "BEFORE" BRAIN SPECT SCAN

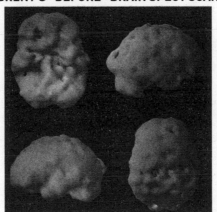

Damage to multiple areas

In July 2007, Anthony Davis, another former NFL player, came to see me as well. He was concerned about the cognitive problems he saw in other retired professional football players, and he was struggling with his own memory, as well as periods of confusion and irritability. AD, as he is called by most who know him, was a College Football Hall of Fame running back for the University of Southern California who scored six touchdowns against the University of Notre Dame in 1972, earning him the nickname the Notre Dame Killer. He then went on to play professional football for eight years.

Because AD's brain showed clear evidence of trauma to his left prefrontal cortex and left temporal lobe, we recommended a number of interventions to him. He faithfully followed through on all of them and reported significant improvements in memory, energy, focus, and judgment. Ten years later, I used SPECT imaging to rescan his brain, which showed remarkable improvement. Usually, as we age, our brains become less and less active. This is especially true for damaged brains, but as I've said, it doesn't have to be the case. Your brain can be better, even if it has suffered.

DR. AMEN AND ANTHONY DAVIS

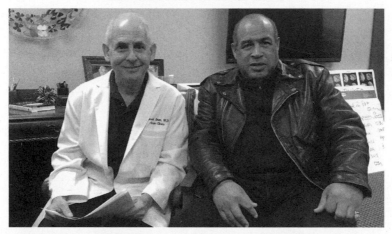

| **ANTHONY'S "BEFORE"** **BRAIN SPECT SCAN** | **TEN YEARS LATER** |

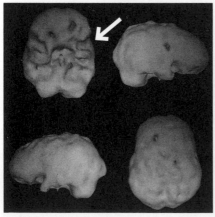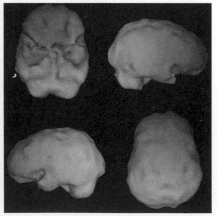

Damage to left prefrontal and temporal lobe   Marked improvement

The Amen Clinics National Football League (NFL) Study

As AD improved, he started to tell other football players that brain rehabilitation might be possible. He referred many other players to us and then asked me to speak to the Los Angeles chapter of the NFL Retired Players Association. At the meeting in January 2009, I was horrified by the levels of depression and dementia in the retired players I met. One player asked me the same question six times. From this encounter, I knew someone desperately needed to study brain damage and football. My research team at Amen Clinics, together with scientists from the University of California, Irvine, and Thomas Jefferson University, decided to tackle the issue with the help of the LA chapter's outgoing president, Reggie Berry, and incoming president, Marvin Smith.

Now we just needed to find funding. It is a myth that retired players are wealthy. A large percentage file for bankruptcy, face sustained joblessness, or divorce within a few years of retirement. Most of the players, especially the ones who needed the most help, could not afford to get help, so all of us scientists donated our time and resources to do a pilot study on 30 players—a number that our statistician said was likely to show scientifically valid results. We fell in love with the players, who, as a group, were kind, grateful, gentle giants. We now have a database of nearly 200 players from 27 teams and all positions, including many Hall of Famers, such as Terry Bradshaw. Chris Borland also saw us; he made national headlines in 2015 when he retired from the San Francisco 49ers after his successful rookie season because he was worried about the long-term consequences of repetitive brain trauma.

For the study, we took detailed histories, had the players perform cognitive tests, and did both brain SPECT scans and QEEG studies on each of them. The results were very clear: Playing football had damaged multiple areas of the brain in more than 90 percent of the players.[8] There was persistent damage to the following areas of the brain:

- prefrontal cortex (judgment, planning, forethought, and impulse control)
- temporal lobes (learning, memory, and mood stability)
- cerebellum (mental agility and processing speed)

Our group was not the only one reporting these problems. In 2002, neuropathologist Bennet Omalu, MD, autopsied Pittsburgh Steeler Hall of Fame center Mike Webster and was the first to discover chronic traumatic encephalopathy (CTE) or "football dementia." Omalu then saw this disease of excessive tau protein deposits in many other football players who suffered with depression, violent outbursts, cognitive impairment, and suicidal thoughts. Dr. Omalu's discovery was celebrated in the movie *Concussion*, starring Will Smith.

Researchers from the Department of Veterans Affairs and Boston University reported that 96 percent (87 of 91) of former NFL players autopsied had clear evidence of CTE; a study from the Mayo Clinic found that 32 percent of males who played football and other contact sports, *even at an amateur level*, had CTE as well.[9] Even a study sponsored by the National Football League itself found that retired players ages 30 to 49 were given a dementia-related diagnosis at 20 times the rate of age-matched populations, while players over the age of 50 received a dementia-related diagnosis five times the national average.[10] At this point, there is little doubt that playing football at any level can cause long-term cognitive and emotional trouble.

Recently, the *Los Angeles Times* reported that some of the powerhouse high school football programs in Southern California were having trouble fielding teams.[11] Mater Dei's freshman team dropped by 30 percent, Loyola had the fewest number of freshman players in two decades, and significant drops were also seen at Notre Dame, Alemany, and Crespi, where I played football 48 years earlier. Nationally, participation in football has declined in six of the past eight years. This is bad news for high schools, colleges, and the NFL, which make billions of dollars each year at the expense of the health of millions of children, teenagers, and young adults. But it is good news for millions of lives.

If you have children or teens who want to play football, first tell them why it is a terrible idea and then tell them no. Your children's brain health will take them through the rest of their lives either as happy, healthy, effective adults, or as ones more prone to depression, dementia, relationship problems, and legal trouble. September 2016 was the first month since 2009 that an NFL player had not been arrested.[12] Previously, each of 72 straight months saw the arrest of a professional football player. Does anyone think brain damage may be at least partially involved? In our study, football players had more than four times the level of depression (28 percent) suffered by the general population (6 percent).

As hard as you may try to justify the benefits of football—and there are many, including hard work, teamwork, strategy, and lessons in dealing with adversity—it's impossible to ignore the physics. The brain is soft and housed in a really hard skull with sharp, bony ridges. It is not anchored to the skull, so the brain floats in cerebrospinal fluid. This means that helmets, which can do a good job of preventing skull fractures, cannot protect the brain from being damaged. Powerful hits propel delicate brain tissue against hard, knife-like edges, causing bleeding, bruising, tearing, and scarring, especially to the prefrontal cortex and temporal lobes. *These hits can cause trouble even without a loss of consciousness or any outward symptoms of concussion.* In our study, the number of concussions a player had was not associated with the level of brain damage. Brain damage may be occurring insidiously without your brain ever telling you it is in trouble, and it can ruin your life.

Once we saw the high levels of damage in our NFL players, we put them on the same Memory Rescue program I am giving you in this book, including the supplements listed on page 136. Eighty percent of our players showed significant improvement in blood flow to the prefrontal cortex, as well as improvements in overall cognitive functioning, processing speed, attention, reasoning, and memory.[13] In this table, you can see the improvements on the cognitive testing, known as MicroCog.

"BEFORE" AND "AFTER" SCORES ON MICROCOG IN 30 NFL PLAYERS

MICROCOG DOMAINS	"BEFORE" MEAN	"AFTER" MEAN	P VALUE	# OF PLAYERS WITH > 50% IMPROVEMENT
General cognitive functioning	31.8	43.4	<0.000	14
General cognitive proficiency	24.7	35.2	<0.000	14
Processing speed	33.1	39.3	0.026	12
Processing accuracy	40.9	48.5	0.012	13
Attention	38.4	48.7	0.025	9
Reasoning	32.7	41.6	0.006	11
Memory	33.8	42.9	0.022	17
Spatial processing	69.0	74.3	0.154	3
Reaction time	70.2	74.67	0.669	6
MicroCog is a computerized neuropsychological battery of tests that looks at nine different areas of cognitive functioning. Scores are presented as a percentage from 0 (worst) to 100 (best).				

As we saw our football players getting better, often decades after their last concussions, we knew this work was incredibly important for members of the armed forces, firefighters, and police officers—anyone who is at risk for brain trauma. In addition to the supplement protocol below, we often use neurofeedback and hyperbaric oxygen therapy to help rehabilitate head trauma. You can find out more about these interventions in chapter 19.

 ## CHECKUP FOR HEAD TRAUMA ISSUES

Know if you have had a concussion

Take some time to remember whether you ever sustained a concussion or a blow without a concussion (subconcussive impact). Think back (or ask your parents). Did you ever

- fall out of a tree or down stairs?
- fall off a horse or roof?
- dive into a shallow pool?
- fall off a fence headfirst?
- have a car accident (as a driver or passenger)?
- have whiplash?
- sustain a work-related head injury?
- suffer a concussion or head injury playing sports?

Consider getting a functional imaging study

A functional imaging study, such as SPECT or QEEG, may help pinpoint injured areas and is worth investigating if your memory is not what you want it to be or if you have signs of cognitive impairment.

Check for loss of smell (anosmia)

Loss of smell, or anosmia, is a common consequence of head trauma, and it could indicate a serious problem. The olfactory cortex, the area of your brain involved with your sense of smell, is near your memory centers, and these regions tend to deteriorate and die together. Having trouble smelling peanut butter, lemons, strawberries, or natural gas is associated with a higher incidence of significant memory problems. Scoring poorly on the University of Pennsylvania Smell Identification Test strongly predicted those who would be diagnosed with Alzheimer's disease later in life.[14] Of course, if you can't smell a natural gas leak in your home, you may not live long enough to have memory problems!

Lab tests

Be sure to assess all the other BRIGHT MINDS risk factors that pertain to you, especially through these blood tests:

- **Omega-3 Index:** Brains with a higher index[15] heal better. (See page 102 in chapter 7 for more information.)

- **HbA1c and fasting blood sugar:** Higher levels impair healing. According to a study from UCLA, rats that were given sugar after a head injury experienced delayed healing.[16] It is time to get Gatorade off the sidelines of sporting events. It is a weapon of mass destruction! (See pages 233–234 in chapter 14 for more information.)

- **Thyroid, DHEA, and testosterone levels:** Because of where it sits in the skull, the pituitary gland (the master hormone gland) is often damaged when the brain is injured. Testing and treating any hormone deficiencies is important to help heal from TBIs. (For more information, see page 217 in chapter 13.)

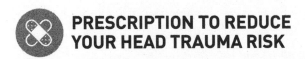

PRESCRIPTION TO REDUCE YOUR HEAD TRAUMA RISK

The Strategies

1. **Reduce your risk of head injury.** Protect your head, wear your seat belt, and avoid high-risk activities if you care about your quality of life. Besides football, sports such as hockey, soccer,[17] horseback riding, auto racing, and skiing can be dangerous.

    The effects of head injury can often be eased with appropriate treatment, providing you offer your brain the support it needs and attack the risk factors for memory decline. I believe the secret to our success with active and former NFL players, as well as other patients with TBIs, is that we use a BRIGHT MINDS approach in all areas, including nutraceuticals. Consider neurofeedback and

HBOT, which have also helped some patients. See more about these treatments in chapter 19.

BRIGHT MINDS TIP

As you age, protect yourself from falls, one of the greatest risk factors for head injuries. (See the BRIGHT MINDS habits list on the next page.)

---

2. **Go and smell the roses.** I mean that literally. There is evidence that repeated exposure to certain odors can improve one's ability to smell.[18] In a study from Aristotle University in Greece, 111 patients with anosmia repeatedly trained their sense of smell twice a day using four odors (phenyl ethyl alcohol, eucalyptol, citronellal, eugenol). Compared to a control group, after eight weeks participants noticed significant improvement that lasted up to a year. If anosmia is an issue for you, put your nose to work. Research shows that sniffing certain essential oils, including rose, lemon, cloves, and eucalyptus, may help restore the sense of smell.[19]

The Nutraceuticals

The following nutraceuticals are essential to help support the brain's healing process.

- *Multivitamin/mineral complex:* A high-dose supplement, with higher doses of vitamin B6, vitamin B12, folate, and vitamin D3 for nutrient support

- *Omega-3 fatty acids:* Highly concentrated and purified, with 2.8 grams of total EPA plus DHA

- *A combination of ginkgo biloba extract* (to support blood flow), *acetyl-L-carnitine* (to support mitochondrial energy), *huperzine A* (to support acetylcholine), *N-acetylcysteine* and *alpha-lipoic acid* (for antioxidant support), and *phosphatidylserine* (for nerve cell membrane support)

The Foods
AVOID (OR LIMIT):

> *Alcohol*

> *Caffeine*, which constricts blood flow

> *Sugar*, which promotes inflammation and prevents healing

> *Fried foods*

> *Processed foods*

CONSIDER ADDING:

> *Spices and herbs to support brain healing*, particularly turmeric and peppermint[20]

> *Choline-rich foods* to boost acetylcholine, such as shrimp, eggs, scallops, sardines, chicken, turkey, tuna, cod, beef, collard greens, and brussels sprouts

> *Omega-3-rich foods* to support nerve cell membranes: See page 107 in chapter 7.

> *Other anti-inflammatory foods, such as prebiotic- and probiotic-rich foods:* See page 107 in chapter 7.

> *Zinc-rich foods:* See page 200 in chapter 12.

 ## PICK ONE HEALTHY BRIGHT MINDS HABIT TO START TODAY

1. Always wear your seat belt when you drive or ride in a vehicle.

2. To prevent falls or other injuries, do not try to carry too many packages or boxes at one time.

3. Wear a helmet when skiing, biking, etc.

4. Avoid going up on the roof or climbing ladders.

5. **Slow down.**

6. **Do not text and walk or drive.**

7. **Be careful when going up and down stairs; hold the handrail.**

8. If you have had a head trauma, have your hormone levels checked and optimize any that are low.

9. Take the herb peppermint to help with healing.

10. Eat eggs to boost acetylcholine.

CHAPTER 10

T IS FOR TOXINS
IS YOUR MEMORY BEING POISONED?

Men who use aftershave, cologne, deodorants, or body washes to
make themselves smell "sexy" are actively decreasing testosterone
activity and thereby making themselves less manly.

JOSEPH PIZZORNO, ND, *THE TOXIN SOLUTION*

LEW: MOLD AND THE MIND

Lew, 67, had been a navy pilot and instructor for 40 years when he had to stop flying because he was unable to think through his flight plans. He and his wife were shocked when he made a mistake regarding some finances, potentially losing $100,000. He did not remember conversations; was unable to keep track of schedules, appointments, and everyday tasks; and forgot the names of people he'd recently met. Lew also had some difficulties with balance, and he felt tingling, numbness, and coldness in his fingers.

His memory problems had begun approximately two years before he came to see Kabran Chapek, ND, at our clinic in Bellevue, Washington. By this point, his wife was afraid to leave him alone. Lew had seen several other doctors, but he felt "they were just throwing meds" at him before any tests were performed. Later, an MRI and EEG showed "age-related atrophy in brain volume and enlarged ventricles." This was very disheartening to him: "I used to have an amazing memory, better than average." His previous doctor had diagnosed him with dementia and gave him a prescription for Namenda, a dementia medication, which did not help.

Our laboratory testing revealed evidence that he had mold (mycotoxin) exposure. Lew and his wife found water damage in their home and had the affected area remediated. Through a cleansing program that included nutrition, supplements, meditation, and exercise (he hikes two to three miles every day with 30 pounds of rocks in a backpack), Lew's memory began to improve. After five months on our program, he said, "I am so much better"— and his brain is better too. His wife said she noticed a huge improvement and was not afraid to leave him alone any longer.

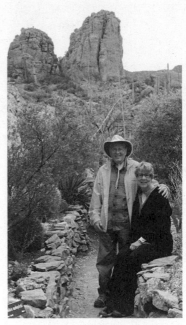

Lew and his wife following his treatment

Lew also had blood sugar issues, which improved over time as he cut out the "little chocolate doughnut" he had with his coffee every morning. That was a sacrifice for him, but as Dr. Chapek explained, "It's your chocolate doughnut or your brain!"

Lew's initial SPECT scan looked toxic (with a bumpy, scalloped pattern), which we've observed in many of the pilots we've scanned. Several months later, his follow-up SPECT showed remarkable improvement.

LEW'S BRIGHT MINDS RISK FACTORS AND INTERVENTIONS

BRIGHT MINDS	LEW'S RISK FACTORS	INTERVENTIONS
Blood Flow	Low blood flow on SPECT	Exercise, diet, ginkgo biloba
Retirement/Aging	Age 67	
Inflammation		
Genetics		
Head Trauma	Dropped on his head while wrestling and injured his neck in high school; neck surgery 16 years later	

BRIGHT MINDS	LEW'S RISK FACTORS	INTERVENTIONS
Toxins	Mold exposure, flying planes, general anesthesia	Stop mold exposure; treat for mold
Mental Health		
Immunity/Infection Issues	Low zinc	Begin zinc supplements
Neurohormone Deficiencies		
Diabesity	High fasting blood sugar	Giving up his little chocolate doughnut in the morning
Sleep Issues		

LEW'S "BEFORE" BRAIN SPECT SCAN

AFTER TREATMENT

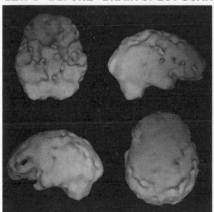

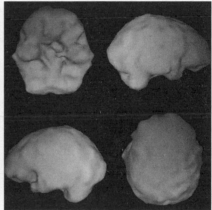

Damage from exposure to mold

Overall improvement

LET'S PLAY 20 QUESTIONS (PLUS 2): WHICH OF THESE STATEMENTS APPLY TO YOU?

1. Do you smoke or are you around secondhand smoke?
2. Do you smoke marijuana?
3. Do you use conventional cleaning products and inadvertently breathe their fumes?
4. Have you been exposed to carbon monoxide?

5. Do you travel on planes more than three to four times a year?
6. Do you pump your own gas or breathe automobile exhaust?
7. Do you live in an area with moderate to high air pollution?
8. Have you lived or worked in a building that had mold in it?
9. Do you come in contact with flame-resistant clothing or carpet, or with furnishings sprayed with chemicals to resist stains?
10. Do you spray your garden, farm, or orchard with pesticides or live near an area with pesticides?[1]
11. Do you paint indoors without excellent ventilation?
12. Do you drink unfiltered water?
13. Do you have more than four glasses of alcohol a week?
14. Do you regularly eat processed or fast foods?
15. Do you regularly eat conventionally raised produce, meat, or dairy, or farm-raised fish?
16. Do you eat large (i.e., mercury-contaminated) fish, such as swordfish?
17. Do you regularly eat nonorganic fruits and vegetables?
18. Do you consume foods with artificial colors or sweeteners, such as diet sodas, or add artificial sweeteners, such as aspartame (NutraSweet), sucralose (Splenda), or saccharin (Sweet'N Low) to your beverages or food?
19. Do you use more than two health and/or beauty products per day without reading and understanding their labels?
20. Does your house contain lead pipes or copper plumbing soldered with lead?
21. Do you have mercury amalgam fillings? How many?
22. Do you work in a job such as firefighting, painting, welding, or working in a shipyard, where you are exposed to environmental toxins?

If you answered yes to more than two questions, this chapter could be very important to the rest of your life.

THE IMPACT OF TOXINS ON YOUR BRAIN AND MEMORY

As a classically trained psychiatrist, I received virtually no training on the impact of toxins on the brain or as a cause of brain fog, memory problems, anxiety disorders, depression, ADHD, autism, temper outbursts, psychotic behavior, obesity, and diabetes. It wasn't until I started looking at the brain that I started to realize the connection between toxins and health problems.

Research now shows that many people with allergies, autoimmune diseases, neurodegenerative diseases, diabetes, and cancers have one thing in common: exposure to environmental toxins. Our bodies have systems in place to get rid of toxins (through the gut, liver, kidneys, and skin), but when our detoxification systems are overwhelmed, we experience brain fog, fatigue, and life-threatening illnesses.

Toxins in any form damage the brain and increase the risk of memory problems and dementia. On SPECT scans, toxins show a pattern I call "scalloping"—overall low activity that leaves the brain looking irregular and bumpy.

"I don't do that anymore"

About 10 years ago, I gave a lecture to a thousand people at Skyline Church in San Diego. The next year I was invited back. As often happens when I speak at a place for the second time, a number of people approached me with their SPECT scans because my first lecture had motivated them to come to one of our clinics to have their own brains evaluated. On this occasion, a 35-year-old man, Scott, came up to me to show me his scan, which looked awful. The Swiss cheese appearance indicated seriously low overall activity, the same pattern we often see in our drug or alcohol abusers. As I looked at the scan, Scott said, "You think I am a drug addict, don't you?"

"The thought had crossed my mind," I replied.

"I have never used drugs," Scott said, "and I don't drink. But before I came to your clinic, I used to paint cars in my garage without much ventilation. I don't do that anymore."

"That is the sign of intelligent life," I replied. "New information caused you to change your behavior."

He went on to tell me that he and his wife had been in marital therapy for several years without any benefit. After his visit to our clinic in Costa Mesa, he started to live a brain-healthy life, taking a multivitamin, fish oil, and the other brain-healthy supplements we recommended. He also ate better and exercised regularly. The difference, he said, had been life changing. After his brain got better, he was a better husband. I wonder how many marriages are suffering because one partner has a brain problem that no one is aware of. How do you do marital therapy with the brain on the next page? It won't work until you help heal that brain.

SCOTT'S "BEFORE" BRAIN SPECT SCAN

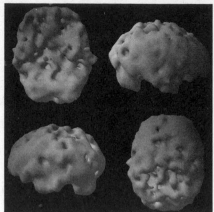

Note the overall bumpiness or "scalloping"
associated with toxic exposure

Toxins: the poisoning of the brain

Common toxins associated with memory loss can be absorbed through the skin (say, when you rub in a cream), ingested when you eat or drink, or inhaled as you breathe. Check these lists to see which toxic substances you may have been exposed to, either now or in the past.

TOXINS THAT CAN BE INGESTED OR ABSORBED

- Polluted or tainted water (including lead and arsenic)
- BPA (bisphenol A, found in plastics, food and drink containers, dental sealants, and the coating of cash register receipts)
- PCBs (see "Gone—But Not Forgotten" on page 146)
- Heavy metals, such as

  - mercury: in "silver" dental fillings (which are 50 percent mercury) and contaminated fish. (The Environmental Protection Agency recommends pregnant women eat fish no more than two or three times a week; limit the consumption of certain varieties, such as grouper and albacore tuna; and avoid the big seven: king mackerel, marlin, orange roughy, swordfish, shark, bigeye tuna, and tilefish from the Gulf of Mexico.)[2]
  - lead: in paint, pipes, aviation fuel, and lipstick (see page 149).
  - cadmium: in cigarettes, soils treated with synthetic fertilizers, and industrial and hazardous waste sites. Cadmium is highly toxic and accumulates in the liver and kidneys. It is linked to

osteoporosis, heart disease, cancer, and diabetes. Once it is in your body, it takes 16 years to get rid of just half of it!

- Excessive alcohol
- Marijuana
- Many medications, such as benzodiazepines (for anxiety or insomnia) or narcotic pain medications
- Chemotherapy
- General anesthesia in some patients
- Silicone breast implants that have leaked
- MSG
- Artificial food dyes, preservatives, and sweeteners
- Herbicides such as glyphosate (the active ingredient in Roundup weed killer, with residue present in genetically modified crops) disrupt the body's endocrine or hormonal system, affecting both testosterone and estrogen.[3] Herbicides may also damage DNA, making cells age faster and increasing their susceptibility to cancer.
- Pesticides, such as organochlorines and organophosphates (neurotoxins), stimulate enzymes that turn calories into fat, which is where toxins are stored. In one study, people in the top 5 percent of exposure to the organochlorine pesticide DDT had a 650 percent increase in dementia.[4]
- Apples sprayed with diphenylamine, which makes them shiny and slows discoloration but breaks down into cancer-causing nitrosamines, associated with Parkinson's and Alzheimer's[5]
- Foods manufactured with plastic equipment, leaking plasticizers
- Health and beauty products absorbed through the skin[6]

DISTURBING FACT: *One of the most effective ways for a woman to decrease her toxic load is through breastfeeding, which decreases the risk of breast cancer. Unfortunately, the baby gets the brunt of it.*

TOXINS THAT CAN BE INHALED
- Air pollution
- Cigarette smoke, secondhand smoke, marijuana smoke
- Automobile exhaust
- Gasoline fumes
- Toxins in the air near high-traffic areas (air pollution, auto exhaust)[7]

- Cleaning chemicals
- Welding,[8] soldering fumes
- Fire retardant fumes
- Carbon monoxide
- Asbestos
- Aviation fumes
- Fire toxins inhaled by firefighters during fires
- Fireplace fumes
- Paint and solvent fumes
- Pesticide or herbicide residues near farms, also backyard applications
- Mold

||||||||||||||||||||||||||||||||||||||||||||||||||||||||||||||||||||||||||||||||||

Gone—but Not Forgotten

Remember PCBs (polychlorinated biphenyls)? These industrial chemicals were banned 50 years ago, but they are still ubiquitous in the environment in rivers and coastal areas, as well as in paints, plastics, rubber products, and other materials manufactured before the ban. PCBs inhibit the workings of the thyroid, leading to constant tiredness. Because the body has a hard time eliminating PCBs, they can accumulate over time and have been linked to heart attacks,[9] diabetes,[10] and cancer. In addition, PCBs can build up in the fatty tissue of fish that live in contaminated rivers or coastal areas. When you eat those fish, PCBs can accumulate in your fatty tissue as well. Limit your exposure by trimming the skin and fat from raw and cooked fish, and avoid eating fried fish.

||||||||||||||||||||||||||||||||||||||||||||||||||||||||||||||||||||||||||||||||||

Toxins poison your brain in 10 ways, both directly and indirectly.[11] They

1. **Harm enzyme systems**, which disrupts many biological processes, including the production of energy and the ability to fight free radicals.

2. **Lower cerebral blood flow**, which makes it harder to think and make good decisions.

3. **Damage organs**, including those in the digestive tract, the liver, kidneys, and brain. This damage reduces the body's ability to detoxify and get rid of the toxins.

4. **Damage DNA**, which can accelerate aging.

5. **Change gene expression**, which not only hurts affected individuals, but can also hurt their children, grandchildren, and even great-grandchildren.

6. **Damage cell membranes** and communication between cells.

7. **Disrupt, suppress, or block hormones**, causing serious imbalances.

8. **Impair the immune system**, increasing the risk of autoimmune disorders and cancer.

9. **Disrupt the intestinal microbiome**, resulting in leaky gut and accompanying problems.

10. **Increase the risk of diabetes and obesity** as the internal toxic load rises. Toxins are also called "diabesogens" and "obesogens" because they can make us diabetic and obese.

Because toxins can affect so many parts of the body, they are associated with a wide range of symptoms. Those that are more directly associated with the brain include poor memory and concentration, word confusion, mood issues, headaches, vertigo, and cravings. Other problems range from abdominal pain, diarrhea, smelly stools, bad breath, low appetite, and weight issues to skin rashes, fatigue and weakness, aches and muscle cramps, numbness and tingling, tremors, sweats, and problems with temperature regulation—and there are more.

Here are some of the most common toxic issues we see at Amen Clinics.

Health and beauty aids: the price of looking good

The average American woman uses about 12 personal care and cosmetic products daily; the average man, about six.[12] The chemicals in these products are easily absorbed into your skin and are transported to every organ in your body. That means you may be working hard to look good on the outside but poisoning yourself on the inside in the process. In 2016, Johnson & Johnson was ordered to pay $72 million to the family of a woman whose death from ovarian cancer was associated with the daily use of Johnson's Baby Powder, among other company products.[13]

The Environmental Working Group's Skin Deep database (http://www. ewg.org/skindeep/) contains information on many products with toxic ingredients and provides healthier options. Below is a chart of chemicals commonly found in personal care products, along with descriptions of the havoc they wreak, from a book I highly recommend—*The Toxin Solution* by Joseph Pizzorno, ND, a founder of Bastyr University.

COMMON CHEMICALS FOUND IN HEALTH AND BEAUTY AIDS

CHEMICAL	PURPOSE	TOXICITY
Acrylates	Artificial nails	Neurotoxins[14]
Aluminum	Antiperspirant	Potential connection to Alzheimer's disease[15]
Formaldehyde	Shampoos, nail polish, hair gel, nail and eyelash glue, body wash, color cosmetics	Cancer,[16] allergic reactions[17]
Fragrance	Shampoos, liquid baby soap, nail polish, glues, hair smoothing, body wash, color cosmetics	Cancer, endocrine disruption, allergic reactions
Oxybenzone	Sunscreen	Endocrine disruption, lowers sperm count, skin allergies
Parabens	Preservative, fragrance in cosmetics (eye shadow, foundation, mascara), shampoos, conditioners, lotions, facial/body cleansers	Endocrine issues, breast cancer,[18] developmental problems in kids, reproductive problems, allergies
Phthalates (banned in Europe)	Fragrances in cosmetics *Also used in plasticizers (plastic wrap, packaging)*	Endocrine disruption;[19] lower IQ;[20] decreases BDNF in males,[21] which helps neurons grow and connect
Polyethylene glycols (PEGs)	Create suds in shampoos, bubble baths, liquid soap	Cancer,[22] birth defects,[23] hair loss, allergies
Triclosan	Antimicrobial cleanser, toothpaste	Endocrine disruption,[24] harmful to the microbiome[25]
Lead	Lipstick (kiss of death)	Neurotoxin, damage to hippocampus and prefrontal cortex[26]
See also: *The Toxin Solution* by Joseph Pizzorno, ND		

Lead: the kiss of death

Lead exposure is related to learning problems in children, lower IQ, speech problems, cancer, cardiovascular problems, arthritis, seizures, headaches, anemia, kidney disease, a metallic taste, and death from all causes. The "safe" level of lead, measured in the bloodstream, used to be less than 60 mcg/dL (micrograms per deciliter), according to the US government. That number has since been lowered to under 10 mcg/dL, and in July 2012, the Centers for Disease Control and Prevention determined that lead in the range of 5 to 10 mcg/dL is particularly problematic for children. Many scientists believe lead is unsafe for humans at any level.

To protect Americans from lead poisoning, the government had the metal removed from gasoline and paint, but it was left in small plane aviation fuel. When we scanned 100 pilots at Amen Clinics, we saw evidence of significant brain toxicity in two-thirds of them. Could it be caused by lead and other toxins they are exposed to when they fly? As for paint problems, any house painted white before 1978 has high levels of lead, which can pose a problem when the paint chips or peels. And houses built or remodeled before 1986 have lead in the pipe solder.

No regulation has required that lead be removed from one of the most widely used cosmetics: lipstick. When lipstick was tested in 30 national brands, lead was found in 60 percent of them.[27] In 2013, researchers at the University of California, Berkeley, found lead in 24 of 32 lip products tested. A number of the products also had high levels of eight other metals, such as cadmium and chromium.[28] To avoid buying and ingesting lead-contaminated lip products, know your lipstick brands and go to www.safecosmetics.org to learn more.

Smoking

When you look at the studies that are not sponsored by the tobacco industry, you can see that smoking clearly increases the risk of dementia—that is, if it doesn't kill you first.[29] Smoking has serious negative health effects. Cigarettes, including tobacco, marijuana, and electronic nicotine and caffeine delivery systems, are efficient ways to inhale into your lungs a host of fine and ultrafine toxic junk that then gets to your brain. Does size matter? Yes! The smaller the particle you inhale, the greater its ability to cause inflammatory reactions and damage your brain.

In 2014, the World Health Organization concluded that tobacco use and exposure to secondhand smoke increased incidence rates for all types of dementia, including Alzheimer's.[30] Smoking is thought to cause dementia in the same way it contributes to vascular diseases: by bombarding the brain with hundreds of different toxins, increasing homocysteine (high levels trigger inflammation), accelerating blood vessel damage (which deprives your brain of oxygen and nutrients), and increasing inflammation and the particulate toxic load in your brain.

Alcohol and marijuana

In recent years, these two hugely popular drugs have become tricky issues. I have a different perspective from most, having worked as an ambulance driver, in emergency rooms, and as a psychiatrist for the past 35 years. I have seen how alcohol devastates families and examined thousands of brain SPECT scans of "moderate" drinkers and pot smokers. Overall, I have seen much more harm than good from these substances.

We've all heard the reports that alcohol is a health food and marijuana is harmless. Indeed, large-scale studies seem to indicate that mild to moderate alcohol use may be good for your heart and mind.[31] Yet the results from a 30-year study of 550 men and women that was published in the *BMJ* (formerly the *British Medical Journal*) suggest that even moderate drinking—one or two glasses of wine a day—leads to atrophy in the hippocampus.[32]

This same study showed no protective effect from drinking one to seven small glasses of wine per week, so you shouldn't feel you have to drink to improve your brain. In a 43-year follow-up study of more than 12,000 people,[33] nondrinkers and light drinkers had a comparable dementia risk, while heavy and very heavy drinkers had an increased risk. Drinking more hard liquor (gin, rum, vodka, tequila, whiskey, brandy) increased the odds of dementia, whereas imbibing wine in moderate amounts is associated with a lower risk (although those who drink large amounts of wine are also at increased risk). Relative to nondrinkers and light drinkers, moderate to heavy drinkers have a 57 percent higher risk of dementia—and they develop it earlier.

A study at Johns Hopkins found that people who drink every day have smaller brains.[34] In addition, alcohol is related to seven different types of cancer, including those involving the mouth, throat, esophagus, liver, colon, rectum, and breast.[35] Why do nurses rub alcohol on your skin before they give you a shot or insert an IV needle? To kill bacteria. Why is alcohol used to preserve dead specimens? To kill all the cells and tissues in the specimens. This should make you wonder what alcohol is doing to your gut.

Alcohol can decrease judgment and decision-making skills, increase cravings, and make you less coordinated. Excessive alcohol is related to high blood pressure, stroke, irregular heartbeat, heart disease, and a weakening of the immune system. To detoxify alcohol, your liver uses glutathione and other essential antioxidants. This can make you more vulnerable to other toxins or weaken your liver function and immunity to infection. Alcohol is associated with a fatty liver and damaged neurons, and it lowers blood flow to the cerebellum, an amazing part of the brain that is associated with physical and thought coordination. Alcohol interferes with the absorption of vitamin B1 and is a common cause of nerve pain. Excessive drinking is listed as the fourth leading cause of preventable death. In the United States, there are about 30 million children of alcoholics, many of whom suffer from post-traumatic stress disorder as a result of growing up in an unpredictable, abusive alcoholic home. Excessive alcohol use is a major cause of divorce, incarceration, and financial problems. If you want a better brain, less is more. For people who want to drink, I recommend no more than two to four servings a week.

BRAIN SPECT SCAN OF HEAVY ALCOHOL USE

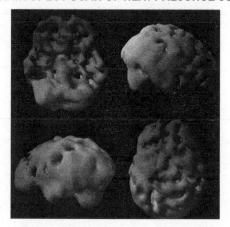

I'm also not a fan of recreational marijuana use. In 2016, we published the largest brain imaging study to date on marijuana users showing overall decreased blood flow in 982 of them compared to 92 healthy nonusers.[36] Blood flow was decreased the most in the right hippocampus, an area commonly involved with Alzheimer's disease and memory loss of all types.

Many years ago, I was on Michael Savage's radio show in San Francisco. We were discussing my observations on marijuana and the brain. Michael predicted that many recreational users would call in to the show wanting to challenge me. I told him that almost everyone calling would be concerned about memory issues. We were both right.

Here is an image of a young daily marijuana user. If the drug does this when you are young, imagine the issues it can cause as you age!

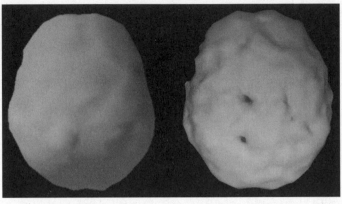

Healthy   Age 18, daily user

The impact of mold

One of the early lessons from our brain imaging work was that many substances are toxic to brain function, and one that is particularly toxic is mold. Here's just one example: In 2003, after reading my book *Change Your Brain, Change Your Life*, Bulletproof 360 CEO Dave Asprey got a brain SPECT scan. It changed everything for him. He was struggling with focus and memory and barely able to pass his classes at Wharton. It turned out that Dave had been exposed to toxic mold in his home. After he underwent healing protocols, his life dramatically improved, and he went on to produce *Moldy: The Toxic Mold Movie* (watch it online at https://moldymovie.com).

A young man I'll call George came to see us at Amen Clinics complaining of sleep disturbance, anxiety, memory problems, and brain fog. After taking a careful history, we learned that George's symptoms started when he moved back home from college into his parents' basement apartment. The whole family seemed to have forgotten that the basement had flooded on several occasions. Mold diagnostic testing revealed George had high levels of mold toxins in his body.

In such cases, the first step is always to remove the affected person from the moldy environment and then to begin treatment—consisting of binding agents and other medications, such as antifungals, as well as metabolic support supplements. For information on mold testing and cleanup, visit https://www.epa.gov/mold and https://www.cdc.gov/mold/. I recommend that you consult an integrative medicine doctor if you suspect a mold exposure problem. George improved with proper treatment and remediation of the mold problem. He did not need psychiatric medications; he simply needed the correct diagnosis and appropriate treatment. What would have been the outcome for him without a proper diagnosis? He almost certainly would have been diagnosed with a mental illness and treated (unsuccessfully) with psychiatric medications.

General anesthesia: cause for concern

I first became aware of the potentially toxic risk of general anesthesia[37] when a patient of mine called me in tears after knee surgery. She said she was having difficulty thinking and remembering and thought she was getting Alzheimer's disease. Since I had done a prior SPECT scan on her, I rescanned her and found that her brain looked toxic and was dramatically worse in her frontal and temporal lobes, which are both involved in memory. It was clear that something bad had happened to her brain since the first scan was taken. She improved after following the BRIGHT MINDS approach to rescue her memory.

Current research on general anesthesia is mixed, with some studies showing no lasting negative effects and some showing toxic effects, but two recent studies stand out: Children who had undergone general anesthesia before the age of four had lower IQ, diminished language comprehension, and decreased gray matter in the back of their brains.[38] That is very concerning. Also, a before-and-after SPECT study of patients who underwent coronary artery bypass surgery showed that 68 percent had diminished blood flow, which was linked to decreased verbal and visual memory six months later.[39] I recommend local or spinal anesthesia whenever possible. If it is not possible, make sure to do everything else right for your brain.

High risks for first responders

Firefighters, police officers, and emergency medical technicians—aka first responders—are the everyday heroes in our society. These brave men and women are involved in dangerous professions that pose many health risks and can have a long-lasting negative impact on their brain function. They are exposed to environmental toxins such as carbon monoxide, benzene, asbestos, and diesel exhaust; head injuries; and emotional trauma. (After taking one dead baby from a burning car or seeing someone who has shot himself in the head, a first responder isn't likely ever to be quite the same again—and these professionals experience many emotional traumas over their careers.) The need for early brain health intervention programs among these professions is critical because studies show an elevated risk of post-traumatic stress disorder and suicide in first responders.[40]

Adam: the trauma of fighting fires

Adam, 33, a firefighter for six years, came to see me for depression, insomnia, and poor concentration. He was struggling in his relationship with his wife and felt distant from his two small children. He cried as he related the many traumas he had seen, especially the first one, when he arrived at a home where a teenage boy had shot himself at point-blank range. He said he could still hear the boy's mother screaming. On other occasions while on the job, Adam also suffered two concussions and a bout of smoke inhalation while battling a Southern California fire.

His lab tests showed low testosterone and vitamin D levels. His scan showed overall low activity in his brain. Adam was one of the most compliant and motivated patients I have ever helped. Within six months his depression had lifted, his brain was better, and he had more skills to deal with the inevitable emotional trauma in his profession.

FIREFIGHTER ADAM'S "BEFORE" BRAIN SPECT SCAN

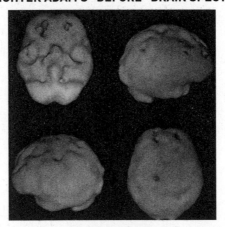

Overall low activity

ADAM'S BRIGHT MINDS RISK FACTORS AND INTERVENTIONS

BRIGHT MINDS	ADAM'S RISK FACTORS	INTERVENTIONS
Blood Flow	Low blood flow on SPECT	Exercise, diet, ginkgo biloba
Retirement/Aging		
Inflammation		
Genetics		
Head Trauma	Two concussions at work	Nutraceuticals and HBOT
Toxins	Multiple toxins from firefighting	Strengthen all detox systems
Mental Health	Depression, emotional trauma, stressful job	Nutraceuticals and psychotherapy
Immunity/Infection Issues	Low vitamin D	Vitamin D3 supplements
Neurohormone Deficiencies	Low testosterone	Limited sugar, DHEA supplementation
Diabesity		
Sleep Issues	Insomnia after accident	Sleep strategies

Other toxins

At Amen Clinics, we have also seen many patients with a history of cancer chemotherapy. Chemotherapy kills cancer cells, but unfortunately it can kill healthy brain cells too.[41] Likewise, excessive exposure to heavy metals, including arsenic, lead, mercury, iron, aluminum, and bismuth (found in Pepto-Bismol—but you have to take a lot of it) can cause significant memory problems. *Screening tests can be very helpful to discover what your heavy metal load is.* If it is elevated, I suggest you consult an integrative medicine doctor.

||||||||||||||||||||||||||||||||||||||||||||||||||||||||||||||||||||||||||||||||||||||||||

Should We Be Concerned About GMOs?

Genetically modified organisms (GMOs) were engineered to resist herbicides or weed killers. Unfortunately, those herbicides affect not only weeds; they may damage us as well. Unlike the regulatory bodies in 64 other countries, the Food and Drug Administration (FDA) does not require labeling of GM foods. But in 2015, two things occurred that should concern us.

First, an editorial in the *New England Journal of Medicine* noted that "there have been sharp increases in the amounts and numbers of chemical herbicides applied to GM crops, and still further increases—the largest in a generation—are scheduled to occur in the next few years."[42]

And second, glyphosate, the herbicide most widely used on GM crops, was classified as a probable human carcinogen by the International Agency for Research on Cancer (IARC). IARC has also classified a second herbicide, 2,4-dichlorophenoxyacetic acid (2,4-D), which will be used on crops in combination with glyphosate in 34 states in 2017, as a possible human carcinogen.[43]

If you have a choice, I recommend that you avoid GMOs by buying organic produce or looking for products labeled "Non GMO." I hate the argument that since they have not been proven dangerous, why worry? If my grandchildren are going to eat something, I want it proven safe before they eat it.

||||||||||||||||||||||||||||||||||||||||||||||||||||||||||||||||||||||||||||||||||||||

CHECKUP FOR TOXINS ISSUES

Your detoxification organs, including your gut, liver, kidneys, and skin, need to be healthy to do their job. Your liver, for instance, filters blood to identify and hold toxins. Its enzyme systems then break them down and produce bile to excrete them. Your kidneys filter all of your blood a remarkable 60 times per day. However, kidney function decreases by 50 percent from age 20 to age 85,[44] so they need your support!

For a gut checkup, see chapter 7. For information on how to protect your other organs, keep reading.

BRIGHT MINDS TIP

If you have limited resources, skip the expensive lab tests and spend your money on high-quality detoxifying food.

Lab tests

Your liver has finite toxin-processing capacity; therefore, it is highly vulnerable to toxic overload. The following tests can help determine how strained it is.

LIVER FUNCTION

- **ALT (SGPT):** Normal range: 7 to 56 units per liter (U/L)
- **AST (SGOT):** Normal range: 5 to 40 U/L
- **Bilirubin:** Normal range: 0.2 to 1.2 mg/dL
- **Zinc:** Normal range: 60 to 110 mcg/dL (low zinc will limit detoxification in the liver)

If your liver function tests are high, cut back on your intake of sugar, simple carbohydrates, and alcohol. Also, you and your doctor might consider whether hepatitis or medications that raise liver enzymes, such as acetaminophen (Tylenol), could be affecting your liver's function.

KIDNEY FUNCTION

- **BUN:** Normal range: 7 to 20 mg/dL
- **Creatinine:** Normal range: 0.5 to 1.2 mg/dL.

SKIN

- **Check for rashes, acne, and rosacea.** All are clues to detoxification problems.

TESTING FOR MOLD

- **TGF beta-1:** This blood test measures a protein found throughout the body that plays a role in immune system function and is often high following mold exposure (also called mycotoxin exposure). Certain infections, such as Lyme disease (see chapter 12), may also increase levels of this protein. The normal level is below 2,380; 0 is optimal. Mold exposure can raise this to more than 15,000.

- **Real Time Labs mycotoxin test** (http://www.realtimelab.com/home): Real Time Labs tests human and environmental samples for mold.

TESTING FOR HEAVY METALS

- Hair sample and urinary challenge tests are easy to access through doctors of integrative medicine.

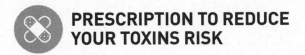

PRESCRIPTION TO REDUCE YOUR TOXINS RISK

The Strategies

You can reduce your toxic load with two simple strategies: (1) limit your exposure to toxins, and (2) strengthen your detoxification systems, especially your gut, liver, kidneys, and skin.

1. **Limit your exposure to toxins.**

   - *Quit smoking.* Try hypnosis, nicotine patches, or bupropion to kick this habit.

   - *Address drug and/or alcohol abuse.* Look for the underlying causes of why you use, such as untreated anxiety or depression. I recommend eliminating marijuana completely.

   - *Slowly replace "silver" dental fillings.* Opt for ceramic fillings rather than amalgams when possible. I suggest removal of amalgam fillings just as soon as feasible, but not all at once because of the risk of releasing toxins into the bloodstream. Removing just one or two at each dental session is best.

   - *Reduce your consumption of toxin-contaminated foods.*

     - Buy organic (and always wash your food). One study found that concentrations of selected pesticides detected in urine samples decreased by 95 percent when a family switched to organic food for two weeks.[45] In another study, the neurotoxic pesticide levels of children who ate conventionally grown foods were nine times higher than those who ate organic.[46] For more information on which foods have the highest and lowest pesticide loads, check out the Environmental Working Group (EWG) website (www.ewg.org).

     - Always read and understand food labels. If you do not know

what is in something, don't eat it or put it on your body. Avoid
the following chemicals, including additives and preservatives:

- Potassium bromate—carcinogen
- BHA, BHT—linked to tumors
- Sodium benzoate—may damage DNA
- Sodium nitrate—linked to cancer
- Tartrazine dye (makes cheese yellow)—linked to asthma
- Monosodium glutamate (MSG and related ingredients,
  including glutamic acid, hydrolyzed protein, autolyzed
  protein, autolyzed yeast extract, and textured protein)—
  linked to seizures and heart issues
- Red dye #40—possible allergen and carcinogen
- Artificial sweeteners—aspartame (blue packets) and
  saccharin (pink packets) are both linked to obesity, diabetes,
  and cancer.[47] Sucralose (yellow packets) is metabolized like
  PCBs and dioxins, both of which have the potential of
  causing direct toxic effects. Sucralose may induce glucose
  intolerance by disrupting the microbiome.[48]

- *Ignore the word* natural *on labels.* When used there, it is
  meaningless.

- *Limit or eliminate conventionally raised produce* (treated with
  pesticides and herbicides), *dairy* (affected by hormones and
  antibiotics), *grain-fed meats, and grain-fed farmed fish.*

- *Avoid aluminum and Teflon cookware.* Teflon may release toxic
  fumes when overheated.

- *Buy and store foods in glass jars* when possible. Plastic containers
  may contain phthalates (a plasticizer) and BPAs. Never reheat
  foods in plastic containers.

- *Avoid processed meats* such as bacon and smoked turkey. They
  contain nitrosamines, which cause the liver to produce fats that
  are toxic to the brain.

- *Limit alcohol consumption* to no more than two to four servings a
  week; choose wine and beer over aged liquors.

- *Add fiber and fiber-rich foods*, which bind to toxins and help your
  gastrointestinal system get rid of them. In the past, humans ate

100 to 150 grams of fiber a day. Americans now eat an average of about 15 grams.[49] Women should consume at least 21 grams; men, 30 grams.

- *Drink eight to ten glasses of clean water a day to stay hydrated.* Water helps flush toxins from your kidneys. Filter your water with charcoal or reverse osmosis. Check the purity of your local water supply with this EPA link: https://ofmpub.epa.gov/apex/safewater/f?p=136:102.

- *Do a food detox.* For two weeks, eliminate the following:

  - Processed foods
  - Glutens, which can increase gut permeability, even in people who are not sensitive to them (found in flour, triticale, triticum, semolina, durum, Kamut, wheat, rye, and barley)
  - Dairy
  - Nonorganic beef and chicken to avoid hormones, antibiotics, and arsenic
  - Farmed fish
  - The "Dirty Dozen" produce items, designated by the EWG (see https://www.ewg.org/foodnews/summary.php)
  - Soy (high levels of arsenic, cadmium; 96 percent of US soy is genetically modified)
  - Artificial sweeteners
  - Alcohol and recreational drugs
  - Water that has not been purified or proven to be clean

- *Breathe clean air.*

  - Check your home for mold and eliminate it whether or not you are symptomatic.
  - Refrain from having wood fires in fireplaces since they release toxic compounds.
  - Change the filters on your heating and cooling systems regularly.

- *Decrease your use of unsafe health and beauty aids.*

  - Do a bathroom cleanse. Download the "Think Dirty" app (www.thinkdirtyapp.com) and then scan all the products in your bathroom. Think Dirty rates products on a scale of 1 to 10 (10 = the most toxic). If you care about your health, throw out toxic products. When I first downloaded this app, I threw out more than 70 percent of the products in my bathroom.

- Use natural products without fragrance that are low in chemicals and free of phthalates. This can really make a difference: 100 teenage girls who avoided these chemicals for just three days had significantly lower levels of toxins in their urine.[50] Natural products may be more expensive in the short run, but they will be cheaper in the long run as you will spend less money on doctor appointments and medicine.

- *Clean the house thoroughly.*

  - Use carbon monoxide alarms and nonradioactive smoke alarms.
  - Use fragrance-free natural household cleansers.
  - Clean, dust, and vacuum regularly.
  - Do not use Scotchgard or any other chemicals that prevent stains on anything in the home.
  - Periodically check for black mold in any potentially wet area of your home.
  - Limit the use of volatile organic compounds (VOCs), often found in cleaning products and air fresheners, by replacing them with VOC-free cleaning products, no- or low-VOC bedding materials made from natural products, low-VOC paints, and throw rugs instead of new carpeting. For more information on the health effects of common household products, see the Household Products Database from the National Institutes of Health/National Library of Medicine at https://hpd.nlm.nih.gov/products.htm.

2. **Strengthen Your Detoxification Systems**

- *Support your gut.* (See chapter 7.)

- *Support your liver and kidneys with the nutraceuticals and food recommendations listed on the following pages.*

- *Support your skin.* Your skin is the largest organ of your body.[51] The state of its health is a reflection of the health of your brain.

  - *Work up a sweat with exercise.* It is one of the best natural ways to cleanse your system. The concentration of most toxins—including arsenic, cadmium, lead, and mercury—is 2 to 10 times higher in sweat than in blood, which indicates that sweating is an effective detoxification process.[52] Boosting sweat with exercise significantly increases glutathione production, one of the most important detoxification nutrients; protects against PCB exposure; helps eliminate phthalates and bisphenol A; and helps keep your skin healthy.[53]

- *Take a sauna.* Saunas have been found to lower toxins in firefighters, which can be an important intervention for this at-risk group.[54] In a follow-up study over 20 years, researchers from Finland found an inverse relationship between sauna bathing and serious memory problems. Compared with men who had one sauna bathing session per week, those who had two to three sessions or four to seven saunas were, respectively, 22 percent or 66 percent less likely to have dementia![55] In other research, those who had frequent sauna baths also had a lower incidence of sudden cardiac death and death from all causes.[56] Saunas have also been found to help depression in cancer patients; increase feel-good endorphins, testosterone, and growth hormone; lower the stress hormone cortisol; and lower blood sugar.[57] According to the research, the goal should be to sweat profusely for 20 to 30 minutes.[58]

- *Take nutraceuticals and eat foods that are good for your skin.* Refer to the lists of nutraceuticals and foods below and on the following pages.

The Nutraceuticals

TO SUPPORT YOUR LIVER

- *NAC (N-acetylcysteine):* 600 mg twice a day. NAC raises blood, liver, cellular, and mitochondrial levels of cysteine and the super-antioxidant glutathione. NAC has also been shown to help decrease the toxicity of chemotherapeutic drugs used to treat cancer and of antibiotics used against infections.[59]

- *Vitamin C:* 1,000 mg twice a day

- *Selenium:* 200 micrograms (mcg) a day

- *Zinc:* 20 to 30 mg a day

- *Folate* (MTHF, methylfolate): 400 mcg a day

- *Vitamin B12* (methyl cobalamin): 500 mcg a day

- *Curcumin* (in a bioavailable form like Longvida): 300 mg twice a day for excellent liver protection; increases bile excretion and decreases cholesterol

- *Artichoke extract:* significantly increases bile excretion from the liver for two to three hours[60]

TO SUPPORT YOUR KIDNEYS

- *Magnesium glycinate, citrate, or malate:* 200 mg twice a day

- *Curcumin:* 300 mg twice a day

- *Ginkgo biloba extract:* 60 mg twice a day; increases blood flow to brain and kidneys[61] and helps protect against glyphosates[62]

- *Fiber:* seven grams (women) or ten grams (men) three times a day combined in food and supplements

- *NAC (N-acetylcysteine):* 600 mg twice a day

- *Omega-3 fatty acids:* 1.4 grams (or more) of a combination of EPA and DHA in about a 60/40 ratio per day

TO SUPPORT YOUR SKIN

- *Vitamin D3:* 2,000 IUs a day or more, depending on your level

- *Vitamin E:* 60 mg of mixed tocopherols a day

- *Omega-3 fatty acids:* 1.4 grams (or more) a day of a combination of EPA and DHA in about a 60/40 ratio

- *CoQ10:* 100 mg a day

- *Alpha-lipoic acid:* 300 to 600 mg a day

- *Grapeseed extract:* 100 to 300 mg a day

- *EGCG:* 600 mg a day

- *Curcumin:* 500 mg a day

- *Selenium:* 150 micrograms (mcg) a day

- *Zinc:* 25 mg a day

- *Astaxanthin:* 4 to 12 mg a day

The Foods
CONSIDER ADDING:
TO NOURISH YOUR LIVER

- *Green leafy vegetables for folate*, an essential detoxification nutrient

- *Protein-rich foods*, including eggs

- *Brassicas:* any color cabbage, brussels sprouts, cauliflower, broccoli, kale for detox; consuming more brassicas also has been found to lower breast cancer risk.[63]

- *Oranges and tangerines:* vitamin C/d-limonene, many beneficial flavonoids

- *Berries:* wide diversity of flavonoids

- *Sunflower and sesame seeds:* high in cysteine

- *Caraway and dill seeds:* d-limonene[64]

TO NOURISH YOUR KIDNEYS

- *Water*

- *Spices to support detoxification:* clove, rosemary, turmeric[65]

- *Nuts and seeds:* cashews, almonds, and pumpkin seeds for magnesium

- *Green leafy vegetables*

- *Citrus fruits, except grapefruit*

- *Beet juice* for circulation and endurance

- *Ginger* for its anti-inflammatory properties

- *Blueberries* (increase filtration rate in kidneys), *raspberries, strawberries, blackberries*

- *Garlic*

- *Sugar-free chocolate:* increases blood flow

TO NOURISH YOUR SKIN

- *Water*

- *Green tea*

- *Colorful fruits and vegetables for antioxidants:* especially organic berries, kiwifruit, oranges, tangerines, pomegranates, broccoli, and peppers

- *Avocados*

- *Olive oil*

- *Almonds, walnuts, sunflower seeds*

- *Wild salmon*

- *Sugar-free chocolate*

AVOID (OR LIMIT):

FOODS AND MEDICATIONS THAT INHIBIT LIVER DETOXIFICATION

- *Processed meats* such as bacon and smoked turkey, that contain nitrosamines, which cause the liver to produce fats that are toxic to the brain

- *Grapefruit* (juice may interfere with medications)

- *Capsaicin* from red chili peppers

- *Conventionally raised produce; dairy; grain-fed meats; and farmed fish*

- *Medications* such as antihistamines, acetaminophen, stomach acid blockers, some antidepressants (such as fluoxetine), and anti-anxiety medications (such as diazepam). Be sure to consult with your doctor before discontinuing any medication.

Note: If you do a liver detox, keep in mind that it is common to feel worse for a week or so while your body unloads toxins. These reactions include feeling tired, achy, irritable, and/or dizzy, and having skin rashes, smellier urine or stools, a stuffy nose, or headaches. Be patient: Those symptoms will likely subside quickly.

FOODS THAT INHIBIT KIDNEY DETOXIFICATION

- *Too much animal protein*

- *Excess salt*

- *Excess phosphates:* processed cheeses, canned fish, processed meats, flavored water, sodas, nondairy creamers, bottled coffee drinks, and iced teas

 ## PICK ONE HEALTHY BRIGHT MINDS HABIT TO START TODAY

1. Buy organic.

2. When pumping gas, be cautious not to breathe in any fumes.

3. Quit smoking and avoid secondhand smoke.

4. Limit alcohol to two glasses a week.

5. Take N-acetylcysteine (NAC).

6. Eat brassicas (cruciferous vegetables) for their detoxifying ability.

7. Avoid handling cash register receipts because the plastic coating contains BPA that can get through your skin.

8. Don't drink or eat out of plastic containers.

9. Eliminate MSG and artificial dyes and preservatives from your diet.

10. **Use apps like Think Dirty or Healthy Living (EWG.org) to scan your personal products and eliminate as many toxins as possible.**

CHAPTER 11

M IS FOR MENTAL HEALTH
YOUR MIND IS ESSENTIAL TO YOUR BRAIN

*Do not conform to the pattern of this world, but be
transformed by the renewing of your mind.*
ROMANS 12:2, NIV

DAVID: A TOXIC STEW OF MIND MEDS

When my wife, Tana, and I met 12 years ago, her 62-year-old father, a pastor and seminar leader, lived about four hours away and had become a recluse. After his mental state began deteriorating, his doctor diagnosed him with Alzheimer's disease and prescribed a new medication, but it just seemed to make him more confused. Tana was deeply concerned about him, so I suggested she let me evaluate him.

David's scan showed that he did not have Alzheimer's disease, but rather a condition called pseudodementia, which is depression that masquerades as Alzheimer's disease. He was also on a toxic combination of psychiatric medications, including Xanax (for anxiety), which can accelerate memory loss. I was alarmed for him and convinced Tana to move him nearby for a few months. When David began our Memory Rescue: BRIGHT MINDS program, he had his important numbers checked—he was overweight; low in thyroid, vitamin D, testosterone, and omega-3s; and had high blood sugar, ferritin, CRP, and homocysteine. Plus he wasn't sleeping well.

DAVID'S BRIGHT MINDS RISK FACTORS AND INTERVENTIONS

BRIGHT MINDS	DAVID'S RISK FACTORS	INTERVENTIONS
Blood Flow		
Retirement/Aging	62, no new learning, social isolation	Reengaged in teaching
Inflammation	High CRP and homocysteine; low Omega-3 Index	Omega-3 fatty acids
Genetics	Family history of depression and suicide	
Head Trauma		
Toxins	Toxic combination of psychiatric medications	Slowly stopped medications
Mental Health	Major depression	Nutraceuticals for depression
Immunity/Infection Issues	Low vitamin D	Vitamin D3 supplements
Neurohormone Deficiencies	Low testosterone and thyroid	Treat thyroid; weight training; decreased sugar
Diabesity	Overweight, high blood sugar	Weight loss and dietary changes
Sleep Issues	Chronic insomnia	Sleep strategies

DAVID'S "BEFORE" BRAIN SPECT SCAN

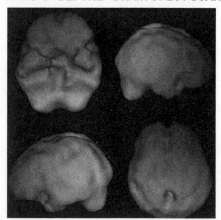

Pseudodementia masquerading as Alzheimer's disease

With targeted treatment—including nutraceuticals to treat his depression and balance his hormones, vitamin D, and blood sugar levels—and support from his daughter, David blossomed. He felt a fresh connection to God when he prayed, and he began to enjoy studying the Bible again. Six months later he taught an all-day seminar at a nearby church. He told me it was as if he had been raised from the dead. We helped him get his life back by taking a BRIGHT MINDS approach to treating his brain. The big benefit to me was that Tana saw firsthand the power of our work and has become a passionate brain warrior for what we do.

BRAIN, MIND, AND MEMORY

Getting your mind right is a critical piece of the puzzle in rescuing and strengthening your memory. Studies have shown that depression, bipolar disorder, schizophrenia, post-traumatic stress disorder (or PTSD) in both veterans and civilians, attention deficit disorder/attention deficit hyperactivity disorder (ADD/ADHD), and chronic stress significantly increase the risk of memory problems, inflammation, and vascular and immunity issues.[1] Poor mental health can be very potent. In fact, new research indicates that men who are depressed have as great a risk of suffering a heart attack or heart disease as men who are obese, and people with mental health issues die an average of 10 years earlier than their mentally healthy counterparts.[2]

Anything that negatively affects your mind also negatively affects your brain. Virtually all psychiatric illnesses have a significant brain component to them. Schizophrenia, for example, has been shown to affect the frontal and temporal lobes; depression has been associated with decreased activity in the frontal lobes; and ADD/ADHD is associated with lower activity in the prefrontal cortex, basal ganglia, and cerebellum.

For many years, I suspected there was a link between untreated ADD/ADHD and memory problems. The hallmark symptoms of ADHD are short attention span, distractibility, disorganization, procrastination, restlessness, and impulsivity; those lifelong traits make people vulnerable to important risk factors for memory problems, such as traumatic brain injury (TBI), obesity, depression, alcohol and drug abuse, and smoking.[3] A recent Argentinian study noted a significant increase in adults diagnosed with ADHD and Lewy body dementia, which is also associated with Parkinson's disease.[4] Both ADHD and Parkinson's disease are associated with lower levels of the neurotransmitter dopamine. Treating ADHD, naturally or with medication, may decrease these risk factors and help save your memory.

Depression doubles the risk of cognitive impairment in women and quadruples it in men. Kristine Yaffe, MD, and her colleagues at the University of California, San Francisco, School of Medicine studied the association between depression and cognitive decline. They evaluated 5,781 elderly women with tests of mood and memory. At the beginning of the study, 211 had six or more depressive symptoms, but only 16 of those 211 (7.6 percent) were receiving treatment, which meant more than 92 percent of the depressed women were not being treated.[5] Increasing symptoms of depression were associated with worse performance at baseline and follow-up on all tests four years later. Women with three to five depressive symptoms were at 60 percent greater odds for cognitive deterioration, and women with six or more depressive symptoms were 230 percent more likely to have problems! The researchers concluded that depression in older women is associated with both poor cognitive function and subsequent cognitive decline. Some researchers believe that late-life depression may, in fact, be a precursor to Alzheimer's disease, and one-third of all patients with mild cognitive impairment (MCI) are reported to suffer from depression, which then accelerates the progression to full-blown dementia.[6] It is critical to get depression treated in order to keep your mind.

||||||||||||||||||||||||||||||||||||||||||||||||||||||||||||||||||||||||||||||||||||||||||||||

Is It Depression—or Dementia?

This is an important question because these two illnesses can masquerade as each other. In a study of more than 4,500 patients that my colleagues and I published in the *Journal of Alzheimer's Disease*, we saw overall lower blood flow to the brains of people with dementia, especially in the hippocampus.[7]

Since most people will never get a brain SPECT or QEEG scan, here are a number of traits you can use as a guide to distinguish between depression and dementia.

MORE LIKELY TO BE DEPRESSION

1. Prior history of depression or family history of depression
2. Presence of physical symptoms, such as aches and pains
3. Pervasive sad or negative feelings
4. Excessive worry; anxiety and panic
5. Feelings that life is pointless and not worth living

6. Loneliness or boredom
7. Crying for no apparent reason
8. Difficulty completing simple chores
9. Lower energy
10. Suicidal thoughts common

MORE LIKELY TO BE DEMENTIA

1. Difficulty performing familiar tasks
2. Problems with words and language; using the wrong words
3. Disorientation of time and place
4. Decreased judgment
5. Memory loss that comes on gradually
6. Misplacement of things
7. Problems with abstract thinking
8. Changes in personality
9. Loss of initiative, apathy
10. Suicidal thoughts uncommon

One additional sign: Depression tends to come on more quickly than dementia.

IIIIIIIIIIIIIIIIIIIIIIIIIIIIIIIIIIIIIIIIIIIIIIIIIIIIIIIIIIIIIIIIIIIIIIIIIIIIIIIIIIIIIIIIIIIIIIIIII

Chronic stress in midlife has been associated with memory problems later on. Brain circuits involved in chronic anxiety and fear extensively overlap in areas associated with Alzheimer's disease, and chronic stress has been shown to decrease the size of the hippocampus and prefrontal cortex, except when it is paired with a low or low-normal level of the hormone DHEA. Stress is considered a normal part of life when it is occasional and temporary, such as when you feel anxious before an exam or a job interview. When it becomes frequent or chronic, as in prolonged grief, however, it needs to be treated.

 # CHECKUP FOR <u>M</u>ENTAL HEALTH ISSUES

Screen for problems

Given that ADHD, PTSD, depression, bipolar disorder, schizophrenia, and chronic stress are risk factors for memory problems as we age, it is important to screen for them. Older people with depression, unlike younger ones who may complain of a sad or depressed mood, may also show signs of cognitive impairment, such as confusion, memory disturbance, and attention deficits, which may be mistaken for dementia. Complicating the picture, depression may coexist with dementia and exacerbate the problem, increasing the disability.

The questionnaires we use at Amen Clinics will help you determine whether you have the common symptoms of ADHD, depression, bipolar disorder, or PTSD.

Please rate yourself on each of the symptoms listed below using the following scale. If possible, to give yourself the most complete picture, have another person who knows you well (such as a spouse, partner, or parent) rate you as well.

0	1	2	3	4	NA
Never	Rarely	Occasionally	Frequently	Very Frequently	Not Applicable/ Not Known

ADHD: *If you have four or more symptoms with a score of 3 or 4, consider seeking an evaluation from a psychiatrist or licensed counselor.*

____ 1. trouble sustaining attention or easily distracted

____ 2. difficulty completing projects

____ 3. overwhelmed by the tasks of everyday living

____ 4. trouble maintaining an organized work or living area

____ 5. inconsistent work performance

____ 6. poor attention to detail

____ 7. impulsive decision making

____ 8. difficulty delaying what you want; having to have needs met immediately

____ 9. restlessness, fidgeting

____ 10. comments made to others without considering their impact

____ 11. impatience; frustration

____ 12. frequent traffic violations or near accidents

Depression: *If you have four or more symptoms with a score of 3 or 4, consider seeking an evaluation from a psychiatrist or licensed counselor.*

____ 1. depressed or sad mood

____ 2. decreased interest in things that are usually fun, including sex

____ 3. significant weight gain or loss without trying, or appetite changes

____ 4. recurrent thoughts of death or suicide

____ 5. sleep changes, lack of sleep, or marked increase in sleep

____ 6. physical agitation or feeling "slowed down"

____ 7. low energy or feelings of tiredness

____ 8. feelings of worthlessness, helplessness, hopelessness, or guilt

____ 9. decreased concentration or memory

Bipolar disorder: *Includes periods of depression (see questions above) that tend to cycle with the manic symptoms below. If you have three or more of these symptoms along with a score of 3 or 4 in depression, consider seeking an evaluation from a psychiatrist or licensed counselor.*

____ 1. periods of an elevated, high, or irritable mood

____ 2. periods of very high self-esteem or grandiose thinking

____ 3. periods of decreased need for sleep without feeling tired

____ 4. periods of talkativeness or pressure to keep talking

____ 5. racing thoughts or frequent jumping from one subject to another

____ 6. frequent distractions because of irrelevant things

____ 7. marked increase in activity level

____ 8. excessive involvement in pleasurable activities with painful consequences (affairs, gambling, etc.)

PTSD: *If you have four or more symptoms with a score of 3 or 4, consider seeking an evaluation from a psychiatrist or licensed counselor.*

____ 1. recurrent and upsetting thoughts of a past traumatic event (flashbacks of an accident, fire, molestation, etc.)

____ 2. recurrent distressing dreams of a past upsetting event

____ 3. a sense of reliving a past upsetting event

____ 4. a sense of panic or fear of events that resemble an upsetting past event

____ 5. effort spent avoiding thoughts or feelings associated with a past trauma

____ 6. persistent avoidance of activities/situations that cause remembrance of an upsetting event

____ 7. inability to recall an important aspect of a past upsetting event

____ 8. marked decreased interest in important activities

____ 9. feelings of detachment or distance from others

____10. feelings of numbness or restrictions in your feelings

____11. feeling that your future is shortened

___12. quick startle

___13. feeling like you're always watching for bad things to happen

___14. marked physical response to events that remind you of a past upsetting event (e.g., sweating when getting in a car if you have been in a car accident)

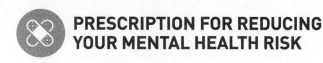

PRESCRIPTION FOR REDUCING YOUR MENTAL HEALTH RISK

The Strategies

1. **Get treated.** Early treatment is essential to stave off the ravages of psychiatric illnesses. Our work with SPECT teaches us that with appropriate treatment, the brain becomes more balanced and works much more efficiently. Treatment does not necessarily mean psychiatric drugs. At Amen Clinics, we prefer natural treatments whenever possible. A healthy diet; exercise; omega-3 fatty acids EPA and DHA and other supplements; as well as meditation and cognitive-behavioral therapy have been shown to help a wide variety of mental health issues. But if these strategies don't work or faster results are needed, medications are important to consider. Work with a skilled mental health professional—because your brain depends on it. Here are potential treatments to boost mental health if you are suffering from one of these issues:

    -   *ADHD.* See my book *Healing ADD* for more detailed information on the seven types of ADD/ADHD, and take our free online test at www.ADDTypeTest.com.
        -   Brain-healthy habits
        -   Exercise[8]
        -   Higher-protein, lower-carbohydrate diet:[9] see the Memory Rescue Diet, page 255.
        -   Work with an ADD/ADHD coach
        -   Medication, if necessary

    -   *Depression.* See my book *Healing Anxiety and Depression* for more detailed information on the seven types of anxiety and depression.

- Brain-healthy habits
- Exercise[10]
- Antioxidant-[11] and tomato-rich diet[12]
- Cognitive-behavioral therapy (CBT)[13]
- Acupuncture[14]
- Medication, if necessary
- Methylfolate (as an add-on treatment to antidepressant medication)[15]

- *Bipolar disorder*
  - Brain-healthy habits
  - Exercise[16]
  - Medication, if necessary

- *PTSD*
  - Brain-healthy habits
  - EMDR (eye movement desensitization and reprocessing;[17] www.emdria.org)
  - Loving-kindness meditation[18] (see page 178)
  - Medication, if necessary

- *Stress*
  - Brain-healthy habits
  - Exercise[19]
  - Prayer and mindfulness meditation[20]

2. **Try these 25 research-proven tips.** Use them to lower stress and boost your level of happiness and overall mental health.

- Start every day with the words "Today is going to be a great day." Your mind makes happen what it visualizes. When you start the day by saying these words, your brain will find the reasons it will be a great day.

- Write down three things you are grateful for every day. Researchers found that people who did this significantly increased their sense of happiness in just three weeks.[21]

- Write down the name of one person you appreciate every day. Then tell him or her. Appreciation is gratitude expressed outwardly and builds positive bridges between people.

- Pray about your concerns. When you pray, you turn over your worries to God, who is sovereign, loving, and active in our lives: "Give all your worries and cares to God, for he cares about you" (1 Peter 5:7). You might also read a few Scripture passages that remind you of God's faithfulness and love before you ask him to help you find solutions for your problems.

- Limit screen time. Studies report a higher level of depression and obesity with increased time spent with technology.

- Exercise. It is the fastest way to feel better. Go for a walk or a run.

- Enjoy some dark chocolate. It can boost blood flow to your brain,[22] help improve your mood, and decrease anxiety. In one study, seniors who ate more of it had a lower incidence of dementia than those who ate less. Don't overdo it, however. Dietitians generally recommend eating no more than one ounce per day.

- Listen to music. Just 25 minutes of Mozart or Strauss has been shown to lower blood pressure and stress. Listening to ABBA has also been shown to lower stress hormones—Mamma Mia![23]

- Choose experiences that give you a sense of awe, such as looking at a sunset or something beautiful in nature.[24]

- Drink green tea, which contains L-theanine, an ingredient that helps you feel happier, more relaxed, and more focused.[25]

- Read an inspiring, powerful novel.[26]

- Take a walk in nature, which is also associated with reducing worry.[27]

- Go barefoot outside. It decreases anxiety and depression by 62 percent, according to one study.[28]

- Listen to a sad song. Really. It was found to increase positive emotions.[29] Listening to lullabies and soothing music also decreased stress and improved sleep.[30]

- Stop complaining! It rewires your brain to see the negative far too often.[31]

- Spend time with positive people if you want to feel happy.[32] People's moods are contagious. (If you want to feel depressed, hang out with gloomy people.)

- Do something you love that brings you joy. For me, it is playing table tennis or spending time with my wife, kids, or grandkids.

- Write down your five happiest experiences; then imagine reliving them.

- Engage in activities that make you feel competent.[33]

- Be patient. People tend to be happier with age, especially if they take care of their brains.[34]

- Learn to forgive. It can help reduce negative feelings.[35]

- Help someone else or volunteer. In one study, people who did felt happier.[36] Make time for friends, too.[37]

- Get intimate with your spouse. Making love increases overall happiness and decreases stress hormones. In mice, it helped boost the hippocampus.[38]

- Journal your feelings. Not only does it help get them out of your head, it helps you gain perspective.[39]

- Learn to kill the ANTs (automatic negative thoughts). Remember that thoughts aren't necessarily accurate. Whenever you feel sad, mad, nervous, or out of control, write down your negative thoughts. Next, ask yourself if they are true or if they are distorted to make you feel worse. Focusing your mind on positive, rational thoughts will help you feel much better.

BRIGHT MINDS TIP

Do a loving-kindness meditation (see page 178). It's a proven way to improve your mood and memory.

||||||||||||||||||||||||||||||||||||||||||||||||||||||||||||||||||||||||||||||||||||

Loving-Kindness Meditation

Loving-kindness meditation (LKM), which aims to foster feelings of goodwill, kindness, and warmth toward others, boosts positive emotions and decreases negative ones,[40] according to scientific studies. LKM has also been shown to decrease pain, migraine headaches, and symptoms of PTSD and social prejudice.[41] It also increases gray matter in the emotional processing areas of the brain and expands social connectedness.[42]

Meditation and prayer are my two favorite things to combat stress. They only take a few minutes. While prayer is addressed to God, LKM is first practiced toward yourself and then toward other people. If you have difficulty loving yourself, it will be harder to be loving and compassionate toward others.

Let me walk you through a loving-kindness meditation. Sit quietly in a comfortable position, close your eyes, breathe naturally, and repeat phrases such as:

- May I be happy.
- May I be healthy.
- May I be at peace.

After you repeat the phrases several times, direct them to someone you are thankful for:

- May you be happy.
- May you be healthy.
- May you be at peace.

Next, visualize someone you feel neutral about and repeat the phrases again.

Finally, visualize someone you don't like or are angry with, such as an ex-spouse or someone who has hurt you, and repeat the phrases again.

As difficult as this exercise can be, it can lead to forgiveness and love, two healing emotions.

||||||||||||||||||||||||||||||||||||||||||||||||||||||||||||||||||||||||||||||||||||

The Nutraceuticals

TO ADDRESS ADHD

- *Omega-3 fatty acids* (higher in EPA than DHA)[43]

- *Zinc*[44]

- *Magnesium*[45]

- *Iron* (if ferritin levels are low)[46]

- *Phosphatidylserine*[47]

TO ADDRESS DEPRESSION

- *Omega-3 fatty acids* (higher in EPA than DHA),[48] especially when inflammation markers, such as CRP,[49] are high

- *SAMe* (s-adenosyl methionine) especially in males[50]

- *Saffron*[51]

- *Optimize vitamin D levels*[52]

- *Magnesium*[53]

TO ADDRESS BIPOLAR DISORDER

- *Omega-3 fatty acids EPA and DHA*[54]

TO ADDRESS STRESS

- *Optimize your DHEA level* to the high-normal range.[55] (See chapter 13, page 218.)

- If you struggle with worry (the inability to let go of bothersome thoughts), consider supplements to raise the neurotransmitter serotonin, such as *5-hydroxytryptophan (5-HTP)* or *saffron*.[56]

- If you struggle with anxiety (a pervasive sense of tension and nervousness), consider supplements to boost GABA, such as *GABA* itself, *magnesium*, and *theanine* from green tea.[57]

The Foods

AVOID (OR LIMIT):

Pro-inflammatory foods: See chapter 7, page 98.

Alcohol[58]

Aspartame[59]

Caffeine[60]

CONSIDER ADDING:

Spices to support mental health: saffron, turmeric (curcumin), saffron plus curcumin, peppermint (for attention problems), and cinnamon (for attention problems, ADHD, irritability)[61]

Dopamine-rich foods for focus and motivation: turmeric, theanine from green tea, lentils, fish, lamb, chicken, turkey, beef, eggs, nuts, seeds (pumpkin and sesame), high-protein veggies (such as broccoli and spinach), and protein powders[62]

Serotonin-rich foods for mood, sleep, pain, and craving control: Combine tryptophan-containing foods, such as eggs, turkey, seafood, chickpeas, nuts, and seeds (building blocks for serotonin) with healthy carbohydrates, such as sweet potatoes and quinoa, to elicit a short-term insulin response that drives tryptophan into the brain. Dark chocolate[63] also increases serotonin.

GABA-rich foods for anxiety: broccoli, almonds, walnuts, lentils, bananas, beef liver, brown rice, halibut, gluten-free whole oats, oranges, rice bran, and spinach

Choline-rich foods: See chapter 9, page 137.

Fruits and vegetables for mood: Eat up to eight servings a day.[64]

Green tea

Maca: a root vegetable/medicinal plant, native to Peru, that has been shown to reduce depression[65]

Omega-3-rich foods to support nerve cell membranes and serotonin:[66] See chapter 7, page 107.

Antioxidant-rich foods: See chapter 6, page 93.

Magnesium-rich foods for anxiety: See chapter 5, page 77.

Zinc-rich foods: See chapter 12, page 200.

Vitamin B6, B12, and folate-rich foods: See chapter 5, page 77.

Prebiotic-rich foods: See chapter 7, page 107.

Probiotic-rich foods: See chapter 7, page 107.

 ## PICK ONE HEALTHY BRIGHT MINDS HABIT TO START TODAY

1. Start every day with the phrase "Today is going to be a great day."

2. Write down three things you are grateful for each day.

3. **Take saffron, which has been found to help both mood and memory.**

4. If you have trouble focusing, consider a high-protein, lower-carbohydrate diet.

5. Eat up to eight fruits and vegetables a day; there is a direct correlation between eating more produce and feeling happier. Tomatoes, for instance, have been shown to help mood.

6. Begin practicing the loving-kindness meditation.

7. Take a walk in nature.

8. **Pray to release your worries and to rejoice over the good things around you.**

9. If natural interventions are not effective, work with a local therapist or psychiatrist.

10. **Kill the ANTs. Whenever you feel mad, sad, nervous, or out of control, write down your negative thoughts and learn to talk back to them.**

CHAPTER 12

I IS FOR IMMUNITY/ INFECTION ISSUES
STRENGTHEN YOUR INTERNAL DEFENDERS

My strategy is to stop the assaults—to reduce the number of factors your immune system has to deal with by cleaning up your diet, healing your gut, lightening your toxic burden, treating your infections, and reducing your overall stress.

AMY MYERS, *THE AUTOIMMUNE SOLUTION*

JESSE: AN IMMUNE SYSTEM GONE HAYWIRE

Jesse, 42, was raised on a farm in the Northwest. She became a successful news reporter, which led to promotions in bigger and bigger cities. She was under chronic stress, dieted constantly to keep her weight low for her television appearances, and rarely got a full night's sleep. While on a work trip to London, she lost her sight for three hours and was incredibly frightened. She hid the incident from her husband and work supervisor, hoping it was a fluke. Three weeks later, feeling weak on one side, she went to her doctor, who referred her to a neurologist. After a physical exam, MRI, and other tests, Jesse was diagnosed with multiple sclerosis (MS), a disorder in which the body's immune system attacks the lining of the spinal cord and brain cells (called the myelin sheath). She was put on immune-suppressing drugs, and their side effects made her feel awful.

Deciding there had to be a better way to deal with her illness, Jesse took time off work and came to our clinic for evaluation. Her SPECT scan revealed overall low blood flow to her brain. She had high levels of C-reactive protein and mercury, and her vitamin D level and Omega-3 Index were both extremely low. She told me that her family's farm had often been sprayed with pesticides and herbicides.

To get healthy, Jesse had eight silver fillings removed and began treatments to support detoxification. She also went on an elimination diet and found she was very sensitive to gluten, dairy, soy, and corn. She was so excited about the improvements she saw from these dietary changes that she became certified in integrative nutrition.

Within six months, Jesse was symptom-free and has remained so for six years. Her initial MRI showed bright white-matter lesions throughout her brain, typical of MS. Her follow-up scan four years later showed that they had significantly decreased—something her neurologist had a hard time explaining.

JESSE'S "BEFORE" AND "AFTER" BRAIN SPECT SCANS

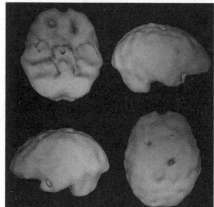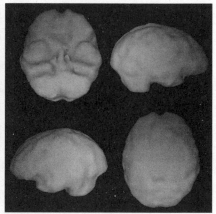

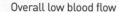

Overall low blood flow　　　　Significantly improved blood flow

JESSE'S BRIGHT MINDS RISK FACTORS AND INTERVENTIONS

BRIGHT MINDS	JESSE'S RISK FACTORS	INTERVENTIONS
Blood Flow	Low blood flow on SPECT	Hydration, exercise, and ginkgo biloba
Retirement/Aging		
Inflammation	High CRP, low Omega-3 Index	Limited omega-6 foods; omega-3 fatty acid supplements; elimination diet
Genetics		

BRIGHT MINDS	JESSE'S RISK FACTORS	INTERVENTIONS
Head Trauma		
Toxins	Pesticides, mercury	Organic diet, detoxification treatments (including N-acetylcysteine), brassicas
Mental Health	Chronic work stress	Stress management tools, saffron
Immunity/Infection Issues	Multiple sclerosis, low vitamin D	Vitamin D3 supplementation, raw garlic and onions, shiitake mushrooms
Neurohormone Deficiencies		
Diabesity		
Sleep Issues	Insomnia	Sleep strategies

YOUR BODY'S DEFENSE SYSTEM

It is important to constantly strengthen and build up your immunity. Why? Think of the infamous December 1981 trash collectors' strike in New York City. Suddenly, the city's rats got to join in the Christmas spirit with plentiful meals on the sidewalks. But not everyone was as happy as the rodents. Tempers flared. Where did the vermin come from? It turns out they were always there, but when the streets were swept clean of junk, the rats were kept under control. They stayed hidden because there was nothing in plain sight to eat. During the sanitation department's strike, however, garbage was everywhere, so the rats wound up running rampant, multiplying and spreading disease. So, too, when you put trash in your body or don't regularly keep your immune system healthy, you become vulnerable to "vermin": serious illnesses, immune dysfunction, and brain disease.

Immunity is your body's natural defense system. In a general sense, it has two broad duties: *defense* and *tolerance*. For the first, it helps to defend against invaders from outside your body, such as bacteria, viruses, and parasites. Your immune system also patrols your body, looking for troublemakers, such as cancer cells. Second, the immune system helps determine your tolerance of potential triggers from the outside world, such as allergens (including pollen, bee stings, wheat, peanuts, and corn), as well as internal attacks, such as autoimmune disorders (including rheumatoid arthritis and lupus).

When your defenses break down, you are more vulnerable to infections and cancer. When your body's tolerance is overwhelmed, you have more issues with allergies and autoimmune disorders, in which your body attacks itself. Both autoimmune disorders and infections (especially when they become chronic) increase your risk of brain fog, memory issues, and dementia.

||||||||||||||||||||||||||||||||||||||||||||||||||||||||||||||||||||||||||||||||||||||

THE FOUR BASIC IMMUNE SYSTEM FUNCTIONS	
Defense against external environment If it fails, you get an **infection**.	**Defense** against internal environment If it fails, you get **cancer**.
Tolerance against external environment If it fails, you get **allergies**.	**Tolerance** against self If it fails, you get an **autoimmune disease**.

||||||||||||||||||||||||||||||||||||||||||||||||||||||||||||||||||||||||||||||||||||||

In a very simple sense, your immune system

- identifies invaders or parts of your own body that have gone awry
- calls for help from your white blood cells
- tags and destroys the troublemakers
- remembers them if and when they resurface

There are five categories of immune disorders:

1. Immune deficiency disorders: These arise at birth because of an ineffective immune system or are acquired as an illness, like human immunodeficiency virus (HIV) or acquired immune deficiency syndrome (AIDS), which damages the immune system.

2. Allergies: Neutral "visitors," such as grass, cat dander, or peanuts, are viewed as foes by the body, causing asthma, eczema, or worse. Asthma has been shown to increase the risk of dementia by 30 percent.[1]

3. Cancers of the immune system, such as leukemia and lymphomas.

4. Autoimmune disorders: Think of these as friendly fire; the immune system attacks its own tissues.

5. Persistent infections, due to a weakened immune system.

This chapter will focus on the last two categories, autoimmune disorders and infections, because when left untreated, they have been associated with serious memory problems and dementia. With treatment, however, there can be significant improvement.

AUTOIMMUNE DISORDERS

When the body's immune system erroneously attacks and destroys healthy body tissue, the result is an autoimmune disorder. White blood cells, an important part of the immune system, help protect against harmful substances, such as bacteria, viruses, toxins, and cancer cells. These substances contain antigens, or foreign substances, that the immune system recognizes as troublemakers and then tries to destroy by producing antibodies against them. When you have an autoimmune disorder, your immune system doesn't distinguish healthy tissue from these antigens. As a result, your body sets off a reaction that destroys normal tissues.

We still do not know all of the causes of autoimmune disorders, but as in Jesse's case, it is likely that many factors may contribute to them, including

- Leaky gut: See chapter 7, page 98.
- Allergens: These may be environmental (trees, grasses, flowers) or milk, eggs, fish, shellfish, tree nuts, peanuts, wheat, or soybeans. (These last eight are the primary food allergens, according to the US Food and Drug Administration.)
- Toxins
- Stress
- Obesity
- Sleep disorders
- Lack of exercise or excessive exercise
- Poor diet
- Nutrient deficiencies
- Hidden infections
- Head trauma

More than 100 different autoimmune disorders affect 50 million people in the United States, including multiple sclerosis, rheumatoid arthritis,[2] systemic lupus erythematosus,[3] Crohn's disease,[4] psoriasis,[5] Hashimoto's thyroiditis, and type 1 diabetes. Many of these double or triple the risk for serious memory problems.

The conventional approach to treating many of these disorders is to shut down the immune system with powerful medications, such as nonsteroidal anti-inflammatory medications, steroids, or anticancer drugs like methotrexate. But my friend and colleague Mark Hyman, MD, director of Cleveland Clinic's Center for Functional Medicine, thinks it is a mistake to think of these as separate disorders requiring distinct treatments. A far better approach is to address them as one disorder in which the immune system begins to attack itself. If you suffer from one of these disorders, he believes the first question to ask yourself is *What is making my immune system so angry at me?* The best defense is to address all of your BRIGHT MINDS risk factors discussed in the book.

INFECTIOUS DISEASES: BRAIN TROUBLE TOO

In a 2016 *Journal of Alzheimer's Disease* editorial,[6] an international consensus group of 33 scientists expressed concern that infectious diseases were being overlooked as a major cause of memory problems and dementia. Presenting evidence from more than 100 research studies, they argued that viruses, usually dormant in the brain, can become active again after significant stress or when the immune system is suppressed. Even something as common as cold sores can have consequences: In a review of 35 studies, people testing positive for herpes simplex 1 (cold sores) or herpes simplex 2 (genital herpes) had an increased risk of memory problems, and having both increased the risk further.[7] Be careful whom you kiss!

Not everyone exposed to infectious diseases gets sick from them. Your vulnerability to illness often has to do with the strength of your immune system and your exposures, stress level, and habits. Yet based on the evidence of tens of thousands of brain scans I have examined, I believe that "infectious disease" will be an important subspecialty in psychiatry within the next twenty years. Infectious illnesses including Lyme disease, toxoplasmosis, syphilis, *Helicobacter pylori* (*H. pylori*), HIV/AIDS, herpes, and others are a major cause of psychiatric and cognitive problems that few medical professionals recognize.

When I first started performing SPECT scans in 1991, I saw a number of patients who had been diagnosed with chronic fatigue syndrome and fibromyalgia. They were often dismissed by the medical community as "psychiatric patients," which was almost like classifying them as hysterical or exhibiting a stress reaction, and then referred to me. (I have always been frustrated by physicians who, when they don't know what is going on with a patient, label them as "psychiatric." *Hey,* I think, *that's my job!*). Many of these patients' scans looked truly awful, revealing overall low blood flow caused by undiagnosed infections. Of course these people appeared hysterical, unhappy, angry, or anxious! The organ behind their behavior—the brain—was being ravaged by an infection. The scan below is an example.

CHRONIC FATIGUE SYNDROME BRAIN SPECT SCAN

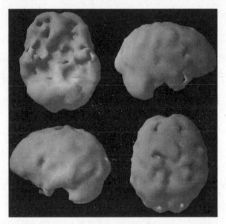

For a look at the connection between an infectious illness and a serious mental health issue, see the image on the next page, which compares the states in the United States with the highest incidence of schizophrenia with those that have the highest incidence of Lyme disease (and the highest prevalence of ticks carrying the disease).

At Amen Clinics we've seen hundreds of patients with resistant complex psychiatric symptoms or cognitive problems who tested positive for Lyme disease and got significantly better when it was treated. Interestingly, a 2014 study reported that the antibiotic minocycline, used to treat Lyme disease, was found to decrease symptoms of schizophrenia in a 12-month study.

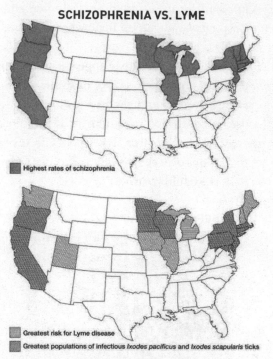

SCHIZOPHRENIA VS. LYME

■ Highest rates of schizophrenia

▨ Greatest risk for Lyme disease
▨ Greatest populations of infectious *Ixodes pacificus* and *Ixodes scapularis* ticks

Source: J. S. Brown Jr., "Geographic Correlation of Schizophrenia to Ticks and Tick-Borne Encephalitis," *Schizophrenia Bulletin* 20, no. 4 (1994), 755–75; used with permission

It was widely reported that Kris Kristofferson was diagnosed with Alzheimer's disease. He was symptomatic for a decade and fading fast when he saw Mark Filidei, DO, at the Whitaker Wellness Clinic. (Mark also works with us at Amen Clinics as our director of integrative medicine.) After extensive testing, Dr. Filidei diagnosed the Hall of Fame singer with Lyme disease and treated him with antibiotics and hyperbaric oxygen therapy. After a few treatments, Kristofferson reportedly told his wife, "I feel like I'm back" and has done much better.[8]

If no one suspects that an infectious illness may be attacking the brain, many doctors settle on the most common diagnosis for one's age group, such as depression or Alzheimer's, and begin treatments that are ineffective or even toxic. Sadly, it is not just a tragedy for older people.

Jasmine: a young woman robbed of her brain

Jasmine, 26, couldn't get out of the funk she had been in for more than a year. She was depressed, anxious, and obsessive. She couldn't focus or remember—all new symptoms for her. Her condition became so bad that she had to drop out of her doctoral program in clinical psychology. Five antidepressants had no effect, three different therapists could not help her, and changes to her diet didn't work. Jasmine was giving up hope when her mother brought her to our clinic.

Her SPECT scan had an overall toxic appearance, even though she said she had never used drugs and didn't smoke or drink alcohol. Her diet was poor, her sleep was interrupted, and she had low vitamin D and Omega-3 Index. Her blood tests confirmed exposures to Lyme, Epstein-Barr virus, West Nile virus, and cytomegalovirus. By supporting her immune system and treating these infections over the next two years, we were able to help her improve her health so she could return to school.

JASMINE'S "BEFORE" AND "AFTER" BRAIN SPECT SCANS

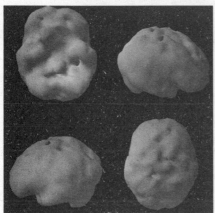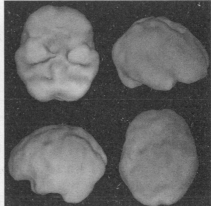

JASMINE'S BRIGHT MINDS RISK FACTORS AND INTERVENTIONS

BRIGHT MINDS	JASMINE'S RISK FACTORS	INTERVENTIONS
Blood Flow	Low blood flow on SPECT	Hydration, exercise, and ginkgo biloba
Retirement/Aging		
Inflammation	Low Omega-3 Index	Limited omega-6 foods; omega-3 fatty acids EPA and DHA supplements; elimination diet
Genetics		
Head Trauma		
Toxins		

BRIGHT MINDS	JASMINE'S RISK FACTORS	INTERVENTIONS
Mental Health	Depressed and anxious	Stress management tools, saffron
Immunity/Infection Issues	Low vitamin D; positive for Lyme, Epstein-Barr virus, West Nile virus, and cytomegalovirus	Supplemental vitamin D3, raw garlic and onions, shiitake mushrooms
Neurohormone Deficiencies		
Diabesity		
Sleep	Insomnia	Sleep strategies

A really bad cat

Question: What do the following have in common: house pets, traffic accidents, bipolar disorder, Alzheimer's disease, reckless behavior, schizophrenia, cancer, and suicide?

Answer: *Toxoplasma gondii*. This devious parasite is carried by cats and infects an estimated one-third of the world's population with toxoplasmosis. It has a strong link to schizophrenia, bipolar disorder, reckless behavior, and suicide. It is also implicated in Alzheimer's and Parkinson's disease, cancer, heart disease, and autoimmune disorders.[9] Women who become infected during pregnancy can pass the infection to their developing infant, which can lead to blindness or mental disability later in life; sometimes there is brain damage at birth.

In a fascinating TED talk,[10] science writer Ed Yong eloquently told this love story:

> Toxo infects . . . a wide variety of mammals, but it can only sexually
> reproduce in a cat. . . . If Toxo gets into a rat or a mouse, it turns
> the rodent into a cat-seeking missile. If the infected rat smells
> the delightful odor of cat piss, it runs towards the source of the
> smell rather than the more sensible direction of away. The cat eats
> the rat. Toxo gets to have sex. It's a classic tale of Eat, Prey, Love.
> . . . Toxo releases an enzyme that makes dopamine, a substance
> involved in reward and motivation. We know it targets certain parts
> of a rodent's brain, including those involved in sexual arousal.

The parasite is controlling the host. Maybe we don't have as much control over our behavior as we think we do.

TOXOPLASMA GONDII

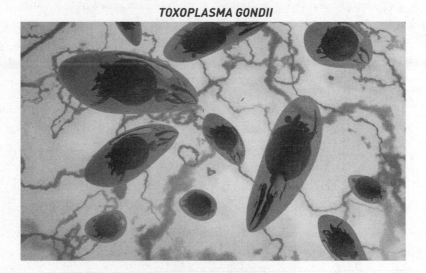

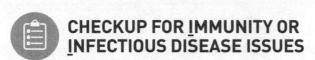

CHECKUP FOR IMMUNITY OR INFECTIOUS DISEASE ISSUES

Know your personal history

If you have a history of allergies, rashes, or repeated infections, it could indicate an immune system vulnerability.

Lab tests

The following blood tests are important to determine the health of your immune system.

- **Complete blood count with differential** to look at the distribution of white blood cells, one of the principal actors of the immune system.

- **Erythrocyte sedimentation rate (ESR):** This common test is a nonspecific measure of inflammation, which is high in autoimmune disorders.

- **Antinuclear antibodies (ANA):** The immune system normally makes antibodies to help fight infection, but antinuclear antibodies often attack the body's own tissues. Test results are often high in autoimmune disorders.

- **Rheumatoid factor (Rh):** Rh is an antibody that is measurable in the blood. It can bind to other antibodies and cause problems.

- **Vitamin D:** The liver and kidneys convert vitamin D into a hormone that regulates almost all organs. Two-thirds of the US population is low in vitamin D. The blood test to get: 25-hydroxyvitamin D level. A normal level is 30 to 100 ng/mL; an optimal level is 50 to 100 ng/mL.

- **Screening for common infections:** When we see evidence of infectious disease on SPECT scans, we look for it with additional testing. At Amen Clinics we often use Medical Diagnostic Laboratories (www.mdlab.com) to screen for possible infectious diseases. If your memory is not what it once was and you don't have the benefit of a SPECT scan, consider getting screened for infectious diseases that commonly affect memory, such as:

  - *Borrelia burgdorferi*[11] (the spirochete that causes Lyme disease)
  - HIV/AIDS[12]
  - syphilis[13]
  - herpes simplex 1 and 2[14]
  - cytomegalovirus[15]
  - Epstein-Barr virus[16]
  - *Toxoplasma gondii*[17]
  - *Helicobacter pylori*[18]
  - *Chlamydophila pneumoniae*[19]

||||||||||||||||||||||||||||||||||||||||||||||||||||||||||||||||||||||||||||||||||||||||||||||

Symptoms to Investigate

If you suffer from one or more of the following symptoms— especially if they have lasted more than two weeks—think of it as a serious reason to investigate whether the culprit is an infectious disease.

- fatigue
- low-grade fevers, hot flashes, or chills
- night sweats
- sore throat
- swollen glands
- stiff neck
- migrating joint pain
- muscle pain
- unexplained chest pain and palpitations

- unexplained abdominal pain, nausea
- diarrhea
- sleep disturbances
- poor concentration and memory loss
- irritability and mood swings
- depression
- blurred vision and eye pain

- tinnitus (ringing in the ears)
- vertigo (spinning sensation)
- facial numbness, pain, tingling, palsy
- eye pain
- headaches
- light-headedness
- dizziness

|||||||||||||||||||||||||||||||||||||||||||||||||||||||||||||||||||||||||||||||||||||||||||||||||

PRESCRIPTION TO REDUCE YOUR IMMUNITY AND INFECTIOUS DISEASE RISK

The Strategies

1. **Work with a knowledgeable health-care professional.** You need a medical partner to diagnose and treat any immune system issues or infections.

2. **Do an elimination diet for a month.** Try staying away from sugar, gluten, dairy, corn, soy, artificial colors, additives, and preservatives to see if you feel better.

3. **Get tested for heavy metals.** See chapter 10, page 158.

4. **Take steps to fix your gut.** See chapter 7, page 98.

5. **Optimize your vitamin D level.** See "The Sunshine Vitamin" on page 197.

6. **Work on managing stress.** Stress lowers immunity and increases the risk of autoimmune diseases.[20] One of my favorite immunity-boosting stress-management techniques is laughter.[21] "A cheerful heart is good medicine" (Proverbs 17:22). Watching comedies can be healing, literally.

   In 1964, noted journalist Norman Cousins, editor of the *Saturday Review*, was diagnosed with a debilitating autoimmune disease and told that he had a 1 in 500 chance of surviving. Given the odds,

Cousins did three things against the medical wisdom of the day. He took high doses of vitamin C; he moved out of his hospital room and into a nice hotel room; and he procured a projector and hundreds of hours of comedies, including episodes of *Candid Camera* and the Marx Brothers. The first night he laughed so hard at the shows that he was able to sleep better, without pain. Over time, as he continued watching the videos, his ESR level dropped. Soon he was back at work, doing what he loved. Cousins literally laughed himself back to health—and lived to tell the story in his 1979 bestseller, *Anatomy of an Illness*. I read it as a second-year medical student, the year I decided to become a psychiatrist.

BRIGHT MINDS TIP

Pop a mushroom pill. The unique and diverse compounds in these fungi, not found in other plants, have immune-enhancing effects.[22] Studies report they also have antioxidant, antitumor, antivirus, anti-inflammatory, and antidiabetic properties.[23]

The Nutraceuticals

- **Take a therapeutic mushroom.** For their multiple benefits, we recommend taking mushrooms as supplements (as well as eating them; see page 200). Among the most researched are

  - *Lion's mane:* improves mood and memory in patients with mild cognitive impairment[24]

  - *Shiitake:* improves immunity and decreases inflammatory markers[25]

  - *Reishi:* anti-inflammatory, immunity enhancing, and mood promoting[26]

  - *Cordyceps:* a favorite among athletes because it increases ATP production, strength, and endurance, and has anti-aging effects[27]

- **Enhance your immune system to fight infections with these nutrients:**

    - *Aged garlic*[28]

    - *Anthocyanins:* fruit and vegetable extracts, blueberries, cranberries, grapes[29]

    - *Echinacea*[30]

    - *Folate*[31]

    - *Melatonin:*[32] See chapter 15, page 250.

    - *Probiotics*[33]

    - *Selenium*[34]

    - *Vitamin A*[35]

    - *Vitamin C*[36]

    - *Vitamin D:*[37] See "The Sunshine Vitamin," below.

    - *Vitamin E*[38]

    - *Zinc*[39]

||||||||||||||||||||||||||||||||||||||||||||||||||||||||||||||||||||||||||||||||||||||||||||||||

The Sunshine Vitamin

Vitamin D, also known as the "sunshine vitamin," is best known for building bones and boosting the immune system,[40] but it is also essential for brain health, mood, memory, and weight control. In the body, this vitamin is converted into a steroid hormone vital to your health. Low levels of vitamin D have been associated with 200 diseases, including depression, autism, psychosis, multiple sclerosis, rheumatoid arthritis, heart disease, diabetes, cancer, and obesity.[41] Low vitamin D has also been associated with memory problems and dementia.[42]

Emerging research supports the possible role of vitamin D against cancer, heart disease, fractures and falls, autoimmune diseases, influenza, type 2 diabetes, depression, and cognitive function.[43] A meta-analysis showed that vitamin D supplementation was associated with a significantly lower death rate.[44] In a 2017 review of 25 controlled trials (11,321 participants, ages 0 to 95 years) published in the *British Medical Journal*, vitamin D3 supplementation reduced the risk of acute respiratory tract infection among all participants.[45]

Receptors for the vitamin D hormone are found throughout the brain and play a critical role in learning and making memories. Human studies have shown that vitamin D3, the active form of vitamin D, may stimulate the immune system to rid the brain of beta amyloid.[46] In 2009, a team at Tufts University in Boston looked at blood levels of vitamin D and their relationship to cognitive function in more than 1,000 people over the age of 65. Only 35 percent of the participants had adequate vitamin D (20 ng/mL or higher); the rest had either "insufficient" or "deficient" levels. Individuals with optimal levels performed better on tests of executive function (such as reasoning, flexibility, and perceptual complexity), as well as attention and processing speed than their counterparts with suboptimal levels.

The lower your vitamin D levels, the more likely you are to feel blue rather than happy, as low levels of vitamin D have been associated with a higher incidence of depression. In recent years, researchers have been asking if, given this association, vitamin D supplementation can improve moods. One trial that attempted to answer that question followed 441 overweight and obese adults with similar levels of depression for one year. The individuals who took vitamin D (20,000 IU or 40,000 IU per week) compared to a placebo showed a significant reduction in depression. In another study, people who took vitamin D over a month noticed a significant decrease in fatigue.[47]

Unfortunately, vitamin D deficiencies are becoming more and more common, affecting about 50 percent of the world's population.[48] This is in part because we spend more time indoors (sun exposure on skin helps activate the hormone) and use more sunscreen when we're outdoors. The following groups are at special risk of vitamin D deficiency:

- older adults
- people with darker skin (who have a reduced ability to make vitamin D from sunlight)
- people with limited sun exposure (think northern latitudes)

- people taking certain medications, such as antihypertensives, antidiabetics, or benzodiazepines[49]
- people with fat malabsorption syndrome, such as liver disease, cystic fibrosis, and Crohn's disease
- people who are obese or who have undergone gastric bypass surgery

People with Alzheimer's disease who took vitamin D with memantine (a common medication prescribed for AD) did better than those who took memantine alone.[50] Current recommended daily dose: 400 IU of vitamin D3 per day. Most experts agree that this is well below the physiological needs of most individuals and instead suggest 2,000–5,000 IU of vitamin D3 daily. In addition, enjoying a little direct sunlight can significantly help: Twice a week (except in winter), between 10 a.m. and 3 p.m., spend five to 30 minutes exposing your face, arms, legs, or back to the sun.

||||||||||||||||||||||||||||||||||||||||||||||||||||||||||||||||||||||||||||||||||||||||||||||||||||||

The Foods
AVOID (OR LIMIT):

Standard American diet, including fast foods and processed foods[51]

Sodas, including diet sodas

Simple sugars, including table sugar and honey

High amounts of omega-6, which is found in most vegetable oils (corn, soybean, sunflower, safflower)

Fried foods

Pesticide-laden foods: Choose organically grown/raised food whenever possible.

Gluten

CONSIDER ADDING:

Immunity-boosting spices: cinnamon (for its antimicrobial activity),[52] garlic, turmeric, thyme, ginger, coriander[53]

Allicin-rich foods to boost immunity, including raw, crushed garlic, onions, and shallots. Garlic is a triple threat against infections due to its antibacterial, antiviral, and antifungal properties.

Quercetin-rich foods: red onions, red cabbage, red apples, cherries, red grapes, cherry tomatoes, teas, lemons, celery, and cocoa

Vitamin C–rich foods: natural blood thinners to boost circulation, including oranges, tangerines, kiwifruit, berries, red and yellow bell peppers, dark green leafy vegetables (such as spinach and kale), broccoli, tomatoes, peas

Vitamin D–rich foods: fatty fish, including salmon (511 IUs in four ounces), sardines, tuna; eggs; beef liver, cod liver oil

Zinc-rich foods: oysters, beef, lamb, spinach, shiitake and cremini mushrooms, asparagus, sesame and pumpkin seeds

Mushrooms: shiitake,[54] white button, portabella,[55] morel, chanterelle. (Mushrooms are also a good source of vitamin D when they have been exposed to ultraviolet light. An easy way to ensure maximum D: Remove store-bought mushrooms from their packaging and set them outdoors in full midday sun for an hour before consuming them.)[56]

Selenium-rich foods: nuts (especially Brazil nuts), seeds, fish, grass-fed meats, mushrooms

Omega 3–rich foods: See chapter 7, page 107.

Prebiotic-rich foods: See chapter 7, page 107.

Probiotic-rich foods: See chapter 7, page 107.

 ## PICK ONE HEALTHY BRIGHT MINDS HABIT TO START TODAY

1. **If you are struggling with brain fog or memory issues, consider being tested for exposure to infectious diseases.**

2. Do an elimination diet for a month to see if you have food allergies, which could be damaging your immune system.

3. Avoid hiking where you may be bitten by a deer tick.

4. **Know and optimize your vitamin D level.**

5. Add extra vitamin C.

6. Supplement with aged garlic.

7. Add onions to meals.

8. Add shiitake mushrooms to your diet.

9. Decrease alcohol consumption. Drinking excessive alcohol can upset the gut microbiome,[57] which is critical to immunity.

10. Watch a comedy or go to a comedy club. Laughing will boost your immunity.

CHAPTER 13

<u>N</u> IS FOR NEUROHORMONE DEFICIENCIES
BOOST THE SYMPHONY OF A YOUTHFUL MIND

Low thyroid doesn't kill you, it just makes you wish you were dead.
RICHARD AND KARILEE SHAMES, *THYROID MIND POWER*

ANITA: BRAIN FOG, WIRED, AND TIRED

Anita, 38, a second-grade teacher and a mother of three, loved teaching and felt that both her family and her career were growing better every year. But in 2016, out of the blue, she started feeling sad and tired, wired and forgetful; no matter how hard she tried, she couldn't shake her negative feelings. Troubled by disrupted sleep, she started drinking more coffee to boost her energy, but it made her feel more anxious. In addition, she became sensitive to loud sounds, which made teaching little children hard, and she started having afternoon headaches.

When Anita came to Amen Clinics, one of the first things I did was check her important health numbers via lab testing. It turned out her TSH (thyroid-stimulating hormone) was high, and her T4 (the active form of thyroid) was low. She also had very high levels of thyroid antibodies: They were over 1,000; a normal level is less than 35. Having such a high level of thyroid antibodies is associated with an autoimmune condition called Hashimoto's thyroiditis; it appeared that Anita's body was attacking her own thyroid tissue. Her level of vitamin D—essential to the health of the thyroid gland—was low, as was her Omega-3 Index. Anita's SPECT scan showed overall low activity, which is common in hypothyroidism.

ANITA'S BRIGHT MINDS RISK FACTORS AND INTERVENTIONS

BRIGHT MINDS	ANITA'S RISK FACTORS	INTERVENTIONS
Blood Flow	Low blood flow seen on SPECT	Treat thyroid
Retirement/Aging		
Inflammation	Low Omega-3 Index	Omega-3 fatty acids
Genetics	Family history of thyroid disease	
Head Trauma		
Toxins		
Mental Health	Thyroid-related anxiety	Thyroid medication
Immunity/Infection Issues	Low vitamin D	Vitamin D3 supplements
Neurohormone Deficiencies	High thyroid antibodies	Thyroid medication, zinc, L-tyrosine
Diabesity		
Sleep Issues	Disrupted sleep	Sleep strategies

We used the BRIGHT MINDS approach with Anita, which included prescribing thyroid medication, putting her on an elimination diet (many people with thyroid issues are sensitive to gluten), and adding the nutraceuticals L-tyrosine, omega-3 fatty acids, zinc, and vitamin D3. These treatments made a big difference in helping her memory, energy, and mental stability. After three months, Anita told me that she felt back to her old self.

HORMONES: IT'S ALL IN THE BALANCE

When your brain, adrenal glands, sex organs, pancreas, and thyroid gland work together, they produce just the right amounts of hormones: chemical messengers that control many of the body's basic functions. This symphony of hormones can be affected by many factors, both inside and outside your body. When they are working in concert, you feel great. When any of these organs is out of sync, however, you can feel awful. Problems start when too much or not enough of one hormone (or several) is produced, which can throw off the delicate balance.

You can experience two types of problems when your hormones are out of balance:

1. uncomfortable symptoms that can begin to change how you think, feel, and act, affecting your quality of life;

2. an increased risk of illness, such as depression, Alzheimer's, heart disease, osteoporosis, diabetes, and certain cancers.

Communication between hormones and the brain is strongly two-way: The brain produces signals that trigger the release of hormones, and hormones from other parts of the body also influence the brain. When thyroid activity is low, for example, as it was for Anita, brain activity is typically low as well. That's why an underactive thyroid often leads to depression, irritability, and brain fog.

Meet the hormone "family"

There are hundreds of hormones in the body that affect the brain. To keep this discussion practical, I am going to show you how to optimize seven of the most important ones:

- thyroid
- cortisol
- DHEA
- estrogen
- progesterone
- testosterone
- insulin (see chapter 14, page 228)

Thyroid: the energy regulator

The thyroid—a small, butterfly-shaped gland located in your lower neck—produces three main thyroid hormones: TSH, T3, and T4. These hormones are among the most influential in your body, and all have to be in the right balance to keep your brain and body healthy. Too little of any thyroid hormone (hypothyroidism) makes you feel like a slug; you just want to lie on the couch all day with a bag of chips. Everything works more slowly, including your heart, your bowels, and your brain (because the thyroid gland drives the production of many neurotransmitters that run the brain, including serotonin, dopamine, and GABA). SPECT scans of people with hypothy-roidism show overall decreased brain activity, which often leads to depres-sion, cognitive impairment, anxiety, and brain fog. More than 80 percent of people with low-grade hypothyroidism have impaired memory function.[1] One-third of all depressions are directly related to thyroid levels being too high or too low.

An overactive thyroid, or hyperthyroidism, is also a problem, because it makes everything in your body work too fast. It can feel like you're in overdrive—you feel jittery and edgy, as though you've had way too much caffeine.

||||||||||||||||||||||||||||||||||||||||||||||||||||||||||||||||||||||||||||||||||||||||||||||||||

Common Symptoms of Thyroid Lows and Highs

UNDERACTIVE THYROID*
feeling cold when others are hot
weight gain
constipation
fatigue
high cholesterol
high blood pressure
dry, thinning hair or hair loss
   (especially the outer third of
   your eyebrows)
dry skin
dry eyes
thin, cracking, or peeling nails
menstrual irregularities
infertility
recurrent miscarriages
birth defects
terrible menopause

OVERACTIVE THYROID
feeling hot when others
   are cold
weight loss (despite
   increased appetite)
loose stools
sleeplessness
anxiety, irritability
fast pulse
breathlessness
racing thoughts
bulging eyes, intense
   gaze

*NOTE: Even if your thyroid is producing hormones at low-normal levels, you can still have symptoms of what's called subclinical hypothyroidism, which can be treated to help you feel better.

||||||||||||||||||||||||||||||||||||||||||||||||||||||||||||||||||||||||||||||||||||||||||||||||||

Thyroid problems can occur at any time in a person's life, though women are especially prone to problems after having a baby—usually within six months of the birth. During pregnancy, certain parts of the immune system relax so that immune cells and antibodies will not reject the baby's placenta, which is attached to the mother's uterus. This is why many women with thyroid problems feel that pregnancy is the best time of their lives, as it calms those issues. After the baby is delivered, however, everything changes: The placenta detaches and parts of the immune system that were turned down to prevent early rejection of the placenta now surge back.

Postpregnancy is not the only vulnerable time for women's thyroid issues. An estimated one in four postmenopausal women has a thyroid imbalance. Nearly 45 percent of people over 50 have some degree of thyroid gland inflammation, according to Ridha Arem, MD, editor of the journal *Thyroid*. Dr. Arem suggests that minor thyroid problems cause more disability in the elderly population than in the young, who have greater reserves of thyroid function.[2]

Tens of millions of men and women—5 to 25 percent of the world's population—are thought to have thyroid problems. And these issues seem to be increasing: The authors of *Thyroid Mind Power* report that "the last 40 years have witnessed a massive increase in the amount of hormone-disrupting synthetic chemicals finding their way into our air, food, and water. . . . The most sensitive and highly susceptible of human tissues turned out to be the thyroid gland."[3]

Most thyroid issues are autoimmune, which means that the body is attacking itself. This may be due to environmental toxins that are stored in our bodies, food allergies (to gluten and dairy products in particular), or something in the air we breathe. For this reason, many physicians consider the thyroid to be the so-called "canary in the coal mine," alerting us to the dangers of ingested toxins.

Factors that inhibit thyroid production include

- excess stress and cortisol production
- selenium deficiency
- deficient protein
- excess sugar
- chronic illness
- compromised liver or kidney function
- cadmium, mercury, or lead toxicity
- herbicides or pesticides
- oral contraceptives
- excessive estrogen production

Cortisol and DHEA: our lady of perpetual stress

The adrenals, a pair of triangle-shaped glands that sit atop your kidneys, are critically involved in your body's reaction to stress. The adrenals produce the hormones adrenaline, dehydroepiandrosterone (DHEA), and cortisol, which are released in the well-known fight-or-flight response. Here is how it works: Let's say you're hiking through the woods with your children when you see a mountain lion; immediately, your adrenals start producing adrenaline and the other hormones that will give you the burst of energy you need to either fight the lion or pick up the children and run.

The problem is, your body doesn't differentiate among the various kinds of stress you experience. Whether it's physical stress at the sight of the mountain lion or mental stress caused by your raging teenager or catty coworkers, your body reacts the same way, pumping out those chemicals. But when you run away from the mountain lion, your body processes the chemicals and gets them out of your system. This is not the case when you get stressed over the way your coworker looked at you; all you can do is return to your office or cubicle and stew. That leaves a dangerous cocktail of chemicals surging through your body until every one of them is finally metabolized.

In today's world, you're likely faced with that kind of psychological stress on a daily basis. You wake up to a blaring alarm, and the first thing you do is check your e-mail to see what people are demanding of you. On the way to work you get stuck in bumper-to-bumper traffic or sardined on a delayed train and arrive late to face a slew of impossible deadlines. Later your son's school calls to tell you that he has been getting into fights. On and on it goes, and if you are not addressing your stress, your poor adrenals keep pumping out cortisol and other chemicals that can overwhelm your body.

When cortisol is chronically elevated, blood sugar and insulin levels also rise. And your brain doesn't fare well. Serotonin, the calming brain chemical, drops, leading to anxiety, nervousness, or depression. Food cravings increase, your sleep is disturbed, and your health can spiral out of control. Chronic exposure to stress hormones has been shown to kill cells in your hippocampus, a major memory center in the brain, especially when DHEA is also low. If the stress continues for months and years, the adrenal glands finally just get tired. When they do, we call it adrenal fatigue, the point at which your body doesn't have the resources it needs to deal with all that daily pressure. You can barely get out of bed in the morning or make it through the day.

You could also be getting fat. Adrenal fatigue leads to an especially dangerous buildup of fat in your abdomen. Not only do you ruin your chances of having a flat belly, but you're at greater risk of cardiovascular disease and diabetes. Low cortisol also promotes inflammation, affects immune function, and alters blood sugar control and sex hormone production. When the adrenals are busy making stress hormones, they divert your stores of DHEA, which would have eventually been converted to sex hormones.

Lately, doctors have been seeing patients with adrenal fatigue more frequently. A big reason is that so many of us are skimping on sleep. The human body needs about seven to eight hours every night, and if it doesn't get it, your system automatically goes into a stressed state. When you self-medicate to counteract the lack of sleep, you just make things worse. Drinking coffee or caffeinated energy drinks to keep yourself awake adds to the stress load. An alcoholic beverage in the evening to quiet down after all that caffeine may be a temporary fix. But once the alcohol wears off, it puts your body into another stress response that wakes you up at two in the morning and keeps you from being able able to fall back to sleep, ensuring you will need more caffeine to face the next day. Now you're in a never-ending cycle of stress that exhausts your adrenal system and keeps you operating on the edge, never at your best.

‖‖

Common Signs of Adrenal Fatigue

- Decreased ability to withstand stress
- Morning and afternoon fatigue; lack of stamina
- High blood pressure and rapid heartbeat
- Abdominal fat that doesn't go away, no matter what you do
- Mental fog with poor memory and difficulty concentrating
- Low sex drive
- Craving for sweets or salty foods
- Dizziness when getting up from a seated or prone position
- Signs of premature aging
- Lowered resistance to infection
- Poor wound healing

‖‖

Tami Meraglia, MD, an integrative medicine physician in Seattle who sees many stressed-out people, wrote to tell me what advice she gives her patients:

My patients have an aha moment when I explain the difference between stress, lack of stress, and doing things that repair the damage and inflammation created by stress. Most patients think that going home and "relaxing" is healing the stress from the day. It is not. That is merely the lack of stress, if you are lucky. My patients see results when they actively engage in activities like the meditation exercises on your online site (www.brainfitlife.com) to heal and rejuvenate the damage done by the stress of that day. I remember asking my dentist when I was 11 years old if I had to floss all my teeth. He told me only the ones I wanted to keep. I think meditation is similar. Stress damages our health every day. You only need to meditate on the days when you want to heal that damage.

Estrogen and progesterone: the female sex hormones

ESTROGEN: BRAIN FOG ANTIDOTE

Two of the major hormones that drive a woman's menstrual cycle are estrogen and progesterone. They affect many systems in the body, including the skeletal and cardiovascular systems, as well as the brain. And they are not found only in women. Men have these hormones, too, only in much smaller amounts—unless they have significant abdominal obesity, which turns healthy testosterone into unhealthy, cancer-promoting forms of estrogen. (In lectures, I often ask why we have so many pregnant men in our society . . . guys, it's time to deliver the baby!)

A woman's menstrual cycle reflects the natural rise and fall of estrogen and progesterone during a typical 28-day cycle. When everything works correctly, estrogen rises and falls in a gentle rolling motion twice during that time frame, while progesterone rises and falls once. The chart on the following page shows the cycle of estradiol, one of the key forms of estrogen, and progesterone.

Healthy levels of estrogen help women feel good, thanks in part to its involvement in the production of serotonin in the brain. Too much estrogen makes you anxious and irritable, like a wet cat; too little makes you depressed and confused. It's the natural rise and drop in estrogen that affects mood. Problems can worsen during perimenopause and menopause, when estrogen levels wane. Critical thinking, short-term memory, and other cognitive functions are also eroded with the loss of estrogen production.

There are three different kinds of estrogen: estrone (E1), estradiol (E2), and estriol (E3). The health of your liver, gut, and adrenals determines which

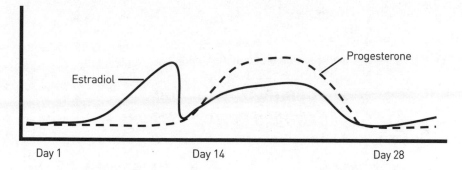

Estradiol

Progesterone

Day 1   Day 14   Day 28

types of estrogen hormones are made. That's one reason why getting healthy is critical to all of your body's systems, including your brain.

- **Estrone** (E1), the main estrogen women's bodies make after menopause, is implicated in breast and uterine cancer. Before menopause, women make all three estrogens plus progesterone. After menopause, the levels of E2, E3, and progesterone drop drastically, and their health-protective effects are lost. It's not surprising that the majority of breast cancer cases occur in postmenopausal women. Obese women are at higher risk because fat turns healthy testosterone and estradiol into estrone.[4] Alcohol consumption also increases estrone, which could be the reason there is an association between alcohol intake and breast cancer.[5] Eating excess sugar, taking the antacid cimetidine or birth control pills, smoking, hypothyroidism, and pesticide exposure also increase estrone production.

- **Estradiol** (E2), the strongest estrogen, helps a female think clearly. It is produced in the ovaries and has many protective effects, including maintaining bone density, improving growth hormone production and cardiovascular function, keeping blood from getting sticky, supporting cognitive function and mood, and improving the lipid profile. Too much estradiol can be associated with estrogen-related cancers, but deficiencies can lead to osteoporosis, heart disease, dementia, and other diseases of aging.

- **Estriol** (E3) is the weakest of the three estrogens and has a protective role in breast tissue. It is believed to protect vaginal tissue too. Estriol helps reduce hot flashes in women, protects the urinary tract, and plays a role in retention of bone density. One compelling study showed that taking estriol can reverse brain lesions in women with multiple sclerosis.[6]

|||||||||||||||||||||||||||||||||||||||||||||||||||||||||||||||||||||||||||||||||||||||||||||

Common Symptoms
of Estrogen Lows and Highs

LOW ESTROGEN
weight gain
bladder incontinence and infection
mood changes/depression
insomnia
heart palpitations
osteoporosis
painful intercourse
foggy thinking
memory and focus problems
irritability
fatigue
weepiness
hot flashes
pain

EXCESS ESTROGEN
puffiness
heavy bleeding
fibrocystic breasts
low libido
weight gain around the
  hips
vaginal or oral yeast
  (thrush)
mood swings/cries
  easily
tender breasts
headaches or migraines
carbohydrate cravings

|||||||||||||||||||||||||||||||||||||||||||||||||||||||||||||||||||||||||||||||||||||||||||||

PROGESTERONE: NATURE'S VALIUM

The other major hormonal player in a woman's menstrual cycle is progesterone. It helps to prepare the uterus for implantation with a healthy fertilized egg and supports pregnancy. If no implantation occurs, progesterone levels drop, and another cycle begins.

However, progesterone, like estrogen, is much more than a sex hormone. Its receptors are highly concentrated in the brain. Progesterone protects your nerve cells; supports the myelin sheath that covers and protects neurons; and can enhance the effect of GABA, the brain's main relaxation neurotransmitter. I like to think of progesterone as the relaxation hormone. It makes you feel calm and peaceful, and it encourages sleep. It's like nature's Valium, only better, because instead of being addictive and making your brain fuzzy, it sharpens your thinking. It has also been shown to help with brain injuries by reducing inflammation and counteracting damage.

Progesterone increases during pregnancy, which is why pregnant women often feel great. Some women with hormonal issues, in fact, feel so much better during pregnancy that they will deliberately get pregnant over and over again to feel normal. Progesterone is low for the first two weeks of the menstrual cycle. It then follows a rolling-hill pattern during the second half of the cycle, rising and falling along with estrogen. A drop in progesterone means the loss of the relaxation hormone. Calmness gives way to anxiety and irritability. Sleep is disturbed. Thinking becomes a bit fuzzy. Along with estrogen, progesterone plummets right before menstruation starts, and for some women, that's when the bottom falls out.

Common Symptoms of Low Progesterone

- anxiety/depression
- trouble sleeping
- fibrocystic breasts
- PMS
- premenstrual headaches
- postpartum depression
- bone loss

Big fluctuations in progesterone can occur in a woman's late thirties and forties, making her feel anxious and out of sorts. A progesterone cream is often very helpful when used under the care of an experienced health-care provider.

Progesterone production can drop with low levels of thyroid hormone; the use of antidepressants; chronic stress; deficiencies in vitamins A, B6, or C; zinc; and a diet high in refined sugar.

The Pill: What Women Need to Know

Millions of women around the world take hormones daily in the form of oral contraceptive pills (OCPs). In the United States, an estimated 10.6 million women of childbearing age who want to avoid pregnancy take OCPs.[7] If you are one of them, you should be aware of the risks. OCPs have been shown to cause problems with blood pressure and blood clots and increase the incidence of strokes, especially in women who smoke or who have a history of migraine headaches.[8] Oral contraceptives may deplete some essential vitamins and minerals, which can lead to deficiencies.

If you are taking birth control pills, be sure to supplement your diet with B vitamins (folate, B6, and B12), vitamin E, and magnesium. Bouts of depression have also been reported by 16 to 56 percent of women on OCPs, which deplete serotonin. (This may also be one reason 23 percent of women ages 20 to 60 are taking antidepressant medication.) Depression increases the risk of dementia in both men and women.

||||||||||||||||||||||||||||||||||||||||||||||||||||||||||||||||||||||||||||||||||||||||||||||||||||

THE BEGINNING OF A NEW PHASE: PERIMENOPAUSE

By the time women reach their thirties or forties, their hormones start undergoing another change as their bodies prepare to leave their childbearing years. It doesn't happen overnight. For eight to ten years before entering menopause (when your menstrual cycle ends completely), women go through a period of adjustment known as perimenopause. Most women don't think about being in perimenopause until their estrogen levels have fallen to the point where they experience hot flashes and night sweats, the most common symptoms. But by the time hot flashes arrive, they've probably been going through perimenopause for up to 10 years.

These years of adjustment can be difficult. The hormone system works less efficiently, and the once (relatively) gentle ups and downs in hormone levels can give way to estrogen spikes followed by a crash right before a period begins. The result may be severe PMS symptoms, even in women who have never experienced them before. When estrogen levels decline during the menstrual cycle, perimenopause, or menopause, short-term memory suffers and crying spells and depression are more likely. Women may forget where they put their house keys or what they came to the grocery store to pick up. Low levels of estrogen can also make women more sensitive to pain. All of these symptoms are exaggerated with the more erratic hormonal shifts of perimenopause as the effect of going from estrogen dominance to withdrawal becomes more pronounced. It isn't fun for anyone, and it can make women feel as though they are literally losing their minds.

To stay on top of the changes, it is a good idea for women to get their hormone levels checked at about age 35 to have a baseline and rechecked every two to three years thereafter. This is much better than waiting—as many women we see in our clinic have done—until they are ten years into the process, have already put on an excess 35 pounds, and are on antidepressant and anti-anxiety medications. Intervening earlier in the process can help avoid a lot of problems. (See "Prescription to Reduce Your Neurohormone Risk," page 219, for healthy strategies to improve your hormonal balance.)

NOT YOUR GRANDMOTHER'S MENOPAUSE

Menopause just isn't what it used to be. My grandmother Marcella, my father's mother, whom I adored, was an old woman in her fifties and sixties. She was overweight and often appeared tired and out of breath. She died at age 62. Contrast her with my mother, who at 85 remains vibrant and active. She still plays golf and is often at the mall with one of my sisters, daughters, or nieces. Today many women in menopause are at the peak of their careers and social lives.

Technically, menopause is the one-year mark after the last menstrual period. Since estrogen and progesterone have fallen to very low levels, women no longer benefit from their protective qualities and are more vulnerable to conditions such as osteoporosis, heart disease, stroke, and Alzheimer's. When estrogen levels go low, so does blood flow to the brain, which is associated with depression, anxiety, insomnia, weight gain, and problems with concentration and memory.

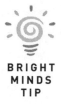

BRIGHT MINDS TIP

It is even more critical after menopause to take brain health seriously, as your brain's reserves of tissue and function have declined.

As I have said throughout this chapter, sex hormones are critical for brain health. Studies of women who had complete hysterectomies (with ovary removal) showed that without hormone replacement, they had double the risk of Alzheimer's disease. Recently, researchers studied the brain scans of women who were either on or off hormone replacement.[9] Over a period of two years, the women who did not take hormones showed decreased activity in the posterior cingulate gyrus, an area of the brain that is one of the first to die in Alzheimer's disease. Those who took replacement hormones showed no reduced activity in that area of the brain.

This is consistent with a prospective study of more than 3,000 women that showed women on hormone replacement therapy (versus those who weren't) scored significantly better on tests of verbal fluency, working memory, and psychomotor speed.[10] The researchers found no evidence that hormone therapy needed to be initiated close to menopause to have a beneficial effect on cognitive function in later life; they also found that it may decrease the risk of dementia even in women with the *APOE* e4 gene. In a 20-year follow-up study of 230,000 women, long-term self-reported postmenopausal estrogen replacement was associated with a 47 percent reduced risk of Alzheimer's disease.[11]

Testosterone: it's not just a guy thing

Most people think of testosterone as the male hormone. That's true in the sense that an infusion of testosterone during a critical time of fetal development creates the male brain, and another at puberty leads to the deepening voice, facial hair, and many other features we associate with maleness. But females have testosterone too (just as males have some estrogen). In both men and women, testosterone helps protect the nervous system and wards off cognitive impairment, depression, and Alzheimer's disease. It also seems to protect cells from inflammation, which some researchers believe is why men (who naturally have more of the hormone) are less susceptible than women to inflammatory diseases like rheumatoid arthritis, psoriasis, and asthma, and even why men suffer less from depression.[12] Men who have low testosterone are more likely to suffer from chronic pain, which is more common in women.

Although testosterone is very important to the health of men's brains, energy, strength, motivation, and sex drive, it's unwise to overdo it. Excessively high testosterone levels are associated with lower empathy and a high sex drive, which could be the prescription for having an affair, getting divorced, and losing half your net worth. For these reasons, I like to keep my male patients in the high-normal range.

A new analysis of medical records from two large hospital systems has shown that men taking testosterone-lowering therapy for prostate cancer were almost twice as likely to be diagnosed with Alzheimer's disease in the years that followed than those who didn't undergo the therapy.[13] If you elect this type of treatment for prostate cancer, make sure to do everything else you can to keep your brain healthy.

BRIGHT MINDS TIP

To keep your testosterone at an optimal level, take steps to reduce abdominal fat; stress; alcohol consumption; and unhealthy foods like excess sugar and processed foods that cause insulin spikes, while correcting any zinc deficiency.

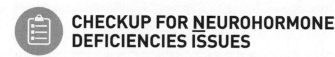

CHECKUP FOR NEUROHORMONE DEFICIENCIES ISSUES

Lab tests

After age 40, be sure to undergo yearly testing of the following hormones for men and women. Note that each lab determines what readings fall in the normal range, so ask for a lab's standards if they don't provide them.

- **Thyroid panel (blood test):** If you have symptoms, don't settle for just a TSH test, which measures your thyroid-stimulating hormone. TSH levels can be normal even when you have an undiagnosed thyroid problem. Instead, insist that your doctor order all of the following:

  - *TSH:* Anything over 3.0 is abnormal and needs further investigation.
  - *Free T3:* Active thyroid; see the normal ranges for the individual laboratory you use.
  - *Free T4:* Inactive thyroid; see the normal ranges for the individual laboratory you use.
  - *Thyroid antibodies*
    - thyroid peroxidase (TPO) antibodies
    - thyroglobulin antibodies (TG); see the normal ranges for the individual laboratory you use.

  An important note: While thyroid tests can be helpful, *your doctor should treat you, not the blood test.* I've seen too many hypothyroid patients who haven't been treated because their thyroid numbers were low but "within normal limits." That's a little like saying a vitamin D level of 31 is normal (the normal range is 30 to 100). I have never wanted to be at the bottom of any class I was in. How a patient feels and functions (e.g., low energy, constipation, dry hair, dry skin, poor cognition, body temperature) is more important in assessing thyroid function than using arbitrary normal ranges on blood tests. All of the above tests could be normal and someone could still have a problem.

- **Liver function tests:** Ninety-five percent of T4 is "activated" in the liver, so having a healthy liver is essential. See chapter 10, page 157, for more on these tests.

- **Ferritin level:** Ferritin is like the bus that drives active T3 into the cells; ferritin needs to be above 50 for this to occur. See page 88 for more on this test.

- **Cortisol (saliva):** This is best done four times, at intervals throughout the day (to track your daily cycle): when you first wake up, around lunchtime, around dinnertime, and just before you go to sleep. Ideally, your cortisol levels are high in the morning (to wake you up) and taper off slowly during the day and evening, allowing you to fall into a restful sleep at night. When cortisol levels are too high, you feel wired. When they are too low, you feel exhausted, spacey, or sluggish.

- **DHEA-S (blood test):** Normal blood levels of DHEA-sulfate can differ by sex and age.

  Typical normal ranges for females:

  - Ages 18–19: 145–395 mcg/dL (micrograms per deciliter)
  - Ages 20–29: 65–380 mcg/dL
  - Ages 30–39: 45–270 mcg/dL
  - Ages 40–49: 32–240 mcg/dL
  - Ages 50–59: 26–200 mcg/dL
  - Ages 60–69: 13–130 mcg/dL
  - Age 70 and older: 17–90 mcg/dL

  Typical normal ranges for males:

  - Ages 18–19: 108–441 mcg/dL
  - Ages 20–29: 280–640 mcg/dL
  - Ages 30–39: 120–520 mcg/dL

- Ages 40–49: 95–530 mcg/dL
- Ages 50–59: 70–310 mcg/dL
- Ages 60–69: 42–290 mcg/dL
- Age 70 and older: 28–175 mcg/dL

- **Free and total serum testosterone (blood test):** Having an optimal level of testosterone is important for your health and well-being. Too much can cause behavioral problems, such as aggression, but too little is associated with depression, poor memory, and low libido.

    Normal levels for adult males:

    - Total testosterone (280–800 nanograms [ng]/dL; 500–800 ng/dL is optimal)
    - Free testosterone (7.2–24 picograms [pg]/mL; 12–24 pg/mL is optimal)

    Normal levels for adult females:

    - Total testosterone (6–82 ng/dL; 40–82 ng/dL is optimal)
    - Free testosterone (0.0–2.2 pg/mL; 1.0–2.2 pg/mL is optimal)

- **Estrogen and progesterone for women:** These levels can be measured in blood or saliva. Women who have menstrual periods are usually tested on day 21 of their cycle; postmenopausal women can be measured anytime. See the normal ranges for the individual laboratory you use.

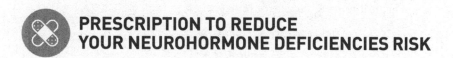

PRESCRIPTION TO REDUCE YOUR NEUROHORMONE DEFICIENCIES RISK

The Strategies

1. **Love your hormones.** To have a great brain, you have to care about the health of your hormones. Make optimizing them a priority, and your life will be much happier.

2. **Limit the bad; expand the good.** To keep your hormones healthy, it is critical to avoid or limit anything that hurts or diminishes them, including smoking (which lowers the age of menopause),[14] stress, processed food, too much sugar, high amounts of unhealthy fats,

wheat, lack of sleep, excessive caffeine, more than a few glasses of alcohol a week, and obesity.[15] To expand the good, engage in these healthy behaviors: exercise, lift weights, get adequate sleep, eat a healthy diet, and manage your stress.

3. **Steer clear of endocrine disrupters.** Pesticides are known to cause hormonal imbalances, and some pesticides have been shown to act as endocrine disrupters, interfering with the body's natural hormone systems and causing an array of health problems.[16] (See chapter 10, pages 158–159, for more on how to avoid these chemicals.)

4. **Use hormone supplements and medications wisely.** When possible use bio-identical hormones, as they mimic the molecular structure of the hormones your body makes. Bio-identicals generally have fewer side effects.

The Nutraceuticals

- *L-tyrosine* to support thyroid function

- *Zinc* to help support healthy testosterone levels

- *DHEA* can be taken over the counter but is best done under the supervision of your health-care professional. Generally, I start patients on 10 mg and go up from there, depending on what each individual patient needs. DHEA is usually well tolerated, but there can be some unpleasant side effects, like acne and facial hair, due to the tendency of DHEA to increase testosterone levels. These can be avoided by using a specific metabolite of DHEA called 7-keto-DHEA, which is more expensive but may be preferable in some cases. The dose of 7-keto-DHEA is typically 50 to 100 mg.

- *Diindolylmethane (DIM)* is a phytochemical found in cruciferous vegetables like broccoli and cauliflower. It shifts estrogen metabolism to favor the friendly or harmless estrogen metabolites.[17] DIM can significantly increase the urinary excretion of the "bad" estrogens in as little as four weeks.[18] The typical dose of DIM is 75 to 300 mg per day.

- *Omega-3 fatty acids (fish oils)* contain eicosapentaenoic acid (EPA), which laboratory studies show helps control estrogen metabolism and decrease the risk of breast cancer.[19]

- *Calcium D-glucarate*, a natural compound found in fruits and vegetables like apples, brussels sprouts, broccoli, and cabbage, inhibits the enzyme that contributes to breast, prostate, and colon cancers. It also reduces the reabsorption of estrogen from the digestive tract. The dose for calcium D-glucarate is typically 500 to 1,500 mg per day.

- *Probiotics* help maintain healthy intestinal flora and hormone levels.

||||||||||||||||||||||||||||||||||||||||||||||||||||||||||||||||||||||||||||||||||||||||

Key Vitamins, Minerals, and Herbs for Hormone Balance

TO SUPPORT MULTIPLE (OR ALL) HORMONES
- Multivitamin/mineral complex
- Omega-3 fatty acids EPA and DHA
- Probiotics for gut health
- Magnesium, 200–300 mg once or twice a day, to keep nerves calm. It is an essential cofactor for enzymes that make energy; is involved in blood sugar regulation; helps fight fatigue, including in fibromyalgia patients; and helps maintain healthy blood pressure and blood vessel tone.
- Vitamin D, generally 2,000–5,000 IUs of vitamin D3 daily, but need should be determined based on lab testing
- Zinc, 20–30 mg, to support optimum levels of testosterone and thyroid in both men and women
- Melatonin: 1–6 mg
- Selenium: 200 mcg

ESTROGEN (FEMALES)
- DIM: 100–200 mg a day
- Calcium D-glucarate: 500 mg a day
- Plant phytoestrogens, including black cohosh, 20–80 mg twice daily
- Evening primrose oil: 500 mg twice a day

PROGESTERONE (FEMALES)
- Chasteberry: 160–400 mg a day

TESTOSTERONE

- DHEA: need determined by lab testing
- Zinc: 20–30 mg daily

THYROID

- Zinc: 20–40 mg daily
- L-tyrosine: 500 mg two to three times a day
- Chromium: 100–1,000 mcg/day
- Iodine: up to 150 mcg a day
- Vitamins A (5,000 IU), B2 (50 mg), B3 (50 mg), B6 (25 mg), C (200–1,000 mg), D3 (2,000–5,000 IU) per day
- Edible seaweed, labeled for iodine and selenium content, maximum 150 mcg iodine and 200 mcg selenium per day
- *Sensoril ashwagandha* extract: 250–500 mg once or twice a day

CORTISOL

- L-theanine: 200 mg two or three times a day
- Holy basil: 300–600 mg two to three times a day
- Relora: a combination of *Magnolia officinalis* and *Phellodendron amurense*, 250 mg two times a day with meals
- *Sensoril ashwagandha*: 250 mg one or two times a day (Those with both thyroid and cortisol issues should not exceed the 250–500 mg dosage once or twice a day.)
- Rhodiola: 200 mg one or two times a day
- Magnesium: 200–300 mg twice a day, to keep your nerves calm

DHEA

- DHEA: need determined by lab testing
- 7-Keto-DHEA: need determined by lab testing

IIIIIIIIIIIIIIIIIIIIIIIIIIIIIIIIIIIIIIIIIIIIIIIIIIIIIIIIIIIIIIIIIIIIIIIIIIIIIIIIIIIIIIIIIIII

The Foods
AVOID (OR LIMIT):

Sugar and simple carbohydrates cause unfriendly flora to grow in the GI tract and disrupt estrogen metabolism. These foods also raise blood sugar and insulin levels, adversely influencing sex hormone balance.

Protein from animals raised with hormones or antibiotics. Instead look for grass-fed, hormone-free, antibiotic-free organic beef and chicken; they are richer in omega-3 fatty acids, which will reduce inflammation and help your hormone receptors to function properly. Also eat organic vegetables, fruits, nuts, seeds, beans, and grains.

Processed foods

Gluten

Soy protein isolate

Excitotoxins, substances that can kill neurons, including MSG, aspartame, hydrolyzed vegetable protein, sucralose, and "natural flavors" (these often contain MSG)

Foods and drinks that lower testosterone levels, including soy, licorice, and spearmint tea

CONSIDER ADDING:

Fiber-rich foods, including those that contain lignin: green beans, peas, carrots, seeds, Brazil nuts.[20] Lignin binds harmful estrogens in the digestive tract so they can be excreted in the feces rather than be reabsorbed. Dietary fiber also improves the composition of intestinal bacteria so the body can excrete harmful estrogen metabolites. It also decreases the conversion of testosterone into estrogens, maintaining a healthy testosterone level.

Hormone-supporting spices: garlic, sage, parsley, anise seed, red clover, hops (see below)

Eggs. Many hormones are made from cholesterol, so make sure you have enough cholesterol in your diet.

Testosterone-boosting foods: pomegranates, olive oil, oysters, coconut, brassicas (including cabbage, broccoli, brussels sprouts, cauliflower), whey protein, garlic

Estrogen-boosting foods: soybeans, flaxseeds, sunflower seeds, beans, garlic, yams, foods rich in vitamins C and Bs, beets, parsley, aniseed, red clover, hops, sage

Thyroid-boosting (selenium-rich) foods: seaweed and sea vegetables, brassicas, maca

Progesterone-boosting foods: chasteberry, plus magnesium-rich foods: See chapter 5, page 77.

Zinc-rich foods to boost testosterone: See chapter 12, page 200.

Prebiotic- and probiotic-rich foods: See chapter 7, page 107.

 PICK ONE HEALTHY BRIGHT MINDS HABIT TO START TODAY

1. Get your hormones tested on a regular basis.

2. **Avoid hormone disruptors, such as BPA, phthalates, parabens, and pesticides.**

3. Avoid animal protein raised with hormones or antibiotics, which can disrupt your hormones.

4. Eat more fiber (to eliminate unhealthy forms of estrogen).

5. Lift weights to boost testosterone.

6. **Limit sugar.**

7. Take zinc to help boost testosterone.

8. Take cortisol-reducing supplements, such as ashwagandha (which also supports the thyroid).

9. For women, make sure to optimize estrogen for overall brain health.

10. Consider hormone replacement when necessary.

CHAPTER 14

D IS FOR DIABESITY
KILL THE SUGAR BEFORE
IT KILLS YOU

Don't dig your grave with your own knife and fork.

ENGLISH PROVERB

Both my wife, Tana, and I know what it is like to have loved ones die of "diabesity," the double-barreled threat of diabetes and obesity. It robbed Tana of one of the most important people in her life: her grandmother Abla. From a young age, I also observed the devastating toll these conditions took on family members and friends. For that reason, rather than beginning with a case study from the Amen Clinics, I want to go further back and introduce you to two people affected by diabesity, both of whom helped steer Tana and me toward careers in the health profession.

GRANDMOTHER ABLA:
THE DEVASTATION OF DIABETES

One of Tana's first—and fondest—memories of her grandmother was of her large, soft belly. When she cuddled with her grandmother, Abla's ample lap and infectious giggles gave Tana a sense of comfort and security. Everything on Abla's four-foot-eleven, 200-pound body was round and soft. As a child, Tana found Abla's plumpness endearing.

Tana also loved the comfort foods her grandmother prepared for the two of them. She savored the warm Syrian bread smothered in butter and dripping with honey. (In a pinch, they'd substitute tortillas slathered with butter and sugar.) In this way, her grandmother passed along her unhealthy attachment to food. As a lonely latchkey child, Tana learned to comfort herself with the same warm, sugary foods her grandmother ate.

As a girl growing up in what is now Lebanon, Abla had been terrorized by Turkish soldiers. The emotional trauma caused her lasting pain, and sugar was one of the ways she medicated herself. Sugar and other simple carbohydrates increase serotonin in the brain and help people feel happier and more relaxed. Unfortunately, they also predispose people to diabetes and obesity and can cause serious mental health crises; Tana's grandmother had several.

Abla had been diagnosed with type 2 diabetes before Tana was born. At the age of 11, Tana started administering Abla's insulin shots because diabetes had compromised her grandmother's eyesight, so she could no longer be trusted to give herself the correct dose. The responsibility fell to Tana because her mother was working three jobs.

By the time Tana was 12, Abla spent her days staring at the television set in her bedroom, even though she could barely see it. She was legally blind and had heart disease as well as significant neuropathy (pain, numbness, tingling, and ulcerations) in her hands, feet, and eyes. Neuropathy made it a struggle for her to walk, even just from her bed to the bathroom. She finally gave in to using a bedside commode, a humiliation for this proud, modest woman. The tips of her toes turned black, sores oozed on her legs, and she sometimes cried from the pain. Had she not died of heart disease, Abla's toes would have had to be amputated.

Tana mourned not only the loss of this sweet woman, but all that diabetes had stolen from her grandmother. Her experience helping administer Abla's insulin shots and caring for her physical needs was part of the reason Tana became a nurse—and became serious about guarding her own health.

Sam: addicted to sweets

Sam was the father of one of my best friends when I was a teenager. I knew him for more than 30 years. Sam struggled with alcoholism, temper problems, and his weight, and at age 55, he was diagnosed with type 2 diabetes. When I was in medical school, Sam confided in me that if his doctor told him he'd have to take insulin shots, he would kill himself. Thankfully, when

FROM *THE BRAIN WARRIOR'S WAY* LIVE CLASS

"It is very interesting when I go to the grocery store. There are whole sections of the store I don't even go through anymore because they no longer apply to my life. At the checkout stand there is always a variety of junk food to tempt people on the way out. It's funny that my eyes see the candy bars, but I am not tempted to eat them because they register in my head as nonfood items. It's like [I'm] looking at a candy bar, but it registers in my head is if it were tape or razor blades or something. I am not tempted on a whim to buy tape or razor blades and run home and eat them in the closet. . . . The candy no longer calls my name! Mr. Snickers and I are officially divorced. Yeah!"

"My husband looks great! And he is no longer prediabetic! Thank you."

"My husband's A1c went from 9.4 to 6.2 since we started The Brain Warrior's Way. *How's that for success! I realize that so many of the things you've taught us are now part of my regular routine and my mind-set. My cabinets have only good-for-us foods. My comfort food recipes have changed. Even things you and Tana have said keep popping into my head. . . . A friend was complaining about loving a food that bothers her. I said to her, 'Why would you eat something that doesn't love you back?' Oh, my goodness! I am a Brain Warrior!"*

he learned he had to get the injections, he didn't commit suicide, but over the next 20 years, his uncontrolled diabetes killed him, slowly and painfully, organ by organ. Even though he was repeatedly counseled to stop eating sugar, Sam was addicted. He would sneak out for doughnuts, sugary pastries, ice cream, and candy. Even though his wife and children were furious with him, he just couldn't stop himself. Sam was able to give up alcohol, but not sugar. Over time, he lost his eyesight and both his legs, and he died with dementia. It was tragic to watch, especially because it didn't have to be that way.

Both diabetes and obesity are independent risk factors for memory problems and several forms of dementia. In this chapter, we will explore these two risk factors, why they cause problems, and what you can do about them.

||||||||||||||||||||||||||||||||||||||||||||||||||||||||||||||||||||||||||||||||||||||

Insulin: The Blood Sugar Hormone

Think of the hormone insulin as a fuel regulator that unlocks cell membranes so they can absorb glucose (sugar) and other nutrients from the bloodstream. The pancreas secretes insulin whenever you eat carbohydrates. Simple sugars and highly processed carbohydrates, such as baked goods, candy, bread, pasta, and crackers demand a large release of insulin and can cause significant blood sugar highs and lows. One consequence of high insulin levels is that the body switches from breaking down dietary fat to storing it, which, over time, can lead to weight problems.

One of the biggest consequences of aging is a loss of insulin sensitivity in the muscles and a decrease in insulin's ability to regulate blood sugar, leading to prediabetes and diabetes. Eliminating sugar and other simple carbohydrates from your diet can help regulate your body's production of insulin; allow fat to be broken down for energy; and prevent the depletion of chromium, a mineral required by insulin receptors.

||||||||||||||||||||||||||||||||||||||||||||||||||||||||||||||||||||||||||||||||||||||

DIABETES: BLOOD SUGAR BLUES

Diabetes develops when insulin, the hormone that regulates blood sugar levels, becomes deficient or ineffective. The illness has two forms: Type 1 diabetes occurs when the body refuses to make insulin, and type 2 develops when the body mismanages it. (Prediabetes is a precursor of full-blown type 2 diabetes.) In both types, the body is subjected to chronically high blood sugar levels, which damage blood vessels, causing them to become brittle, inflexible, and more likely to break. Damaged blood vessels cannot supply nutrients or take away toxins, which ultimately leads to problems with every organ in the body, including the brain. Recently, scientists reported new evidence linking abnormal insulin levels to Alzheimer's disease and cognitive decline.[1] The correlation is so strong that some researchers have labeled Alzheimer's "type 3" diabetes.[2]

Risk factors for diabetes include aging, a family history of the disease, excessive consumption of sugar and high-glycemic foods, obesity, alcohol abuse, exposure to toxins discussed in chapter 10, and a sedentary lifestyle. Watch for these warning signs: increased urination, excessive thirst, increased appetite, and delayed wound healing.

The negative effects of diabetes include increased inflammation, depression, Alzheimer's disease and vascular dementia, strokes, heart disease, hypertension, and accelerated aging.[3] Diabetes has been linked to decreased blood flow to the brain (the number one predictor of future memory problems), apparent on SPECT imaging,[4] and a smaller hippocampus.

Scientists have been studying whether medications for diabetes might help people with Alzheimer's, and the answer seems to be yes. Medical data from more than 145,000 diabetics treated with two common medications to lower blood sugar—Actos (pioglitazone) and Glucophage (metformin)—revealed that they also lowered the risk of dementia.[5] Another study found that dementia-related changes in the brain could lead to diabetes, instead of the other way around.[6] This is contrary to what had been previously thought—that diabetes begins with trouble in the pancreas or a high-fat and/or high-sugar diet.

Even mildly elevated blood sugar levels and prediabetes are significant problems and are associated with brain atrophy, memory problems, and dementia.[7] In people who didn't have diabetes, for example, the risk for dementia was 18 percent higher for those with an average blood glucose level of 115 milligrams per deciliter compared to those with an average glucose level of 100 mg/dL. (See "Checkup for Diabesity Issues" for information on healthy blood sugar numbers.) And every incrementally higher glucose level was associated with a higher risk of dementia. "High-normal" blood sugar levels have also been associated with shrinkage in the hippocampus (leading to memory problems).[8] The dementia risk was even worse for people who had diabetes, because their blood sugar levels were generally higher: It was 40 percent higher for people with an average glucose level of 190 mg/dL compared to those with an average glucose level of 160 mg/dL. That's a lot of numbers, but the bottom line is that the higher your blood sugar level, the higher your odds of getting dementia.

Here is the scariest part of this story: *Diabetes and prediabetes now affect a horrifying 50 percent of the US population.*[9] Blood sugar problems have dramatically escalated in the last 30 years. One of every 100 people in the United States had type 2 diabetes in 1960; that percentage has increased tenfold to 1 in 10 people today. The rate of type 2 diabetes has increased 700 percent just since the 1980s.[10]

Our sedentary lifestyles and standard American diet (SAD), along with increased toxins, are likely to blame. The great news is that a majority of these cases are preventable. Lifestyle changes have actually been shown to reverse the disease. People of faith may also find motivation in the fact that making better dietary choices honors their Creator, who designed foods that in their natural state can perfectly meet our bodies' needs: "Whether you eat or drink, or whatever you do, do it all for the glory of God" (1 Corinthians 10:31).

OBESITY: THE RISK OF THE "DINOSAUR SYNDROME"

In 2010, my friend Cyrus Raji, MD, PhD, and his colleagues at the University of Pittsburgh (Dr. Raji is now at the University of California, San Francisco) published a study on elderly adults that looked at the relationship between brain volume and body mass index (BMI),[11] a measure of body fat based on weight and height. They found that compared to people who were at a healthy BMI (18.5–25), those who were overweight (with a BMI of 25–30) had 4 percent less brain volume on MRI and their brains looked eight years older; people who were obese (with a BMI greater than 30) had 8 percent less brain volume and their scans looked 16 years older. After I read Dr. Raji's study, our team at Amen Clinics published research that looked at our brain SPECT scan database and found the same trend in our overweight and obese patients.[12] Following the publication of these papers, dozens more have been published with the same finding.

Shortly after we published the paper on obesity, I was flying from Chicago to Des Moines on a small plane to do a public television appearance for my program *Change Your Brain, Change Your Body*. The woman who sat in the seat next to me was extremely obese. Part of her body was in my seat, which made things a bit uncomfortable for both of us. About halfway through the short flight, this thought came to mind: *You should tell her she wants to avoid the "dinosaur syndrome"—big body, little brain—so she doesn't become extinct.*

My next thought was *Shut your mouth! That is so rude.*

Did you have a mother like mine, who used to say, "If you don't have anything good to say, don't say anything at all"?

When I got off the plane in Des Moines, I called my wife, Tana, and told her about the dinosaur syndrome and my crazy thought. She said, "Don't ever say that out loud. That is so rude!" We think alike.

Two weeks later, Tana and I were visiting a health-care company about possibly working together. The marketing director—I'll call him Will—was morbidly obese, which frustrated me. I believe if you don't live the message of your work (his was health), you cannot be a good messenger. But I didn't say anything until that night, when we were out at a restaurant with his marketing group. Whenever I go out to dinner, I try to be thoughtful about what I put in my body. I love my brain and try to protect it. I ordered a salad with blackened wild salmon and grilled asparagus. After Will ordered clam chowder and chicken-fried steak with mashed potatoes, along with wine and two chocolate soufflés for dessert (one for the table), I couldn't take it anymore. I said, "Will, you might want to avoid the dinosaur syndrome." At that point Tana kicked me under the table and gave me the look that only your wife can give you, the one that says, "What's the matter with you?"

But Will was curious. "What do you mean?" he asked. That prompted a long discussion about his goals, weight, brain size, and health.

"How old are you?" I asked.

"Forty-two," he said.

"Are you done with your career? Have you achieved your goals?" I queried.

"Not even close," he said.

"Then you need your brain to be healthy to progress even more," I said, stating what was obvious to me, but unfortunately is not to most people.

He said his cholesterol had been fine and his doctor didn't seem "that concerned" about his weight. He asked why I thought there was a connection between weight and brain size.

I replied, "The fat on your body is not innocuous. It produces inflammatory chemicals that can damage every organ in your body. Depression and dementia are associated with inflammation. Plus, fat stores toxins, so the more fat on your body, the higher your toxic load; and belly fat turns healthy forms of testosterone into unhealthy, cancer-promoting forms of estrogen."

After our conversation, Will vowed to get serious about his health. A month later he wrote to tell me that he was down 17 pounds, and after a year he had lost 80. He has since been promoted multiple times.

With two-thirds of Americans overweight and more than one-third obese, we are seeing the biggest brain drain in the history of our country. It has even become a national security crisis: The military rejects 70 percent of potential new recruits because of health reasons, with weight issues being the most common cause. Obesity has also recently been associated with 11 different types of cancer.[13]

It is critical to get your weight under control because excess pounds can damage your brain. (And if you are also diabetic, the harm may be even worse.[14]) In a study that followed more than 10,000 people for 36 years, being overweight or obese in midlife was shown to be strongly associated with memory problems and dementia in later life.[15] In another study of 408 healthy adults, as BMI went up, cognitive scores went down, especially in decision making (executive function).[16] In yet another, overweight people were less responsive to memory training.[17] With all of this new information, our team at Amen Clinics looked at our NFL player data and found the same correlation: When we paired players by position, the function of their prefrontal cortex went down (as well as their scores for reasoning and memory) as their weight went up.[18]

This information got my attention, too, as I was once overweight myself. Over the course of a year or so, I lost more than 25 pounds, and I have kept it off for the past 10 years. I never want to knowingly do anything that harms my brain. I use all the principles in this book because, like you, I need to live the message.

||||||||||||||||||||||||||||||||||||||||||||||||||||||||||||||||||||||||||||||||||||||||||||||||||

Metabolic Syndrome (MetS)

Five common risk factors raise the odds of heart disease, diabetes, and stroke. When you have at least three, you have a health problem known as metabolic syndrome, which is closely related to insulin resistance. The five risk factors are:

- high fasting blood sugar levels
- a large waistline (abdominal obesity)
- high triglycerides
- low HDL cholesterol
- high blood pressure[19]

Watch out for any combination of these symptoms; MetS increases your overall risk of memory problems and dementia by a whopping 300 percent.[20] It is also associated with low blood flow throughout the brain.[21] If you have or suspect you have MetS, take it as a sign that you need to make a number of lifestyle changes to keep your brain working for you. The good news? You *can* do something about it if you are serious about rescuing your memory. Losing as little as 10 percent of your belly fat can decrease your cardiovascular risk by 75 percent.

||||||||||||||||||||||||||||||||||||||||||||||||||||||||||||||||||||||||||||||||||||||||||||||||||

CHECKUP FOR D̲IABESITY ISSUES

To make sure your weight doesn't become a health issue, you should always know how you stack up on these health numbers.

Body mass index (BMI)

Your BMI is a measure of weight compared to height. An optimal BMI is between 18.5 and 25; the overweight category falls between 25 and 30; over 30 indicates obesity, and over 40 indicates morbid obesity. If you take our free Brain Health Assessment on www.amenclinics.com, we will calculate your BMI.

Waist to height ratio (WHtR)

Another way to measure whether your weight falls in a healthy range is to calculate your waist to height ratio. Some researchers believe this number is even more accurate than BMI because the most dangerous place to carry weight is in the abdomen. Abdominal fat, which is associated with a larger waist, is metabolically active and produces various hormones that can cause harmful health effects, such as elevated blood pressure, high cholesterol and triglyceride levels, and diabetes.

WHtR is calculated by dividing your waist size by your height. A woman with a 32-inch waist who is 5'10" (70 inches) would divide 32 by 70 to get a WHtR of 45.7 percent. Generally speaking, it's healthy to stay under 50 percent—in other words, your waist size should be less than half your height in inches. When measuring your waist size, use a tape measure! Don't hazard a guess or rely on your pants size, which can vary among manufacturers. In my experience, 90 percent of people underestimate their waist circumference.

Lab tests

Get blood tests for your fasting blood sugar, insulin, and hemoglobin every year. If they are abnormal, think of it as a health crisis to be taken very seriously.

- **Fasting blood sugar:** This is one of the tests commonly used to help determine whether a patient has diabetes or prediabetes.

  Normal: 70–105 mg/dL
  Optimal: 70–89 mg/dL

Prediabetes: 105–125 mg/dL

Diabetes: 126 mg/dL or higher

Kaiser Permanente conducted a large study showing that for every point above 85 mg/dL, patients had an additional 6 percent increased risk of developing diabetes within the next 10 years (for example: 86 = 6 percent increased risk; 87 = 12 percent increased risk; 88 = 18 percent increased risk). Those whose fasting blood sugar was above 90 already had vascular damage and were at risk of having damage to the kidneys and eyes.

- **Hemoglobin A1c (HbA1c):** This test reveals your average blood sugar levels over the previous two to three months and is used to diagnose diabetes and prediabetes. Normal results for a nondiabetic person are in the range of 4 to 5.6 percent; under 5.3 percent is optimal. Levels of 5.7 to 6.4 percent indicate prediabetes. Higher numbers may indicate diabetes.

- **Fasting insulin:** High insulin levels, usually due to a diet high in simple carbs, are associated with many negative health consequences. These include fatty liver, abdominal obesity, excessive cravings, elevated blood sugar, acne, polycystic ovarian syndrome, hair loss in women in the male pattern (front and sides), increased risk of gout, high blood pressure, and swollen ankles. A normal level is 2.6–25; less than 10 is optimal. High levels are an early marker for diabetes.

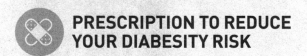

PRESCRIPTION TO REDUCE YOUR DIABESITY RISK

The Strategies

The exciting news about diabesity is that, with a targeted plan, you can significantly decrease your odds of diabetes and related illness.[22] As with all the BRIGHT MINDS risk factors, it is important to take the long view and develop a lifestyle you can live with and feel happy about. Even though you will feel better quickly on the Memory Rescue plan, you need to stay with it for a year to get the long-term benefit for your brain. This recommendation is consistent with the findings of others' research as well.[23]

1. **Follow the Memory Rescue Diet.** It's especially important to limit high-glycemic, low-fiber foods (sugar and foods that turn to sugar),

wheat (including whole wheat), and processed foods, and to eat a diet high in smart carbohydrates, which are high in fiber and low on the glycemic index. This diet will give the pancreas a break from constantly having to secrete high levels of insulin and will make your cells more insulin-sensitive. A Swedish study compared the effects on blood sugar of a grain-free diet (Paleo) and a Mediterranean diet, which relies, in part, on whole grains. After 12 weeks, the blood sugar levels were markedly lower in the Paleo group (down 26 percent) than in the Mediterranean group (down 7 percent). At the end of the study, all patients in the Paleo group had normal blood glucose, which was not true for those in the Mediterranean group.

Grains may impact weight and insulin resistance because they contain proteins called lectins, which some researchers suspect can promote inflammation and halt weight loss efforts. Aside from promoting weight loss and improving blood sugar regulation, avoiding grains is very beneficial for overall intestinal health. Anti-inflammatory in nature, the Memory Rescue Diet promotes a favorable balance of good to bad bacteria in the gut. In addition, many patients feel relief from minor digestive discomforts such as bloating, gas, and indigestion when following a low-sugar, no-dairy, no-grain plan.

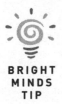

BRIGHT MINDS TIP

A daily glass of fruit juice has been linked to signs of preclinical Alzheimer's disease. Choose whole fruit instead.[24]

---

2. **Lose weight slowly (if you need to lose).** It's the healthiest way to drop pounds and keep them off. A good, safe rule of thumb is one to two pounds a week. Here are more weight-loss tips:

- Drink more water.
- Have protein for breakfast to balance your blood sugar.
- Decaffeinated green tea and coffee have been shown to increase metabolism and decrease the risk of diabetes, and both are loaded with antioxidants. Be careful, though, what you put in them.
- Cook with coconut oil.[25]

- Don't drink your calories. In 1980, Americans drank an average of 225 calories a day; in 2015, it was 450 calories a day. The extra 225 calories a day will put 23 pounds of fat on your body every year! Plus, calories you drink are more quickly absorbed than those you have to chew.
- Find a healthy plan to guide you in healthy food choices for the rest of your life—like the Memory Rescue Diet.
- Take saunas and eat detoxifying foods. Fat stores toxins, so it's critical to detox when you lose weight.
- Don't overdo your weight loss. Being too thin is definitely not the answer. A too-low BMI is associated with cognitive problems.[26]

3. **Exercise!** It's known to improve blood sugar levels and reduce weight, and it also helps with detoxification. Strength training has been shown to be particularly effective. Compared with women who reported no strength training, women engaging in any strength training reduced the incidence of type 2 diabetes by 30 percent.[27] All movement matters, even just walking, but walk as if you are late[28] (see chapter 5, page 67).

4. **Check with your physician to see if other treatment is necessary.** Depending on your personal numbers and your genetic risks, you may be able to improve your health without resorting to taking medication.

The Nutraceuticals

- *Omega-3 fatty acids EPA and DHA* help maintain proper insulin signaling in the brain, counteract nonalcoholic fatty liver (common in metabolic syndrome), and decrease the overall risk of metabolic syndrome.[29] In a large study of older adults, the diabetes risk was 43 percent lower among those with the highest blood concentrations of omega-3 fats compared with those with the lowest concentrations.[30] In a well-designed placebo-controlled trial of overweight type 2 diabetics, supplementing with the omega-3 fatty acid EPA significantly decreased serum insulin, fasting glucose, HbA1c, and insulin resistance.[31] (Check out information on the Omega-3 Index on page 102 in chapter 7, which will let you know if you're on the right track toward omega-3 protection.) The effective daily dose seems to be 1.4 grams (or more) of a combination of EPA and DHA, in about a 60/40 ratio for most adults.

- *Chromium picolinate* can aid in insulin regulation, which enhances the body's ability to metabolize glucose and fat. Supplementation with chromium picolinate has been shown to reduce carbohydrate cravings and binge eating, which helps in managing both blood sugar and weight.[32] In some but not all studies, chromium picolinate has also been shown to significantly lower HbA1c in type 2 diabetics.[33] The typical recommended adult dosage is 200 to 1,000 micrograms a day.

- *Cinnamon*, the savory and sweet spice, has a bouquet of benefits for those at risk of diabetes. It's been shown to lower fasting glucose levels and HbA1c and improve insulin sensitivity.[34] It also reduced cholesterol and improved working memory in older prediabetic adults, while improving blood flow to the prefrontal cortex.[35] It has been shown to decrease abnormal tau protein aggregation, thought to be one of the major contributors to Alzheimer's disease.

  Cinnamon's reputation as an aphrodisiac is centuries old. The Old Testament book of Proverbs extols the spice's love-enhancing qualities: "I've perfumed my bed with myrrh, aloes, and cinnamon. Come, let's drink our fill of love until morning" (Proverbs 7:17-18). In ancient Rome, the word *cinnamon* was equivalent to current endearments like "sweetheart" or "darling."

  When I told my mother about the aphrodisiac power of cinnamon, she hit her forehead and said, "That is why I have seven children. Your father would never leave me alone." Being Lebanese, she cooked with a lot of cinnamon.

  The typical dose for blood sugar control is one to six grams a day as a supplement. Use the spice liberally. However, if you are taking medication to control your blood sugar, talk to your doctor before taking supplemental cinnamon, as it may have an additive effect and lower blood sugar too much.

BRIGHT MINDS TIP

Cinnamon can help your blood sugar levels and spice up your love life.

- *Alpha-lipoic acid (ALA)* is a nutrient vital for our cells' mitochondria to produce energy. ALA has very high antioxidant capacity,[36] so powerful it can help regenerate other antioxidants such as vitamin E, vitamin C, and glutathione. ALA is also an essential cofactor for enzymes that process glucose. Supplementing with ALA, therefore, can improve cellular utilization of glucose and overall blood sugar management.[37] Evidence suggests that the neuroprotective properties of ALA may slow cognitive decline in those with mild dementia.[38] The typical recommended adult dosage is 300 to 600 mg a day. When ALA (600 mg) or testosterone (50 mg) was administered daily for 12 weeks, men who suffered with erectile dysfunction had improved erections, lost weight, and had better blood sugar control, along with improved HDL cholesterol and decreased triglycerides.[39] In women with polycystic ovarian syndrome (PCOS), a condition associated with excess body hair, poor blood sugar control, and obesity, ALA improved weight and blood sugar control.[40]

- *EGCG*, a well-studied catechin from green tea, was shown to reduce glucose and insulin levels and improve insulin sensitivity. In a 16-week placebo-controlled trial of 92 subjects with type 2 diabetes, those who took 500 mg of EGCG three times daily showed significant increases in insulin sensitivity and HDL cholesterol levels, as well as a significant decrease in triglycerides.[41] A two-month trial of 103 healthy postmenopausal women found significant improvements in glucose and insulin levels in a group that took up to 800 mg of EGCG per day compared with a placebo group.[42] Typical dosage is 500 to 800 mg a day. If you take the higher doses, do so under a physician's supervision.

- *Magnesium*, involved in more than 300 biochemical reactions in your body, is vital for your body to make energy and plays a key role in blood sugar regulation. Low magnesium levels are more common in diabetics, while higher magnesium levels correlate with lower HbA1c and decreased risk of developing type 2 diabetes.[43] Low magnesium is also associated with high CRP and inflammation. Given that 68 percent of Americans do not consume enough magnesium, it is no wonder that diabetes is on the rise. The mineral is found in green leafy vegetables, such as spinach, kale, and Swiss chard; legumes; and nuts and seeds. In general, foods that contain dietary fiber provide magnesium. The typical adult dose is 50 to 400 mg a day.

- *Vitamin C* can improve blood sugar and HbA1c. In one study, type 2 diabetics took either 1,000 mg of vitamin C or a placebo, along with the diabetes drug metformin, for 12 weeks. Researchers found that fasting blood sugar and HbA1c were significantly lowered in the vitamin C group.[44]

• *Vitamin D3:* Vitamin D is low in people with diabetes and/or obesity. Test and optimize your level (see page 197 for more information on vitamin D).

The Foods
AVOID (OR LIMIT):

High-glycemic, low-fiber foods such as white and wheat bread, pasta, white potatoes, rice

Sugar, which has no nutritional benefit and depletes chromium and other valuable vitamins and minerals

Corn

Processed foods

Dried fruits, including prunes, dried apricots, cranberries, raisins, dates

High-glycemic fruits, such as pineapple, watermelon, ripe bananas

CONSIDER ADDING:

Spices: cinnamon, turmeric, ginger, cumin, garlic, cayenne, oregano, marjoram, sage, nutmeg[45]

Fiber-rich foods to balance cholesterol and blood pressure: psyllium husk, navy beans, raspberries, broccoli, spinach, lentils, green peas, pears, winter squash, cabbage, green beans, avocados, coconut, fresh figs, artichokes, chickpeas, hemp seeds, and chia seeds

Polyphenol-rich foods/drinks, especially green tea, decaffeinated coffee, and blueberries: See page 118 in chapter 8.

Protein-rich foods: eggs, meats, fish

Vegetables: The best choices have a low glycemic index, such as celery, spinach, and brassicas (broccoli, brussels sprouts, cauliflower).

Fruits: The low-glycemic varieties include apples, oranges, blueberries, raspberries, blackberries, and strawberries.

Omega-3-rich foods: See page 107 in chapter 7.

Magnesium-rich foods: See page 77 in chapter 5.

Vitamin D–rich foods: See page 200 in chapter 12.

 ## PICK ONE HEALTHY BRIGHT MINDS HABIT TO START TODAY

1. **Know your BMI now and check it monthly.**

2. Measure your waist-to-height ratio.

3. Don't drink your calories.

4. **Start the Memory Rescue Diet.**

5. Eat protein and fat at each meal to stabilize blood sugar and reduce cravings.

6. Lose weight slowly if you are overweight, and develop lifelong healthy eating habits.

7. Supplement with chromium picolinate.

8. Take alpha-lipoic acid.

9. Use cinnamon and nutmeg in your cooking.

10. Weigh yourself daily—it will keep you honest and motivated.[46]

CHAPTER 15

S IS FOR SLEEP ISSUES
CLEANSE YOUR BRAIN AND ELIMINATE ITS TRASH NIGHTLY

*That we are not much sicker and much madder than we are is due
exclusively to that most blessed and blessing of all natural graces, sleep.*

ALDOUS HUXLEY, *THEMES AND VARIATIONS*

KYLE: WHY SLEEP MATTERED MOST

A number of years ago, I evaluated a group of seven CEOs who met regularly to support and encourage one another. Every year they took a special "bonding" trip and had some amazing experiences skiing, parachuting from airplanes, and scuba diving. This particular year, their leader wanted them to have the ultimate brain experience, so they were evaluated at our Southern California clinic, where they were assessed as a group. They reasoned that they would learn about one another in a much deeper sense. They would see one another's brains!

One of the group members who needed me most was Kyle, 51, the CEO of his family's meatpacking business. Even though he was successful at work, he was not doing well personally. Several years earlier, he'd had a concussion caused by a car accident, and he felt his concentration was getting worse. He was disorganized, and his office was a mess. He had trouble making simple decisions and really struggled with procrastination and being on time. In order to get things done, he needed last-minute pressure. He told me his wife had noticed he was a poor listener and easily distracted. In meetings, he tended to blurt things out and was restless and fidgety. He was also experiencing increasing anxiety and even a few panic attacks, as well as chronic stress from working in his family business.

Kyle's BMI was 31.5 (in the obese range), and he had been diagnosed with type 2 diabetes and hypertension. His important lab numbers were a mess. His total and LDL cholesterol levels were high; his fasting blood sugar and HbA1c were also high (a sign of uncontrolled diabetes, despite his being on the diabetes medication metformin); homocysteine, high; free testosterone, low; and vitamin D, extremely low (15 ng/mL). Although he had been diagnosed with sleep apnea three years earlier, he had never gotten his continuous positive airway pressure (CPAP) mask to treat it.

Kyle's SPECT scan looked terrible. I could see evidence of his ADHD (the history above is classic for it), concussion, and a vulnerability to Alzheimer's disease. In addition, his QEEG showed excessive theta activity, which is also consistent with ADHD, as well as pending memory problems.

KYLE'S "BEFORE" BRAIN SPECT SCAN

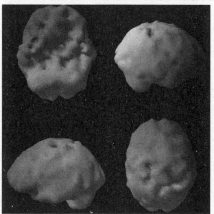

Sleep apnea, head trauma, metabolic syndrome, low vitamin D

KYLE'S QEEG

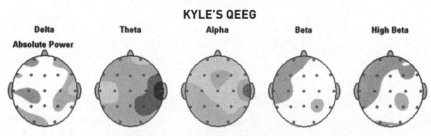

Kyle's summary shows excessive theta (slow-wave) brain activity, evidenced by the deep gray color (the darker the gray, the higher the level of activity).

KYLE'S BRIGHT MINDS RISK FACTORS AND INTERVENTIONS

BRIGHT MINDS	KYLE'S RISK FACTORS	INTERVENTIONS
Blood Flow	Hypertension	Exercise, ginkgo biloba
Retirement/Aging		
Inflammation	High inflammation blood markers (CRP and homocysteine)	Omega-3 fatty acids, limit processed and omega-6 foods
Genetics		
Head Trauma	Recent concussion	Nutraceuticals and HBOT
Toxins		
Mental Health	ADHD, chronic work stress	Treatment for ADHD, stress management tools
Immunity/Infection Issues		
Neurohormone Deficiencies	Low testosterone and vitamin D	Vitamin D3 supplements, limited sugar, weight lifting, hormone replacement if necessary
Diabesity	Obesity and type 2 diabetes (high HbA1c and fasting blood sugar)	Memory Rescue Diet
Sleep Issues	Untreated sleep apnea	Immediate sleep apnea treatment

Providing feedback on Kyle in front of the CEO group was a new experience for me. I had met with countless families but never a support group. However, I loved that Kyle would not be able to procrastinate anymore. His group would pressure him to do the right things for his health. Besides encouraging him to treat his ADHD so he could better follow through on what he needed to do, I impressed upon him the critical importance of getting his sleep apnea under control. Without that one intervention, nothing else would work. Over time Kyle made remarkable progress: He lost 35 pounds, all his important numbers improved, and his energy came back.

After the group's trip, he became more effective in his marriage and at work. He had been blindly headed for a disaster and, at least temporarily, was able to divert it.

SLEEP DISORDERS PUT YOU AT RISK OF COGNITIVE DECLINE

A number of studies link sleep problems, such as insomnia and sleep apnea, to a higher risk of memory problems and dementia, but effectively treating these disorders can have a positive impact on memory and brain function.[1]

Proper sleep is essential for brain health. In fascinating new research, scientists have shown that your brain cleanses or "washes" itself during sleep. The brain has a special waste management system that helps get rid of toxins that build up over the course of a day, including the beta-amyloid plaques associated with Alzheimer's disease. Your brain is so busy managing your life during the daylight hours that this cleaning system is pretty much turned off. One theory about why people with dementia sleep so much is that their brains are trying to clear out the accumulating plaques/gunk.

Insomnia: the health price of sleepless nights

Without healthy sleep, the brain's cleaning crew does not have enough time to do its job, and trash builds up, causing brain fog and memory problems. How would your home look if no one cleaned it for a month? That is the effect chronic insomnia can have on your brain, and unfortunately, it is all too common, affecting about one in four people.[2] There are different types of insomnia, including transient insomnia, which lasts a few days and is caused by such things as short-term stress or time change; acute insomnia, which lasts several weeks and is common during grief or relationship- or work-related stress; and chronic insomnia, which may last for months or years. Chronic insomnia elevates a person's risk of stroke, pain, cardiovascular disease, anxiety, cancer, and death from any cause.[3]

Many lifestyle habits, illnesses, and stresses can trigger insomnia, including poor sleep hygiene (such as drinking caffeine at night or leaving the phone on next to the bed), depression, worry, restless leg syndrome, hormonal imbalances (especially progesterone in women), and shift work. See page 246 for a more complete list of sleep robbers.

With increasing insomnia rates, the sales of sleep-aid medications have skyrocketed, but not without a cost. A well-designed study showed an association between popular sleep medications such as zolpidem (Ambien), eszopiclone (Lunesta), and temazepam (Restoril) and *a more than three-fold increased risk of death.*[4]

Researchers suggest we aim for seven to eight hours of sleep a night; it seems to be the sweet spot for most people. Getting less than seven hours is associated with lower overall blood flow to the brain and a higher risk of dementia, and it can disrupt hundreds of health-promoting genes.[5] In addition, sleep problems in the elderly have been linked to lower brain volume.[6] Sleeping more than eight hours a night was also associated with cognitive problems.[7]

Having too few hours of shut-eye can have catastrophic consequences if you drive afterward. In a new report from the Automobile Association of America (AAA), drivers who got between six and seven hours of sleep were 1.3 times more likely to be involved in a car crash than those who got more than seven hours; those who slept for five to six hours a night were 1.9 times more likely to have an accident; four to five hours, 4.3 times more likely; and those who got fewer than four hours were 11.5 times more likely to crash.[8]

Sleep apnea: killing brain cells

Sleep apnea, which includes loud snoring, short periods in which you stop breathing at night, and chronic tiredness during the day, is terrible for your health as well as for your partner's (he or she is also not getting a good night's sleep). Untreated sleep apnea triples your risk of dementia and depression and makes it hard to lose weight. It looks like early Alzheimer's disease on SPECT scans, with decreased blood flow to the parietal and temporal lobes. Diagnosing and treating sleep apnea is critical to keeping your brain healthy. Too many people find out they have sleep apnea and, like Kyle, never follow through with the treatment because they hate wearing the CPAP mask. Unfortunately, because the brain is so oxygen sensitive, untreated sleep apnea literally kills brain cells. If you are having trouble getting used to the mask, return to your doctor as often as it takes to find a different strategy for treating this condition. A variety of CPAP masks are available; find one that works for you.

BRAIN SPECT SCANS

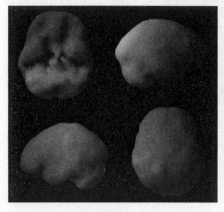 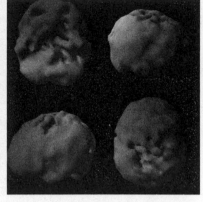

Healthy   Sleep Apnea

 ## CHECKUP FOR <u>S</u>LEEP ISSUES

Get assessed for sleep apnea

If you snore loudly, stop breathing at night, or are chronically tired during the day, get evaluated at a sleep laboratory, or have your health-care professional order a home sleep apnea study.

Determine the number of hours of sleep you need each night

One way to do this: Whenever you are free to experiment (say, on vacation), go to bed at the same time each night without setting an alarm, and see what time you awaken the next morning. Over a week or ten days' time, you will discover what your natural sleep needs are. If you are unable to try this, strive to get seven to eight hours each night, which is a healthy amount for most people.

||||||||||||||||||||||||||||||||||||||||||||||||||||||||||||||||||||||||||||||||||||||||||||||||||||||

Health Problems That Can Steal Your Shut-Eye

The following conditions affect sleep in myriad ways—from preventing sleep to interrupting it to causing early morning wakefulness. If you suffer from one of them and find yourself struggling with getting adequate rest, speak with your health-care provider about possible solutions.

- Sleep apnea. It leads you to stop breathing for short periods throughout the night, which prevents you from getting restful sleep and leaves you feeling sluggish, inattentive, and forget-ful the next day.
- Restless leg syndrome. This nighttime jerking or pedaling motion of the legs drives a person's bed partner crazy, not to mention the person who has it.
- Thyroid conditions. Both hypothyroidism and hyperthyroidism can cause sleep problems. See page 217 to find out about testing for thyroid issues.
- Congestive heart failure.
- Chronic pain.
- Untreated or undertreated psychiatric conditions, such as obsessive-compulsive disorder, depression, or anxiety.
- Alzheimer's disease. Some patients with dementia are more active at night, and they may even wander from their beds.
- Chronic gastrointestinal problems, such as reflux.
- Benign prostatic hypertrophy. Men with this condition may visit the bathroom often at night, which robs them of restful sleep.

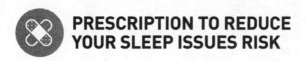

PRESCRIPTION TO REDUCE YOUR SLEEP ISSUES RISK

The Strategies

1. **Treat sleep apnea.** If you have symptoms of the disorder, discuss it with your doctor. Be serious about treatment if you have it.

2. **Avoid sleep robbers.** In our hectic 24-7 society, we could just as eas-ily ask, "What *doesn't* cause sleep deprivation?" There is a seemingly endless number of reasons why millions of us are missing out on a good night's sleep. This list includes some of the most common factors.

- *Environment unconducive to sleep.* The temperature, lighting, and noise (including snoring) in your room may keep you awake.
- *Technological gadgets.*
- *Negative emotions, such as anger and worry.*
- *Medications.* Many drugs, including asthma and cough medications, antihistamines, anticonvulsants, and stimulants (such as amphetamine salts [Adderall] or methylphenidate [Concerta], prescribed for ADHD), disturb sleep.
- *Caffeine.* Too much of this stimulant can disrupt sleep.
- *Women's issues.* Hormone levels are affected by pregnancy, PMS, perimenopause, and menopause. These fluctuations may disrupt women's sleep cycles.
- *Shift work.* Nighttime shift workers, such as health-care workers, truck drivers, and first responders, are particularly prone to irregular sleep patterns, which leads to excessive sleepiness, reduced productivity, irritability, and mood problems.
- *Stress.* Whether caused by a major event, such as the death of a loved one or a divorce, or a temporary situation, such as a major work deadline or another call from your child's teacher, stress may prevent you from falling—or staying—asleep.
- *Eating within two to three hours of bedtime.* Besides keeping your GI tract active, it will cause higher blood pressure at night and increase the risk of heart attack and stroke.
- *Jet lag.* International travel across time zones disrupts sleep cycles.

3. **Adopt these sleep enhancers.** To get a better night's sleep and allow your brain time to clean itself up, try one or more of the following ideas. If something doesn't work, experiment with other techniques until you notice your sleep improving.

- *Set up your bedroom for sleep.* It should be cool, completely dark, and quiet. The ideal sleeping temperature may vary from person to person, but it should be on the cool side. If your room is too light, consider wearing a sleep mask or hanging blackout shades, and try using earplugs if you live in a noisy neighborhood or sleep next to a snoring spouse.
- *Block gadget disruption.* Stash your phone, tablet, and digital watch away from your bed, or at least turn the sound off. Face your digital clock toward the wall so you aren't distracted by luminescent numbers.

- *Ban pets from the bedroom*—or at least keep them off the bed.
- *Try to fix emotional problems before bedtime.* If you are a worrier, devote about 10 to 15 minutes before bedtime to your nagging concerns; then put a stop to them. If you're at odds with someone, send him or her a positive text or e-mail—or determine to deal with the issue in the morning. In other words, "don't let the sun go down while you are still angry" (Ephesians 4:26). Doing so may prevent your anger from festering and growing further.
- *Establish and stick to a regular sleep schedule.* Try to go to bed at the same time each night and wake up at the same time each morning, including on weekends. Getting up at the same time each day, regardless of how long you slept the previous night, will help set your internal body clock, which can keep insomnia at bay.
- *Read a book before bed.* Preferably pick up something thick or tedious, such as Leviticus in the Old Testament. If you read the Acts of the Apostles in the New Testament or the latest Stephen King thriller, it is likely to keep you up. Avoid reading from an e-reader or tablet; its light will keep your brain alert.
- *Don't take daytime naps*—even if you have trouble sleeping at night. Napping is one of the biggest mistakes insomniacs can make since it compounds the nighttime sleep-cycle disruption.
- *Lull yourself to sleep with sound therapy.* Listening to audio of soothing nature sounds or soft music, or taking in white noise from a fan, may enable you to drift off more easily. Studies show slower classical music or any music with a rhythm of 60 to 80 beats per minute may help with sleep.[9] Sleep-enhancing music by Grammy Award–winning producer Barry Goldstein is available at www.brainfitlife.com.
- *Drink a cup of warm, unsweetened almond milk.* Add a teaspoon of vanilla extract (the real stuff) and a few drops of stevia. The combination may increase serotonin in your brain, helping you sleep.
- *Don't exercise within four hours of bedtime.* Regular workouts are a great way to combat insomnia, but vigorous exercise late in the evening may keep you up.
- *Wear socks to bed.* Warm hands and feet are the best predictors of rapid sleep onset, according to researchers.

- *Cut out caffeinated beverages in the afternoon or evening.* Refrain from drinking coffee, tea, or other caffeinated beverages after 2 p.m. Also avoid chocolate, nicotine, and alcohol—especially at night. Although alcohol can initially make you feel sleepy, it actually interrupts sleep.
- *Don't look at the clock if you wake up in the middle of the night.* Checking the time can make you feel anxious, which aggravates the problem of sleeplessness.
- *Use the bed and bedroom only for sexual activity or sleep.* Sexual activity releases muscle tension and a flood of natural hormones. Adults with healthy sex lives tend to sleep better and feel better overall. If you are unable to fall asleep or stay asleep, move to another room.

BRIGHT MINDS TIP

Use the scent of lavender to enhance your slumbers. It has been shown to decrease anxiety and improve mood and sleep.[10]

- *Stay away from benzodiazepines and traditional sleep medications.* When medications are necessary, I often prescribe trazodone, gabapentin, or amitriptyline to my patients.
- *Develop a relaxing nighttime routine that encourages sleep.* Turn off all electronic devices at least an hour before bedtime, and lower the lights in your house. A warm bath or shower, meditation, prayer, or massage may also help you relax. (Download helpful meditations at www.mybrainfitlife.com.)

The Nutraceuticals

- *Melatonin:* 0.3–6 mg a day

- *5-HTP* (especially for worriers)*:* 50–200 mg a day

- *Magnesium:* 50–400 mg a day

- *Zinc:* 20–40 mg a day

- *GABA:* 250–1,000 mg a day

- *Lemon balm* (*Melissa officinalis*): 300–600 mg a day

- *Vitamin D3:* 3,500 IU a day[11]

- My patients tend to like a combination of melatonin, magnesium, zinc, and GABA.

The Foods
AVOID (OR LIMIT):

Alcohol, including wine: Though hard liquor is worse for your brain, snoring can occur after any form of alcohol is consumed. Alcohol can also disrupt sleep.

Caffeine, including dark chocolate (which also contains theobromine), a few hours before bedtime

Energy drinks (duh!)

Spicy foods, especially at night

Grapefruit, due to acidity, which may cause heartburn at night

Foods that contain diuretics (which will keep you up going to the bathroom): celery, cucumbers, radishes, watermelon

Foods that contain tyramine, such as tomatoes, eggplant, soy, red wine, and aged cheeses, which increase norepinephrine, a stimulating neurotransmitter

Unhealthy fatty foods, including burgers, fries, and pizza, which all contain harder-to-digest saturated fats

Black bean chili, which will keep your GI tract rumbling

High-protein foods, which are harder to digest

CONSIDER ADDING:

Sleep-enhancing spices such as ginger root

Foods rich in melatonin (the hormone of sleep): tart cherry juice concentrate[12] (also improves antioxidant status),[13] cherries, walnuts, ginger root, asparagus

Serotonin-rich foods: See page 180 in chapter 11.

Magnesium-rich foods, which reduce anxiety: See page 77 in chapter 5.

Healthy carbohydrates, such as sweet potatoes, quinoa, and bananas (which also are rich in magnesium). These foods can also increase tryptophan, which increases serotonin and improves sleep.

Chamomile or passion fruit tea[14]

 ## PICK ONE HEALTHY BRIGHT MINDS HABIT TO START TODAY

1. **If you snore, get assessed for sleep apnea.**

2. Eliminate caffeine during the day (gradually—to avoid headaches!).

3. Put blue light blockers on your electronic gadgets.

4. Cool your home a bit before bedtime.

5. Darken your bedroom.

6. **Turn off your gadgets so they do not wake you.**

7. Maintain a regular sleep schedule.

8. Take melatonin and magnesium.

9. Listen to audio created to help with sleep.

10. Supplement with 5-HTP if you are a worrier (see pages 179, 250).

PART 3

DAILY FOOD, HABITS, AND MORE TO BOOST YOUR MEMORY

CHAPTER 16

THE MEMORY RESCUE DIET
FOOD FOR BRIGHT MINDS

I visited one of the big box stores for the first time ever this weekend. There was death everywhere (the toxic food), around every corner. Samples of death covered in death. I just kept hearing Dr. Amen in the back of my mind. So I walked past it all! Got my organic goods and left, which is saying a lot because it was nearly lunchtime and it all smelled so good! Thank you for giving me the tools to make good choices.

FROM A PARTICIPANT IN *THE BRAIN WARRIOR'S WAY* LIVE CLASS

To rescue your memory, choosing the right foods is one of the most important strategies of all. Your brain uses 20 to 30 percent of the calories you consume. It is the most energy-hungry organ in your body. If you eat a fast-food diet, you will have a fast-food mind that is less capable of quick thinking and reliable decision making.

The prescriptions at the end of every chapter in part 2 include lists of foods shown to have particular benefit in reducing the various risk factors. In this chapter I want to introduce you to a diet that everyone should follow if they want to protect their memory. Once you commit to the brain-healthy diet I discuss, you will quickly notice that you have more energy; fewer cravings; better focus, memory, and moods; and even a flatter stomach within a matter of weeks.

A number of recent studies report that a healthy diet, like the Memory Rescue Diet, is associated with significantly lower risks of severe memory problems such as Alzheimer's disease, as well as most of the risk factors I've discussed, including heart disease, inflammation, depression, and diabesity.[1] Healthy diets are also associated with bigger brain size.[2] And bigger is better when it comes to the brain.

THE MEMORY RESCUE DIET CHECKLIST

Over the past three decades I have developed a new approach to diet that focuses on changing the way you think about eating as well as the way you actually eat. These two principles form the backbone of the Memory Rescue Diet, and the checklist below provides the specific components of this brain-healthy approach to eating. They are designed to guide you to make the best food choices for your brain for the rest of your life.

1. Change the Way You Think about Eating
   ✓ Get your mind right. Being healthy is about abundance, not deprivation.
   ✓ Think of calories like money; spend them wisely.
   ✓ Beware the standard American diet (SAD).

2. Change the Way You Eat (and Drink)
   ✓ Pick the healthiest protein.
   ✓ Get your fill of the right fats.
   ✓ Go for the greens (and reds, yellows, blues, and other hues).
   ✓ Choose brain-boosting carbohydrates.
   ✓ Say good-bye to sugar.
   ✓ Hydrate with H_2O.
   ✓ Flavor your food with smart herbs and spices.

As you adopt these healthy eating habits, you will begin developing a new, healthy relationship with food. Contrary to what you might think, eating in a brain-healthy way is not more expensive. It is *less* expensive when you consider that your medical bills will be lower and your productivity will go up. And what price can you put on your memory?

In fact, the Memory Rescue Diet includes no gimmicks, and there are no "designer" foods to buy. Plus it is simple. I know you won't follow a program that is complicated or requires you to eat boring foods for the next 40 years. I wouldn't—why would anyone else? The recommended foods are delicious, energizing, and healing.

CHANGE THE WAY YOU THINK ABOUT EATING

✓ *Get your mind right. Being healthy is about abundance, not deprivation.*

Too many patients I've seen start with this attitude: "I don't want to deprive myself. I want what I want when I want it."

My response is, "Which do you want *more*? Your health, a great brain, years added to your life, and freedom from dementia . . . or the nightly alcohol and sugar?"

Most people fail in nutrition programs because they focus on what they cannot have, rather than on what they can have. They have a deprivation mind-set. They focus on the loss of the very foods that drive inflammation and hijack their taste buds—empty-calorie foods, sugary foods, fast foods, and pesticide-laden foods.

> *To rescue your memory, the first thing you must do*
> *is get your mind right.*

In my experience, as people start down the road to getting well, they begin to miss the Rocky Road ice cream, look longingly at the doughnuts, and feel sad about not being able to eat the chicken fried steak, mashed potatoes, and key lime pie. Yet after about 10 days of eating high-quality food, they realize that their taste buds have come alive and food tastes better than ever.

Getting well is about focusing on an abundance of the right nutrients, which will deprive you of illnesses like diabetes, heart disease, cancer, depression, and dementia. This is a critical shift. Those people who continue to follow the Memory Rescue Diet begin to see many unhealthy foods as weapons of self-destruction and avoid them, just as they would avoid shaking hands with someone who was sneezing and coughing up green gunk.

Think of your relationship with food the way you think about your other relationships. Find foods you love that love you back, and stay away from those that abuse you. Just because you "love" something doesn't mean it's good for you. I had a patient tell me she'd rather get Alzheimer's disease than give up sugar. That is an example of an abusive relationship. She was in love with something that hurt her. Fortunately, over time she ended the toxic relationship and helped her whole family get well.

Also lose the idea that you should be able to eat "everything in moderation." It is nothing more than the gateway thought to dementia hell. It gives you an excuse to continue down the wrong path, and before long it becomes your justification for unhealthy eating every day.

✓ *Think of calories like money; spend them wisely.*

Thoughtful, successful people tend to be conscientious with their money; they save for retirement and spend their hard-earned cash wisely. Those who don't are much more likely to experience financial hardship or to file for bankruptcy. I think of calories the same way. They are incredibly important, and you should spend them carefully. That means using your calories on foods that nourish you, rather than on those that steal from your health.

Make no mistake, the quality of your food matters more than the quantity. Compare a 500-calorie blueberry crumb doughnut to a 500-calorie plate of rainbow trout, broccoli, orange bell peppers, raspberries, and almonds. The doughnut will zap your energy and set off an inflammatory response; the fish meal will power your brain and reduce your risk of accelerated aging. You are likely to gulp down the first in a matter of minutes, sending your blood sugar sky-high and teasing your pleasure centers; the second you enjoy at a leisurely pace, and it helps you feel full longer as well as happier and more emotionally stable.

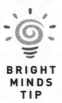

BRIGHT MINDS TIP

Calories are like money. If you overspend, your body will eventually become bankrupt. Some calories have better exchange rates than others.

This is not to say that the quantity of calories you take in is unimportant. On the contrary, substantial research, first in animals and now in humans, indicates that a calorie-restricted (CR) diet can help control weight; decrease the risk of heart disease, cancer, and stroke; and trigger mechanisms in the body that increase the production of nerve growth factors, which are helpful to the brain. A 25-year study on rhesus monkeys found that those that ate 30 percent fewer calories than the others not only lived longer, they also had a lower incidence of diabetes and cancer, and their hair, skin, and brains looked younger (less shrinkage in the hippocampus).[3] Eating too many calories causes waste to build up in the body's cells, making everything look and feel older.

Researchers at Columbia University have found that eating fewer calories may be particularly important for people with the *APOE* e4 gene.[4] They followed 980 elderly individuals for four years, measuring their daily calories. Compared to people with a low calorie intake, those with the highest calorie intake were 2.3 times more likely to develop Alzheimer's disease—but only if they also had the *APOE* e4 gene. In other research on CR, in an ongoing project known as the CALERIE study, volunteers who were normal weight or slightly overweight reduced their calorie intake by 25 percent for two years and had significant decreases in cardiovascular risk factors, including lower blood pressure.[5]

However, calorie restriction has drawbacks: It is hard to maintain long-term and has been associated with decreased testosterone levels, irritability, and a lower sex drive—so there may not be a good reason to live longer. Scientists have looked at other ways to mimic the benefits of CR without these side effects, including the antidiabetic drug metformin, which lowers high blood sugar levels; exercise; stress management; and improved sleep.

CONSIDER INTERMITTENT FASTING AND THE TIMING OF YOUR MEALS

There may be another way to keep your calorie intake in check. As I have discussed, a possible cause of memory loss is the overproduction of beta amyloid and abnormal tau proteins that damage brain cell circuits. One way your brain eliminates these proteins is through autophagy,[6] a process that's like having tiny trash collectors cleaning up the toxins. Nightly 12-to-16-hour fasts turn on this process. That means if you eat dinner at 7 p.m. and don't eat again until between 7 and 11 a.m., you give your brain time for trash cleanup. This "intermittent fasting," as it is called, can significantly improve memory,[7] mood,[8] fat loss,[9] weight, blood pressure, and inflammatory markers.[10] You can also use this method of eating to reduce your calorie consumption—for example, by skipping breakfast and eating only lunch and dinner two or three days each week.

New research also suggests that you should avoid eating within two to three hours of bedtime and that late-night eating puts you at a higher risk of heart attack, stroke, and diabetes.[11] Eating late puts your brain in a "high alert" stress state, causing your body to release stress hormones when it should be winding down. In healthy people, blood pressure drops by at least 10 percent when they go to sleep, but late-night eaters' blood pressure stays high. People whose blood pressure does not fall at night are known as "nondippers," and they have a much higher rate of heart-related death. Research has shown that late eaters are nearly three times more likely to be nondippers. You don't want to be one of them.

Two things seem certain: Consuming too many calories is bad for your brain and body, and if you are going to put something into your body, you want to be sure you are getting the biggest health bang for the cost.

✓ Beware the standard American diet (SAD).

No one makes a *conscious* decision to eat foods that trigger inflammation, but that is exactly what most Americans do in consuming the standard American diet of fast food; sugar; simple carbohydrates; dairy products; trans fats; some animal-derived saturated fats; excess omega-6 fatty acids; nutrient-bankrupt refined and processed foods; and products filled with pesticide residues, antibiotics, and hormones. This type of diet is loaded with chemicals that are unnatural to your body, which causes it to respond as if it has been injured. Inflammation is your body and brain's healing response to that injury. Over time, if your diet doesn't change, the inflammation can become chronic, and as we've seen, that can lead to many health problems. It's enough to make anyone feel *SAD*!

Right now, make a commitment to become more aware of and serious about the foods you put in your body. Aim to eat "clean"—foods that are organically grown or raised and free of hormones, antibiotics, and pesticides. (Even small amounts of pesticides can build up in your brain and body over time.) Whenever possible, choose meat from animals that are free range and/or grass fed, and organically grown nuts and seeds. Start reading food labels, and do your best to avoid food additives and artificial preservatives, dyes, and sweeteners.

Fish is an excellent source of healthy protein and omega-3 fats, but some varieties are more toxic than others. Generally, smaller fish contain lower amounts of mercury than larger fish like tuna, so limit your consumption of the latter. Whenever possible, buy species that are not overfished, and eat a fairly wide variety, preferably those highest in omega-3s, like wild Alaskan salmon, trout, sardines, anchovies, and Atlantic and Pacific mackerel. Learn more about which fish to add to your diet at www.seafoodwatch.org, the website of the Monterey Bay Aquarium in Monterey, California.

Organic and sustainably raised produce can be pricey, so it helps to know which fruits and vegetables carry the highest pesticide loads and to buy organic when it matters most. I consult the Environmental Working Group's annual lists of foods with the highest and lowest levels of pesticide residues and recommend that you do so as well. (Stay updated at www.ewg.org.) Here is the current list of 13 foods with the highest levels of pesticide residue: strawberries, spinach, nectarines, apples, peaches, pears, cherries, grapes, celery, tomatoes, sweet bell peppers, potatoes, and hot peppers. Try to buy organic when purchasing these fruits and vegetables.

The 15 foods with the lowest levels of pesticide residue are sweet corn, avocados, pineapples, cabbage, onions, frozen sweet peas, papayas, asparagus, mangoes, eggplant, honeydew melon, kiwifruit, cantaloupe, cauliflower, and grapefruit. (The EWG notes that because a small amount of sweet corn, papaya, and summer squash sold in the United States comes from genetically modified seeds, if you want to avoid GMOs, buy organic varieties.)

CHANGE THE WAY YOU EAT (AND DRINK)

✓ *Pick the healthiest protein.*

It may come as a surprise to learn that the only component of your body more abundant than water is protein. You need protein in order to keep your cells, tissues, and organs growing and functioning properly. It also contributes to the health of everything from your muscles, hair, and skin to various hormones and neurotransmitters, which all require a steady supply of the 20 amino acids that are the building blocks of protein. A portion of these amino acids are made by your body, but the rest—the essential amino acids—must come from the food you eat.

Protein is also a critical part of your diet because of its role in maintaining a healthy metabolism. It stimulates the release of metabolic hormones that help stabilize your blood sugar levels and stop energy crashes. As a result, eating or snacking on protein helps you feel full longer than you do after a high-carb or sugary snack or meal. And because protein takes more energy to digest, you also wind up burning more calories.

With all these benefits, you might think you need to eat lots of protein to stay healthy, but small quantities are all that is required. In fact, consuming too much can be detrimental, as it accelerates the internal processes (oxidation, inflammation) that contribute to faster aging and disease. Our recommendation at Amen Clinics is to eat a limited amount with every meal and snack, every four to five hours, to help balance your blood sugar and decrease cravings.

Given that small doses are better for you than large ones, it becomes even more important to choose the highest-quality protein. High-quality animal protein, whether lamb, turkey, chicken, beef, or pork, is free of hormones and antibiotics, free range, and grass fed. Though it is more expensive than industrial farm-raised animal protein, it is a good investment in your health. Compared with grass-fed meat, industrially raised meat is about 30 percent higher in palmitic acid (a type of unhealthy saturated fat), which has been linked with cardiovascular disease. And don't forget fish, beans and other legumes, raw unsalted nuts, and high-protein veggies, such as broccoli and spinach. Fish, poultry, and most meats contain *all* the necessary amino acids, while plant foods contain only *some* of them. However, plant foods are an essential part of a healthy diet—not just for their protein, but also for their many disease-preventing phytonutrients. See "Go for the greens (and reds, yellows, blues, and other hues)" for more information.

|||||||||||||||||||||||||||||||||||||||||||||||||||||||||||||||||||||||||||||||||||||||||||||||

Say, What's Wrong with Soy?

One of the more ubiquitous plant-based proteins in America today is soy. Whether in the form of tofu, tempeh, edamame, soy sauce, chips, nuts, or milk, soy is often touted as the ideal protein replacement for meat and dairy—for vegetarians and nonvegetarians alike. But soy can be problematic. Many commercially prepared foods now contain soy, and constant exposure can lead to increased sensitivity. And although moderate amounts of soy in the right form can be beneficial, it has components that are harmful to the health of your brain and body. These include a high concentration of lectins (carbohydrate-binding proteins that can be toxic, allergenic, and inflammatory), large amounts of omega-6 fatty acids, phytoestrogens (which may contribute to the development of cancer, early puberty in girls, and impotence in men), and phytic acid, which is thought to reduce the absorption of vital minerals. For these reasons, I recommend limiting or even eliminating soy.

|||||||||||||||||||||||||||||||||||||||||||||||||||||||||||||||||||||||||||||||||||||||||||||||

✓ *Get your fill of the right fats.*

You may be thinking, *Why is fat so high on this checklist?* It is because healthy fats are essential to keeping your body and brain disease-free. A case in point: A Mayo Clinic study found that the risk of cognitive impairment was 42 percent lower in people who ate a fat-based diet; 21 percent lower in those who ate a protein-based diet; but four times *higher* in those who ate a simple carbohydrate–based diet (think bread, pasta, potatoes, rice, and sugar).[12] It's the sugar, *not* the fat, that's the problem (see more in "Choose brain-boosting carbohydrates" and "Say good-bye to sugar").

The war on fat is over—at least in terms of dietary fat. It is clear that your body needs good fats for a variety of essential functions, from storing energy and maintaining healthy brain function to creating healthy cells and hormones. Eating more of the right fats will also help you lose body fat. Research has shown that eating a moderate-fat versus a low-fat diet (35 versus 20 percent of calories from fat) can mean the difference between losing weight and waistline inches and actually *gaining* both! A moderate-fat diet has another advantage: Healthy fats help with satiety—feeling full. In the study mentioned above, 54 percent of the moderate-fat dieters were able to follow their program for the entire 18 months, while only 20 percent of the low-fat dieters were able to stick with theirs.

Notice that I keep reiterating the terms *good* and *healthy* in describing the fats you should be eating. You still need to avoid the so-called bad fats: fried fats, trans fats, and some saturated fats. Here is a look at how different kinds of fats impact your health.

Unsaturated fats. These are beneficial fats thanks to their role in improving cholesterol levels, easing inflammation, stabilizing heart rhythms, and balancing blood sugar. There are two kinds of unsaturated fats: polyunsaturated and monounsaturated. Commonly referred to as PUFAs and MUFAs (polyunsaturated fatty acids and monounsaturated fatty acids), they are predominantly found in plant foods, such as vegetable oils (like olive oil), nuts, and seeds. Earlier we introduced these two important polyunsaturated fats:

- *Omega-3 fatty acids.* Two types of omega-3s in particular, EPA and DHA, are crucial for optimal brain health and are found in cold-water fish, such as salmon, mackerel, sardines, and trout. Getting inadequate amounts of EPA and DHA (which must come from your diet) puts you at greater risk of cognitive decline in aging, psychological disturbances, depression, and many other illnesses. Higher levels of EPA and DHA are associated with significantly less beta amyloid in the blood, a reduced incidence of Alzheimer's, and slower cognitive decline.[13]

- *Omega-6 fatty acids*, like omega-3s, are essential for health, playing a critical role in brain function as well as in normal growth and development. Sources include most vegetable oils (soybean, sunflower, safflower, corn, canola), many fried foods, cereals, whole-grain breads, and processed foods. However, overconsumption of omega-6 fatty acids can cancel out the benefits of omega-3s, and the standard American diet, with its overabundance of omega-6-rich vegetable oils, puts many people's ratio of omega-6s to omega-3s at a whopping 20 to 1 or even higher (an optimal ratio may be less than 4 to 1). This high ratio is pro-inflammatory and increases the risk of heart disease, cancer, diabetes, and many other health problems.

To reach a more favorable balance of omega-6s to omega-3s, eat fewer foods that contain omega-6s and more with omega-3 EPA and DHA. Taking fish oil supplements can also help maintain a healthy omega balance.

Saturated fats. These fats can be either bad *or* good, depending on their structure. According to cardiologist Mark Houston, MD, from Vanderbilt University,[14] short- to medium-chain saturated fats (4 to 12 carbon triglycerides) tend to be healthier than long-chain ones. Here are a few examples of potentially healthy and unhealthy saturated fatty acids:

- *Butyric* (4 carbon) *acids* are found in fiber-rich foods like sweet potatoes, vegetables, beans, nuts, and fruit, as well as in butter and ghee (clarified butter).
- *Caprylic* (8 carbon), *capric* (10 carbon), and *lauric* (12 carbon) acids are medium-chain triglycerides (MCTs) found in coconut and coconut oil that, although saturated, can be used by the brain to make energy and have shown memory benefits, particularly in people with blood sugar problems.[15]
- *Myristic acid* is a 14-carbon saturated fat found in most animal fats (including dairy foods) and some vegetable oils. These fatty acids may be detrimental to heart health, so they should be consumed only in small amounts.
- *Palmitic acid* is a 16-carbon saturated fat that negatively affects cholesterol and heart health. This fat is created in your liver when you eat a high-sugar, high-carbohydrate diet. It also creates the marbling in the meat of corn-fed cattle.
- *Stearic acid* is an 18-carbon fatty acid found in grain-fed meats, sausage and bacon, cold cuts, peanuts, peanut butter, margarine, fried potatoes, whole milk, cheese, and vegetable oils (it is highest in sunflower oil). Although chocolate is high in stearic acid, it is also high in antioxidants and flavonoids, which help balance its health benefit when eaten in small amounts.

Overall, the healthiest strategy is to cut back on saturated fats like myristic, palmitic, and stearic acids and add more polyunsaturated fats (fish oil, nuts, and seeds) to your diet.

Trans fats. These synthetic fats, or "Frankenfats," are the *worst* fats. They have no place in your diet. They are associated with memory problems, even in young adults.[16] They also decrease healthy blood flow and increase the likelihood of clots, which can cause strokes and heart disease. Partially hydrogenated vegetable oils, shortening, margarine, many processed foods, commercially prepared fried foods, and packaged baked goods, including doughnuts, crackers, and snack foods, contain trans fats.

Beware of the many processed foods carrying a "trans fat–free" label on their packaging. Because current government regulations require that trans fats be listed on a food label only if the level is above the legal limit of 0.5 grams per serving, many products aren't really trans fat–free. One way to know: If the label lists partially hydrogenated oils or vegetable shortening, the food contains trans fats. The FDA has set a deadline of 2018 for companies to eliminate trans fats from their products. Until then, avoid these health-harming fats.

||||||||||||||||||||||||||||||||||||||||||||||||||||||||||||||||||||||||||||||||||||||||||

Sources of the Healthiest Fats and Oils vs. the Unhealthiest Fats and Oils

HEALTHIEST FATS AND OILS

- avocados
- avocado oil
- cocoa butter
- coconuts
- coconut oil
- flax oil
- grass-fed beef, bison, and lamb
- macadamia nut oil
- nuts
- olives
- olive oil
- organic poultry
- seafood: anchovies, arctic char, catfish, herring, king crab, mackerel, wild salmon, sardines, sea bass, snapper, sole, trout, tuna, clams, mussels, oysters, and scallops
- seeds
- sesame oil
- walnut oil

UNHEALTHIEST FATS AND OILS

- canola oil
- corn oil
- excessive omega-6 fats
- industrial farm-raised animal fat and dairy
- processed meats
- safflower oil
- soy oil
- trans fats

||||||||||||||||||||||||||||||||||||||||||||||||||||||||||||||||||||||||||||||||||||

✓ *Go for the greens (and reds, yellows, blues, and other hues).*

If you were to do nothing else to change your diet except eat more colorful fruits and vegetables, you would still get enormous benefits from the nutrients, vitamins, and minerals they contain, which your body needs for robust health. Broccoli and other cruciferous vegetables, for example, as well as various herbs and spices (e.g., curcumin) contain sulforaphane, which powerfully assists in DNA repair. Foods from plants of every color, even white, also help prevent cancer and reduce the inflammation that contributes to Alzheimer's disease, heart disease, arthritis, gastrointestinal disorders, and many other illnesses. Plant nutrients bolster your immune system in its role of fending off attacks and disease. (Just be sure to eat twice as many vegetables as fruits to avoid the extra sugar.)

Some of the most age-defying ingredients in produce are its antioxidants, which decrease the destruction caused by free radicals in the body. A food's antioxidant capacity is measured by its oxygen radical absorbance capacity or ORAC value; see opposite page. Blueberries have a well-deserved reputation for being a brain-healthy food, but it's clear from this chart that acai fruit and raspberries have even more antioxidant clout and that a number of herbs and spices—cloves, oregano, rosemary, thyme, cinnamon, turmeric, and sage— have true antioxidant superpowers. (Read more about them in "Flavor your food with brain-smart herbs and spices," page 275.)

||||||||||||||||||||||||||||||||||||||||||||||||||||||||||||||||||||||||||||||||||

Antioxidant-Rich Foods with ORAC (Oxygen Radical Absorbance Capacity) Ratings

FOOD/SPICE/HERB	ORAC UNITS (PER 100 GRAMS OF WEIGHT)
Cloves	290,000
Oregano	175,000
Rosemary	165,000
Thyme	157,000
Cinnamon	131,000
Turmeric	125,000
Sage	120,000
Acai fruit	102,000
Parsley	73,000
Cocoa powder	55,000
Raspberries	19,000
Walnuts	13,000
Blueberries	9,600
Artichokes	9,400
Cranberries	9,000
Kidney beans	8,600
Blackberries	5,900
Pomegranates	4,400

||||||||||||||||||||||||||||||||||||||||||||||||||||||||||||||||||||||||||||||||||

✓ *Choose brain-boosting carbohydrates.*

It makes perfect sense to discuss the best carbohydrates for your brain right after touting the benefits of fruits and vegetables because some of the healthiest carbs are . . . fruits and vegetables! Veggies like brussels sprouts and asparagus, which are nonstarchy, and fruits like pears and apples are complex carbohydrates, the best kind of carbs to eat as they are high in fiber, slower to digest, and low glycemic (which means they don't cause your blood sugar to shoot up). If you can swap foods like these for the high-glycemic, low-fiber carbs in your diet—the doughnuts, pizza, candy, cookies, French fries, and such—you'll be on a fast track to improving your insulin and blood sugar levels, reducing your cravings, and bettering your memory.

Keeping insulin in check is critical to your overall mental and physical health. It's a hormone that helps determine how the calories you eat are used by your body. It is manufactured in the pancreas, which boosts production when you consume more simple carbs like sugar, processed grains, potato chips, and other foods that are quickly converted to sugar. Research by Harvard endocrinologist and obesity expert David Ludwig, MD, PhD, has shown that insulin tends to increase both the size and number of fat cells. When insulin levels are high, fat cells accumulate more and more glucose and fat. Staying on this kind of diet makes it impossible, practically speaking, to lose weight. The answer? Wean yourself off of the insulin-boosting simple carbohydrates and replace them with hunger-satisfying, high-fiber, low-glycemic carbohydrates.

MEET THE GLYCEMIC INDEX (GI) AND GLYCEMIC LOAD (GL)

These two rating systems can help you make better food choices. The glycemic index (GI) ranks carbohydrates on their effect on blood sugar, using a scale of one to 100+ (glucose is 100). GI foods with a lower number tend to be healthier because they don't spike blood sugar; foods with a higher GI number are generally less healthy because they quickly raise blood sugar. In general, it's healthiest to stick with foods that have a GI value under 60. One surprising finding from the research: Table sugar is ranked lower on the GI than potatoes and bread!

Glycemic load is an even more valuable number because it takes both blood sugar and portion size into account. Pineapple, for instance, has a high GI (66), but a low GL (6). That means you have to eat a lot of pineapple to raise your blood sugar. A low GL is 10 or under (for a comprehensive list of GL foods from the American Diabetes Association, see http://care.diabetes journals.org/content/suppl/2008/09/18/dc08-1239.DC1/TableA1_1.pdf). Don't assume, however, that a food with a low GL is automatically good for you. Milk, for example, has a low GL, but it may be adulterated with antibiotics and hormones. To be sure your diet is healthy, check that the foods you are eating meet all the Memory Rescue Diet principles.

FIBER: A VITAL CARBOHYDRATE

Fiber is an unsung dietary hero. It provides a raft of health benefits, including balancing blood sugar, helping you feel full after a meal, reducing colon cancer risk, and keeping your bowels working smoothly. Yet most of us get far too little. The average American consumes less than 15 grams of fiber a day; compare that to the estimated 135 grams our prehistoric ancestors used to eat! The recommended amounts today are 25 to 30 grams for women, and 30 to 38 grams for men.

There are two types of fiber—soluble and insoluble. Soluble fiber, found in foods such as apples, blueberries, beans, oatmeal, and fiber supplements, helps prevent heart disease and diabetes. It also feeds the good bacteria in your gut, boosting immunity and helping limit the growth of bad bacteria (see chapter 7 for more on the role of gut bacteria in brain and body health). Insoluble fiber—what we think of as roughage—is found in seeds, stems, and skins. It helps keep the intestines cleaned out and distributes the critical by-products of soluble fiber throughout the colon.

Eating lots of vegetables will significantly increase your intake of both soluble and insoluble fiber. Fiber supplements also can be helpful, especially if you are insulin resistant or have high cholesterol.

TROUBLESOME GRAINS

Many people look to breads and pasta as their primary sources of fiber; however, their health benefits are dubious at best. Sadly, the wild grains that our ancestors ate in tiny amounts bear little resemblance to the genetically hybridized grains produced today. I say sadly because our digestive systems are simply not equipped to process these modern grains—especially since the quantity we now consume has increased exponentially since the agricultural revolution began 300 years ago.

Modern grains are problematic in at least two ways. First, many of them turn to sugar in the body. And second, several—wheat, barley, rye, kamut, bulgur, corn, and spelt—contain gluten (the Latin word for *glue*), a sticky substance that gives bread dough its elasticity and helps it rise. Gluten has found its way into commercially made breads, cakes, cookies, cereals, pasta, and other grain-based products, as well as salad dressings, sauces, processed foods, and even cosmetics. And that has given rise to gluten-related health issues, including the autoimmune illnesses celiac disease, type 1 diabetes, and Hashimoto's disease. Gluten can also cause flu-like symptoms, psychological disturbances, acne, arthritis, and food addiction and increase insulin resistance. And it can lower brain blood flow.[17] According to the Center for Celiac Research, 18 million Americans have gluten sensitivity, which can lead to more than 100 symptoms, including chronic diarrhea, bloating, flatulence, nausea, abdominal pain, skin rashes, fatigue, and mental fogginess. Gluten-free diets are associated with a reduction, and even full remission, of symptoms in a subset of schizophrenic patients[18] and improvement in autistic and ADHD symptoms in a subset of patients.[19]

Another troublesome grain is corn. Its unhealthy fatty-acid profile (high levels of omega-6 fats plus very low levels of omega-3s) makes it an inflammatory food that can damage the intestinal lining. Of particular concern is the widespread use of Roundup (a highly toxic glyphosate pesticide that is banned in some European countries) on US corn,[20] most of which is raised from genetically modified seeds. Glyphosate has been associated with ADHD,[21] cancer, depression, Parkinson's disease, MS, hypothyroidism, and liver disease.[22]

Corn is ubiquitous in America, from corn oil to cornstarch to corn syrup and beyond, but you can greatly reduce your intake by avoiding processed foods and recipes containing corn kernels. That was true for Victor, who had suffered with anxiety, depression, and insomnia for decades. He had seen endocrinologists, psychiatrists, cardiologists, and sleep doctors but found no relief.

After a week on the Memory Rescue eating plan, his mood was better than it had been in years. When Victor added corn back into his diet, he said that "within a couple of bites" he knew it was the problem. Although he loved corn chips, corn tortillas, and popcorn, he decided the relationship wasn't worth the pain, so he broke up with corn. He was amazed that after suffering for so long, he could feel happy by doing something so simple.

Animals Need Good Food Too

Getting food right is not just for humans. Aslan, our white shepherd, has a sweet disposition, but from the day we got him, he had chronic diarrhea and ear infections, and he was always anxious.

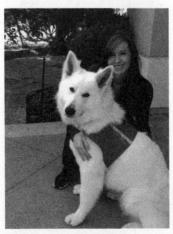

Aslan with Tana

One day we came home and found him bleeding, crying in the corner. He looked like he'd been attacked by another animal, and he wouldn't let me touch him.

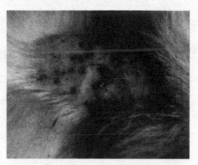

Aslan's macerated skin

We were horrified and spent thousands of dollars to find out he was having severe food allergies to the "high-quality" premium dog food we were feeding him. The vet suggested we put him on an elimination diet, which was funny, because we do that all the time for our patients. His new dog food had just five ingredients—lamb or duck, sweet potatoes, cranberries, blueberries, and kale. Sound familiar?

Within *one* week his skin cleared up, his fur became shiny, and he was happier, calmer, and more playful. Aslan has not been back to the vet for any medical problems in two years. Many people think good food is expensive, but being sick is *way* more expensive and painful. Food is medicine . . . or it is poison!

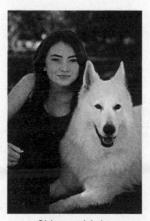

Chloe and Aslan

✓ *Say good-bye to sugar.*

Arguably the worst carbohydrate in terms of your overall health is sugar. Per person, Americans eat about 140 pounds of sugar a year. Refined sugar is 99.4 to 99.7 percent pure calories, with no vitamins, minerals, or other redeeming ingredients. And don't be fooled: Whether it comes from a beehive, a maple tree, or any other natural source, it is still sugar. In the past several years, many sources have suggested that diabetics should use the sweetener agave because of its high fructose content (a staggering 80 to 90 percent). Fructose is often called a low-glycemic sweetener because unlike sucrose it doesn't cause insulin to spike. However, fructose is toxic to the liver and may trigger metabolic syndrome, fatty liver, and insulin resistance.

When you eat any form of sugar, your blood sugar spikes, your pancreas releases insulin, your blood sugar drops, and you long for something sweet . . . which restarts the same cycle. Thus, when you eat sugar and simple carbs, you wind up craving them like a drug addict craves his drug.

Of course, that's just one of sugar's ill effects. Eating sugar and sugary foods increases inflammation and erratic brain cell firing, causes mineral deficiencies and overweight, and has been associated with increased triglycerides, as well as lower HDL and higher LDL cholesterol. As for its impact on the brain, sugar consumption has been linked with depression, ADHD, hyperactivity, and increased slow brain waves in brain imaging studies. Research at UCLA showed that sugar affects learning and memory as well.[23]

||||||||||||||||||||||||||||||||||||||||||||||||||||||||||||||||||||||||||||||||||||||||||||||||

How to Identify Sugar on Food Labels

Because two-thirds of packaged foods contain added sugar, it is critical to read food labels when you shop and know all the different aliases for sugar.[24]

- sugar
- molasses
- caramel color
- barley malt
- corn syrup
- corn syrup solids
- high fructose corn syrup
- honey
- sorbitol
- fructose
- cane juice crystals
- maltose
- fruit juice concentrate
- maltodextrin

||||||||||||||||||||||||||||||||||||||||||||||||||||||||||||||||||||||||||||||||||||||||||||||||

ARTIFICIAL SWEETENERS: NOTHING SWEET ABOUT THEM

Consuming artificial sweeteners regularly is not a recipe for good health. It can contribute to chronically high insulin, which increases your risk for Alzheimer's disease and raises the risk of heart disease, diabetes, metabolic syndrome, and other health problems. It's a fallacy that artificial sweeteners help you lose weight; on the contrary, they may lead to weight gain because they may lower metabolism. Animal research has shown that artificially sweetened food slowed metabolism and led to greater weight gain than sugar-sweetened foods—even though those animals eating the sugary foods consumed more calories. The bottom line: Whether the sweetener is aspartame (NutraSweet, Equal), saccharin (Sweet'N Low), or sucralose (Splenda), it is better to avoid it.

ERYTHRITOL AND STEVIA: BETTER ALTERNATIVES

Erythritol, a sugar alcohol that comes in crystals or powder form, has no calories and doesn't lead to blood sugar or insulin spikes. Use it with caution until you know how you react to it, since most sugar alcohols (such as xylitol and maltitol) cause GI distress.

Stevia, extracted from the leaf of an herb, is 200 to 300 times sweeter than sugar, but it does not affect blood sugar levels the way sugar does. In fact, it may stabilize blood sugar levels, enhance glucose tolerance, and lower blood pressure, but more research is needed. **Note:** Consult with a healthcare provider before using stevia if you take medication for blood pressure or diabetes.

✓ *Hydrate with H₂O.*

If you are a man, roughly 60 percent of your body is water; if you are a woman, about 55 percent. The percentage of your brain that is water is even higher: 80 percent. Water is essential for everything from lubricating your joints, flushing out waste products, and manufacturing hormones and neurotransmitters to regulating body temperature and helping deliver oxygen throughout your body. Not staying adequately hydrated has consequences for both brain and body: Research has shown that performance in tasks requiring attention, memory, and physical performance are diminished when you are just 2 percent dehydrated.[25] The elderly, in particular, need to make a point of drinking water because the mechanism that triggers thirst can become less efficient with age.

Staying adequately hydrated—which I define as drinking eight to ten glasses of clean water a day—is especially important if you are losing weight.

First, it helps prevent overeating. When you think you're hungry, you may actually be thirsty. Second, your body needs water to flush out the toxins released by stored body fat. Finally, if you drink two glasses (16 ounces) of water 30 minutes before a meal or snack, you can eat less and still feel satisfied. But dieting or not, avoid drinking water *with* your meals because it dilutes stomach acid, slowing digestion.

BRIGHT MINDS TIP

Cutting out sweet beverages like soda and fruit juice eliminates an average of 400 calories per day from the typical American diet!

Just as important as downing enough water is limiting liquid calories and dehydrating drinks. Replace sodas (including diet sodas), fruit juices, and other sugary drinks with water. (You can either swap those calories for an equivalent amount of healthier food or cut them entirely and could lose 40 pounds in one year.) Avoid caffeine, alcohol, and other diuretics, and when you sweat during exercise, be sure to replace those fluids.

||||||||||||||||||||||||||||||||||||||||||||||||||||||||||||||||||||||||||||||||||||||

Move on from Cow's Milk

It may have motherhood and childhood memories on its side, but cow's milk appears to be doing us more harm than good, according to accumulating scientific research. Take lactase, the enzyme needed to break down lactose (milk sugar) and digest milk. Much of the world's population is unable to produce the enzyme in their bodies. The resulting lactose intolerance can cause a lot of nasty GI tract troubles. Having the enzyme is no cause for celebration, however, since the products of lactose breakdown, galactose and glucose, elevate blood sugar and can cause inflammation.

Next there's casein, a protein in milk and an excitotoxin that can lead to brain inflammation and neurodegenerative diseases. Casein also binds to beneficial polyphenols found in coffee, tea, berries, and vegetables, making them unavailable when you combine milk with these foods. Several studies also show a link between drinking milk and Parkinson's disease, which may be due to pesticide exposure.[26] And hormones in the milk you drink—both bovine growth hormones and natural estrogens from pregnant cows—can increase the risk of prostate and breast cancers.[27] The natural estrogens are also suspected of contributing to early puberty in children.

If you are worried about where you will get your calcium, eating plenty of green leafy vegetables, exercising, and increasing your protein intake are much more effective ways to get it than drinking milk. Alternative milks (almond, coconut, hemp, or rice) are often calcium fortified, too—though they can be low in protein and high in sugar; choose brands carefully. Or try goat's milk, which has more protein, calcium, and magnesium than cow's milk. It's also naturally homogenized and easier to digest, though it does still contain lactose.

||||||||||||||||||||||||||||||||||||||||||||||||||||||||||||||||||||||||||||||||||||||||||||

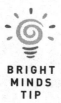

BRIGHT MINDS TIP   Swap regular butter for clarified butter, or ghee. It's the pure butterfat that remains once the allergenic milk proteins, casein and whey, have been removed.

✓ *Flavor your food with brain-smart herbs and spices.*

It's easy to forget that herbs and spices are not just flavor enhancers for food, but promoters of good health too. These plant-derived seasonings have a long history of medicinal uses that you can capitalize on in your cooking. (For ideas on how to incorporate them into your cooking, see *The Brain Warrior's Way Cookbook*.) Here are some of the most powerful memory-enhancing herbs and spices, along with a few of their benefits.

THE HERBS

- *Basil:* This potent antioxidant has been shown to improve blood flow to the brain, as well as improve cognitive function and prevent strokes.

- *Garlic:* Eating this bulbous herb increases blood flow and improves brain function. Regular consumption can help lower the risk of strokes and boost the immune system's ability to ward off colds and flu. Garlic can also help stabilize blood sugar and improve cholesterol levels.

- *Marjoram:* The lineup of nutrients in this pretty, sweet-flavored herb is impressive—vitamin C, beta carotene, vitamin A, lutein, and zeaxanthin, which are known to protect against age-related degenerative diseases and cataracts. Marjoram also has anti-inflammatory and antibacterial properties.

- *Mint:* The scent of peppermint improves memory and focus, and its oils can soothe digestive upsets.

- *Oregano:* A superstrong antioxidant (as its ORAC score attests), oregano protects brain and body cells from free radicals that can cause premature aging. It may also ease insomnia and relieve migraine headaches.

- *Rosemary:* Another ORAC star, this well-known herb has both antioxidant and anti-inflammatory properties. It improves circulation and digestion and offers protection from the cognitive decline associated with dementia. The smell of rosemary alone has been shown to help memory.[28]

- *Saffron:* This herb appears to increase serotonin levels in the brain. Multiple studies at the University of Tehran in Iran found that saffron was as effective as antidepressant medication in treating people with mild to moderate depression. Saffron can also improve memory and the ability to learn.

- *Sage:* Sage enhances memory and decreases the cognitive decline associated with Alzheimer's disease. The herb inhibits an enzyme that breaks down acetylcholine, a neurotransmitter that is memory enhancing at high levels.

- *Thyme:* This herb helps to protect neurons in the brain from premature aging. It also increases the amount of DHA in the brain. Thyme is so densely packed with polyphenols, vitamins, and minerals that it, too, has one of the highest ORAC values of all herbs.

THE SPICES

- *Black pepper:* This spice enhances absorption of numerous compounds, including curcumin (a powerful antioxidant). It also increases hydrochloric acid (stomach acid), which aids in digestion.

- *Cayenne pepper:* The bold taste in cayenne is created by capsaicin, a well-known pain reliever. It, too, increases hydrochloric acid and helps lower inflammation, improve immunity, and stimulate metabolism. A large population study found that people who ate red chili peppers had a 13 percent lower risk of death from heart disease and strokes than those who ate none.[29] Be careful to moderate your intake if you suffer from hypertension.

- *Cinnamon:* This sweet/savory spice has been shown to lower cholesterol, fasting glucose, and HbA1c levels and improve insulin sensitivity. It has also been found to improve working memory in older adults and in prediabetic people, while improving blood flow to the prefrontal cortex.

- *Cloves:* This fragrant super-antioxidant (it tops the ORAC list) has had many medicinal roles over the millennia, from soothing upset stomachs and tooth pain (clove oil) to relieving diarrhea and acting as an expectorant. It also contains eugenol, a potent anti-inflammatory. The familiar dried flower buds of the clove tree are a popular flavoring in many Middle Eastern and Asian cuisines.

- *Coriander:* The phytonutrients in coriander may help control blood sugar and lower cholesterol levels. It is rich in manganese, vitamin C, and vitamin K.

- *Curcumin:* A polyphenol mix from turmeric root that is used in curry, curcumin is the primary curcuminoid in turmeric. (Curcuminoids have been shown to decrease beta-amyloid plaques and inflammation.) In a double-blind, placebo-controlled study,[30] a special curcumin preparation with enhanced absorption (Longvida) improved memory and attention after just one hour. After four weeks, participants' working memory, energy levels, calmness and contentedness (measures of mood), and even fatigue induced by psychological stress all significantly improved.

- *Ginger:* The spice has anti-inflammatory properties that may protect against neurodegenerative diseases and reduce the oxidative stress that causes brain cells to age and die. Ginger contains natural agents to help decrease nausea and vomiting, and it may help lower cholesterol.

Note: Because of ginger's anticoagulant properties, check with your health-care provider before using ginger supplements if you are taking an anticoagulant medication.

- *Nutmeg:* This aromatic spice contains eugenol, a compound thought to protect the cardiovascular system. It also contains myristicin, which helps to prevent the formation of beta-amyloid plaques.

TAKE A BRIGHT MINDS APPROACH TO THE FOOD YOU EAT

Based on these 10 nutrition principles, here is a reminder of what to eat—and what to avoid—from a BRIGHT MINDS viewpoint. Knowing your personal risk(s) will help you choose the areas to focus on.

Blood Flow

FOODS TO CHOOSE	FOODS TO LOSE
Spices: cayenne pepper,[31] ginger, garlic,[32] turmeric,[33] coriander and cardamom,[34] cinnamon,[35] rosemary, and bergamot (for cholesterol-lowering properties)	Caffeine
	Soda, both regular and diet
Arginine-rich foods to boost nitric oxide and blood flow: beets, pork, turkey, chicken, beef, salmon, halibut, trout, steel-cut oats, clams, watermelon, pistachios, walnuts, seeds, kale, spinach, celery, cabbage, and radishes. Drinking nitrate-rich beet juice has been found to lower blood pressure, increase stamina during exercise, and in older people, boost blood flow to the brain.[36]	Baked goods
	French fries and other foods fried in vegetable oils
	Trans fats
Foods rich in vitamin B6, B12, and folate: leafy greens, cabbage, bok choy, bell peppers, cauliflower, lentils, asparagus, garbanzo beans, spinach, broccoli, parsley, cauliflower, salmon, sardines, lamb, tuna, beef, and eggs	Low-fiber "fast" foods
	More than two to four servings of alcohol a week
Vitamin E–rich foods to widen blood vessels and decrease clotting: green leafy vegetables, almonds, hazelnuts, and sunflower seeds	
Magnesium-rich foods to relax blood vessels: pumpkin and sunflower seeds, almonds, spinach, Swiss chard, sesame seeds, beet greens, summer squash, quinoa, black beans, and cashews	

Potassium-rich foods to help control blood pressure: beet greens, Swiss chard, spinach, bok choy, beets, brussels sprouts, broccoli, celery, cantaloupe, tomatoes, salmon, bananas, onions, green peas, sweet potatoes, avocados, and lentils

Fiber-rich foods, which have been shown to lower blood pressure[37] and improve cholesterol levels.[38] See page 239 in chapter 14.

Vitamin C–rich foods: See page 200 in chapter 12.

Polyphenol-rich foods: See page 118 in chapter 8.

Garlic-rich foods, which lower cholesterol

Omega-3-rich foods: See page 107 in chapter 7.

Maca, a root vegetable/medicinal plant native to Peru, which reduces blood pressure[39]

Retirement/Aging

FOODS TO CHOOSE	FOODS TO LOSE
Antioxidant-rich spices: cloves, oregano, rosemary, thyme, cinnamon,[40] turmeric, sage, garlic, ginger, and fennel[41]	**Sugar and foods that turn to sugar**
	Charred meats
Antioxidant-rich foods: acai fruit, parsley, cocoa powder, raspberries, walnuts, blueberries, artichokes, cranberries, kidney beans, blackberries, pomegranates, chocolate, olive and hemp oil (not for cooking at high temperatures), green and dandelion green tea	**Trans fats**
	If ferritin or iron levels are high, avoid foods with high dietary iron: red meat, spinach, chard, cumin, soybeans, collard greens, lentils, chickpeas, broccoli, leeks, beans, sprouts, asparagus, kelp, pumpkin and sesame seeds, olives
Choline-rich foods to support acetylcholine and memory:[42] shrimp, eggs, scallops, chicken, turkey, beef, cod, salmon, shiitake mushrooms, chickpeas, lentils, and collard greens	
Allicin-rich foods: See page 200 in chapter 12.	
Polyphenol-rich foods: See page 118 in chapter 8.	
Foods rich in vitamin B12 and folate: See page 77 in chapter 5.	

Inflammation

FOODS TO CHOOSE	FOODS TO LOSE
Anti-inflammatory spices: turmeric,[43] cayenne, ginger,[44] cloves, cinnamon,[45] oregano, pumpkin pie spice, rosemary, sage, and fennel[46]	**High omega-6 vegetables**: corn and soybeans
Folate-rich foods: spinach, dark leafy greens, asparagus, turnips, beets, mustard greens, brussels sprouts, lima beans, beef liver, root vegetables, kidney beans, white beans, salmon, and avocados	**High omega-6 vegetable oils:** corn, safflower, sunflower, soybean, canola, and cottonseed
Omega-3-rich foods; the best studied to lower cardiovascular risk and inflammation: flaxseeds, walnuts, salmon, sardines, beef, shrimp, walnut oil, chia seeds, and avocado oil	**Sugar and refined grains**
	Wheat flour
Prebiotic-rich foods: dandelion greens, asparagus, chia seeds, beans, cabbage, psyllium, artichokes, raw garlic, onions, leeks, and root vegetables (sweet potatoes, yams, squash, jicama, beets, carrots, and turnips)	**Trans fats:** anything with "partially hydrogenated" or "vegetable shortening" on the label
Probiotic-rich foods: brined vegetables (not vinegar), kimchi, sauerkraut, kefir, miso soup, pickles, spirulina, chlorella, blue-green algae, and kombucha tea	**Processed meats**
	Grain-fed meats
Tart cherry juice, which decreases levels of inflammatory CRP[47]	**Food additives**, such as MSG and aspartame
Magnesium-rich foods: See page 77 in chapter 5.	
Polyphenol-rich foods: See page 118 in chapter 8.	**Gluten and other foods that disrupt the gut lining**
Allicin-rich foods: See page 200 in chapter 12.	
Fiber-rich foods: See page 239 in chapter 14.	

Genetics

FOODS TO CHOOSE	FOODS TO LOSE
Spices to decrease beta amyloid: sage, turmeric, cinnamon, cardamom, ginger, and saffron	**Meals with high GI foods and lots of saturated fat**
Spices to decrease tau aggregation: cinnamon	
Foods to decrease beta amyloid: salmon, blueberries, and curry	**Processed cheeses and microwave popcorn**

Polyphenol-rich foods that contain quercetin and other ingredients that increase circulation, prevent LDL oxidation, and decrease inflammation and beta-amyloid plaques: chocolate, green tea, blueberries, kale, red wine, onions, apples, cherries, and cabbage

Foods rich in vitamin B6, vitamin B12, and folate: See page 77 in chapter 5.

Magnesium-rich foods: See page 77 in chapter 5.

Vitamin D-rich foods: See page 200 in chapter 12.

A ketogenic (very low carbohydrate) diet has been shown to decrease beta amyloid in animal models.[48]

Head Trauma

FOODS TO CHOOSE	FOODS TO LOSE
Spices to support brain healing: turmeric[49] and peppermint[50]	Alcohol
	Caffeine
Choline-rich foods to boost acetylcholine: shrimp, eggs, scallops, sardines, chicken, turkey, tuna, cod, beef, collard greens, and brussels sprouts	Sugar
	Fried foods
Omega-3-rich foods to support nerve cell membranes; see page 107 in chapter 7.	Processed foods
Other anti-inflammatory foods, such as prebiotic- and probiotic-rich foods: See opposite page or page 107 in chapter 7.	
Zinc-rich foods: See page 200 in chapter 12.	

Toxins

FOODS TO CHOOSE	FOODS TO LOSE
Foods that nourish your liver: green leafy vegetables for folate, an essential detoxification nutrient; protein-rich foods, including eggs; brassicas (any color cabbage, brussels sprouts, cauliflower, broccoli, and kale) for detoxification; oranges and tangerines (for vitamin C/limonene); berries; sunflower or sesame seeds (high in cysteine); and caraway and dill seeds (for limonene)[51]	**Foods that inhibit liver detoxification:** processed meats; grapefruit; capsaicin from red chili peppers; conventionally raised produce; dairy; grain-fed meats; and farmed fish

Foods that nourish your kidneys: water (drink 8 to 10 glasses a day); spices to support detoxification, including clove,[52] rosemary,[53] turmeric;[54] nuts and seeds, such as cashews, almonds, and pumpkin seeds for magnesium; green leafy vegetables; citrus fruits, except grapefruit; beet juice for circulation and endurance; ginger for its anti-inflammatory properties; blueberries (which increase filtration rate in kidneys), raspberries, strawberries, blackberries; garlic; and sugar-free chocolate to increase blood flow

Foods that nourish your skin: water; green tea; colorful fruits and vegetables for antioxidants, especially organic berries, kiwifruit, oranges, tangerines, pomegranates, broccoli, and peppers; avocados; olive oil; almonds, walnuts, sunflower seeds; wild salmon; and sugar-free chocolate

Foods that inhibit kidney detoxification: too much animal protein; excess salt; excess phosphates (processed cheeses, canned fish, processed meats, flavored water, sodas, nondairy creamers, bottled coffee drinks and iced teas)

Mental Health

FOODS TO CHOOSE	FOODS TO LOSE
Spices to support mental health: saffron,[55] turmeric (curcumin),[56] saffron plus curcumin,[57] peppermint (for attention problems),[58] and cinnamon (for attention problems,[59] ADHD,[60] and irritability)[61]	**Pro-inflammatory foods**
	Alcohol[68]
Dopamine-rich foods for focus and motivation: turmeric,[62] theanine from green tea,[63] lentils, fish, lamb, chicken, turkey, beef, eggs, nuts and seeds (pumpkin and sesame), high-protein veggies (such as broccoli and spinach), and protein powders	**Aspartame**[69]
	Caffeine[70]

Serotonin-rich foods for mood, sleep, pain, and craving control: combining tryptophan-containing foods, such as eggs, turkey, seafood, chickpeas, nuts, and seeds (building blocks for serotonin) with healthy carbohydrates, such as sweet potatoes and quinoa, elicits a short-term insulin response that drives tryptophan into the brain; dark chocolate[64] also increases serotonin.

GABA-rich foods for anti-anxiety: broccoli, almonds, walnuts, lentils, bananas, beef liver, brown rice, halibut, gluten-free whole oats, oranges, rice bran, and spinach

Choline-rich foods: See page 137 in chapter 9.

Fruits and vegetables for mood: Eat up to eight a day.[65]

Green tea

Maca, which has been shown to reduce depression[66]

Omega-3-rich foods to support nerve cell membranes and serotonin;[67] see page 107 in chapter 7.

Antioxidant-rich foods: See page 93 in chapter 6.

Magnesium-rich foods for anxiety: See page 77 in chapter 5.

Zinc-rich foods: See page 200 in chapter 12.

Foods rich in vitamin B6, vitamin B12, and folate: See page 77 in chapter 5.

Prebiotic-rich foods: See page 107 in chapter 7.

Probiotic-rich foods: See page 107 in chapter 7.

Immunity/Infection Issues

FOODS TO CHOOSE

Immunity-boosting spices: cinnamon (for antimicrobial activity),[71] garlic, turmeric, thyme, ginger, and coriander[72]

Allicin-rich foods to boost immunity: raw, crushed garlic, onions, and shallots

Quercetin-rich foods: red onions, red cabbage, red apples, cherries, red grapes, cherry tomatoes, teas, lemons, celery, and cocoa

Vitamin C-rich foods, which are natural blood thinners to boost circulation: oranges, tangerines, kiwifruit, berries, red and yellow bell peppers, dark green leafy vegetables (such as spinach and kale), broccoli, brussels sprouts, cauliflower, cabbage, tomatoes, and peas

Vitamin D-rich foods: fatty fish, including salmon (511 IUs in four ounces), sardines, tuna; eggs; mushrooms (maitake, morel, shiitake); beef liver; and cod liver oil

FOODS TO LOSE

Standard American diet[75]

Sodas, including diet sodas

Alcohol

Simple sugars

High omega-6s, found in most vegetable oils

Fried foods

Pesticide-laden foods

Dairy

Gluten

Zinc-rich foods: oysters, beef, lamb, spinach, shiitake and crimini mushrooms, asparagus, and sesame and pumpkin seeds

Mushrooms: shiitake,[73] white button, and portabella[74]

Selenium-rich foods: nuts (especially Brazil nuts), seeds, fish, grass-fed meats, and mushrooms

Omega-3-rich foods: See page 107 in chapter 7.

Prebiotic-rich foods: See page 107 in chapter 7.

Probiotic-rich foods: See page 107 in chapter 7.

Neurohormone Deficiencies

FOODS TO CHOOSE	FOODS TO LOSE
Fiber-rich foods, including those that contain lignin: green beans, peas, carrots, seeds, and Brazil nuts[76]	**Sugar and simple carbohydrates**
Hormone-supporting spices: garlic, licorice, sage, parsley, aniseed, red clover, and hops	**Protein from animals raised with hormones or antibiotics**
Eggs: Many hormones are made from cholesterol, so make sure you have enough cholesterol in your diet.	**Processed foods**
Testosterone-boosting foods: pomegranate, olive oil, oysters, coconut, brassicas (including cabbage, broccoli, brussels sprouts, and cauliflower), whey protein, and garlic	**Gluten** **Soy protein isolate**
Estrogen-boosting foods: flaxseeds, sunflower seeds, beans, garlic, yams, foods rich in vitamins C and Bs, beets, parsley, aniseed, red clover, licorice, hops, and sage	**Excitotoxins** including MSG, aspartame, hydrolyzed vegetable protein, sucralose, and "natural flavors" (which often contain MSG)
Thyroid-boosting (selenium-rich) foods: seaweed and sea vegetables, brassicas, and maca	
Progesterone-boosting foods: chasteberry and magnesium-rich foods; see page 224 in chapter 13.	**Foods/drinks that lower testosterone levels**: spearmint tea, soy, and licorice
Zinc-rich foods to boost testosterone; see above or page 200 in chapter 12.	
Prebiotic- and probiotic-rich foods: See page 107 in chapter 7.	

Diabesity

FOODS TO CHOOSE	FOODS TO LOSE
Spices: cinnamon,[77] turmeric, ginger, cumin,[78] garlic, cayenne, oregano, marjoram, sage, and nutmeg	**High-glycemic, low-fiber foods**
Fiber-rich foods to balance cholesterol and blood pressure: psyllium husk, navy beans, raspberries, broccoli, spinach, lentils, green peas, pears, winter squash, cabbage, green beans, avocados, coconut, figs, artichokes, chickpeas, and hemp and chia seeds	**Sugar** **Corn, peas** **Processed foods**
Polyphenol-rich foods/drinks, especially green tea, coffee, and blueberries; see page 118 in chapter 8.	**Dried fruits** **High-glycemic fruits** such as pineapple, watermelon, and ripe bananas
Protein-rich foods: eggs, meats, and fish	
Low-glycemic vegetables, such as celery, spinach, and brassicas (broccoli, brussels sprouts, cauliflower)	
Low-glycemic fruits, such as apples, oranges, blueberries, raspberries, blackberries, and strawberries	
Omega-3-rich foods: See page 107 in chapter 7.	
Magnesium-rich foods: See page 77 in chapter 5.	
Vitamin D–rich foods: See page 200 in chapter 12 or see page 283.	

Sleep

FOODS TO CHOOSE	FOODS TO LOSE
Sleep-enhancing spices, such as ginger	**Alcohol,** including wine
Melatonin-rich foods (melatonin is the hormone of sleep): tart cherry juice concentrate,[79] sour cherries, walnuts, ginger, asparagus, and tomatoes	**Caffeine,** including dark chocolate **Energy drinks**
Serotonin-rich foods: See page 180 in chapter 11.	**Spicy foods**, especially at night
Magnesium-rich foods: See page 77 in chapter 5.	
Healthy carbohydrates, such as sweet potatoes, quinoa, and bananas (which contain magnesium, too)	**Grapefruit**

Chamomile or passion fruit tea

Foods that contain diuretics: celery, cucumbers, radishes, and watermelon

Foods that contain tyramine: tomatoes, eggplant, soy, red wine, and aged cheeses

Unhealthy fatty foods

Black bean chili

High-protein foods, which are harder to digest

NOTE: Eat under low-stress conditions to allow for better digestion/absorption of nutrients.

CHAPTER 17

SHARPEN YOUR MEMORY
BRAIN WORKOUTS FOR
A RICHER LIFE

We must challenge the brain. It gets bored; we know that well.

MARIAN DIAMOND

Use it or lose it. The old adage is as true of your brain as it is of your muscles. When you learn something, new neural connections are created, which improves your capacity to remember. In fact, regardless of your age, mental exercise has an overall positive effect on your brain. On the other hand, when you stop learning, cognitive performance suffers as the internal connections in your brain begin to break apart.

Neuroscientist Marian Diamond, PhD, from the University of California, Berkeley, spent four decades researching the brain, and her findings revolutionized our understanding of brain health and neuroplasticity. In a lecture to the American Society on Aging, she said, "We now know that with proper stimulation and an enriched environment, the human brain can continue to develop at any age."

Diamond and her colleagues reached that conclusion after studying middle-aged rats, comparable to 60-year-old humans, as well as older rats, some equivalent in age to people in their nineties. When the researchers provided the rodents with toys, balls, mazes, and other active rats to provide companionship, the size and cognitive ability of the rats' brains increased. This was evident from the sprouting dendrites, nerve cells, blood vessels, and the thicker cerebral cortex of their brains.

Dr. Diamond, who died in 2017 at age 90, summarized the findings this way: "We can change the brain at any age. We're saying that if you use your brain you can change it as much as a younger brain." Although learning may take a bit more effort as we grow older, our brains can change for the better, especially if we keep them healthy with diet, exercise, challenge, newness, and love.

JIM KAROL: THE BRAIN'S MEMORY MAGIC

Mentalist Jim Karol is the human embodiment of Dr. Diamond's research. Jim grew up in Allentown, Pennsylvania, where he was a mediocre student

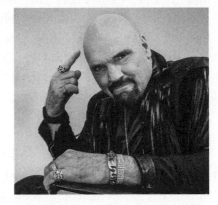

who was bullied because of his large frame. He attended a local college and ended up working in a steel mill. At the age of 29, he hurt his knees and was laid off from his job. It was then that he started working in a magic shop, where he discovered he had a talent for it. At 31, he started performing magic shows, and word spread about this "madman of magic." Before he knew it, Jim found himself on the front pages of newspapers across the country for correctly predicting the Pennsylvania lottery. He was asked to appear on several television shows, and his popularity began to grow. He became a hit on college campuses and was even invited to the White House.

Just before turning 50, Jim had a health crisis and was diagnosed with cardiomyopathy and an enlarged heart. His doctor told Jim that his heart looked like that of his 93-year-old mother, and there was nothing Jim could do but "enjoy the ride." Unsatisfied with the prognosis, Jim started a course of exercise under the direction of a physical therapist. Instead of watching TV as he rode a stationary bike, he started to use his mind. This man with such humble beginnings began memorizing the states and their capitals, more than 80,000 zip codes, every word in the Scrabble dictionary, and thousands of digits of pi. He knows the day of the week for every date from AD 1 on. If handed a just-shuffled deck of cards, he can memorize the order in less than a minute!

Jim was about to head overseas on a USO tour to entertain the troops when I met him through a mutual friend at Andrews Air Force Base. After I watched him memorize a deck of cards and then guess which card I had picked in my mind, I was completely blown away. As I got to know Jim, it became clear that he was focused on growing his brain.

Memory athlete is a term coined for people like Jim who are adept at these kinds of memory feats. Now, exciting new research from Stanford University School of Medicine and the Max Planck Institute of Psychiatry in Munich[1] has shown that mnemonic training, one of the methods favored by memory athletes, can be successfully taught to people without any special memory skills and that it "bulks up the brain's memory networks."[2] First, a group of brain athletes took a 72-word memorization test and, on average, were able to recall 71 words correctly. Then study participants who had no previous training practiced the techniques of these brain athletes and were tested 20 minutes and 24 hours later. They were tested again four months later (with a different set of words) and were able to remember nearly as many words as the brain athletes. (If you want to try some of these mnemonic exercises, see "Memory Strategies" on pages 295–298.)

The best mental exercises involve acquiring new knowledge and doing things you haven't done before. Even if your routine activities are fairly complicated, such as teaching a college course, reading brain scans, or fixing a crashed computer network, they won't help your brain as much as learning something new. Whenever the brain does something over and over, it learns how to do it using less and less energy. New learning, such as memorizing zip codes or learning a new game, helps establish new connections, thus maintaining and improving the function of less-often-used areas of the brain. When scientists tested Jim's hippocampus, it was in the top one percent for a person of his age and size.

The parts of your brain that you use will grow, and the parts of your brain you do not use will atrophy, or shrink. That tells us something about how to exercise the brain. Just doing crossword puzzles or sudoku won't give you the full possible benefits. That's like going to the gym and leaving after doing right bicep curls. Here are some ideas for doing "whole-brain combination workouts."

Prefrontal cortex (PFC) exercises

- *Language games* such as Scrabble (if you memorize the Scrabble dictionary, you will crush your friends), Boggle, and Words With Friends
- *Crossword puzzles*[3]
- *Speech and debate classes* in college; Toastmasters and other public speaking

- *Strategy games* such as chess and Risk
- *Tetris* (which also works the parietal and occipital lobes) can help decrease cravings for drugs (alcohol, nicotine, caffeine), food and drink, and activities (sex, exercise, gaming) after just three minutes.[4]
- *Prayer and meditation* may be the most powerful prefrontal cortex booster of all. I have published several studies on meditation, and I have seen how it reliably activates the PFC.[5] It improves focus, executive function, judgment, and impulse control, which results in more thoughtful and moral decisions. In a study, my friend and colleague Andrew Newberg, MD, a neuroscientist at Jefferson University Hospital, found increased blood flow to the PFC in participants engaged in meditative prayer. The Franciscan nuns in the study performed a practice called centering prayer, in which they focused their attention on a phrase from the Bible or a prayer over a period of time. Their goal was to open themselves "to being in the presence of God."[6]

||||||||||||||||||||||||||||||||||||||||||||||||||||||||||||||||||||||||||||||||||||||||

Soothe and Strengthen Your Brain with Scripture Meditation

Meditation, like prayer, is a well-known form of stress management. What may surprise you is the impact this practice has on your brain. Brain imaging shows that, rather than having a sedating, calming effect, meditating on a phrase or short portion of Scripture actually activates the prefrontal cortex, the most human and thoughtful part of your brain.

If you want to try meditating, first choose a favorite Bible verse. Then sit quietly and spend two to twenty minutes repeating the words over and over. If other thoughts come into your mind, imagine a big broom sweeping them away, so you focus only on the verse. During this time, allow your breathing to become slower, deeper, and more regular.

As an alternative, you might ponder a prayer or quote from a great Christian thinker. One of my favorite prayers for meditation is the Prayer of St. Francis of Assisi, which begins, "Lord, make me an instrument of your peace. Where there is hatred, let me sow love . . ." Meditation isn't a brain teaser; as you ponder and consider these truths, you will gain wisdom, perspective, and fresh insights.

|||||||||||||||||||||||||||||||||||||||||||||||||||||||||||||||||||||||||||||||||||||||||||||||||||||||

- *Weight training and aerobic activity (fast walking)*, when combined, increased executive function—which encompasses complex thought processes such as reasoning, planning, problem solving, and multitasking—in dementia patients.[7]

Temporal lobe exercises

- *Three-dimensional video games*, such as Super Mario 3D World—but not Angry Birds and other two-dimensional games—lead to enhanced hippocampal function.[8] The added complexity and special dimension in 3-D games means players have more to explore and learn than in 2-D games, strengthening the players' learning and memory.
- *Intensive learning*, such as medical or law school, has been shown to increase hippocampal size after just 14 weeks.[9]
- *Memorization of poetry and prose* increases hippocampal size.[10]
- *Memory and mnemonic training* (see page 297)[11]
- *Learning to play new musical instruments* strengthens the PFC, parietal lobes, and cerebellum.[12]
- *Physical exercise* also increases the hippocampus.[13] Learn a new sport as you are exercising for even greater benefit.

Parietal lobe exercises

- *Math games* like sudoku
- *Juggling*, which also involves the PFC, temporal lobes (hippocampus), occipital lobes, and cerebellum[14]
- *Golf, even for novices*; 40 hours of training increases gray matter in the parietal and occipital lobes[15]
- *Dance*, including the tango, even for those with Parkinson's disease[16]
- *Learning to read and play music*[17]
- *Map reading* without a GPS device

Basal ganglia exercises

- *Balancing*
- *Synchronizing arm and leg movements*
- *Manipulating props* like ropes and balls[18]

Cerebellum exercises

- *Coordination games* like table tennis (which also involves the PFC), dancing (and learning new dance steps), yoga, and tai chi
- *Basketball*[19]

MEMORY WORKOUTS BY BRAIN REGION

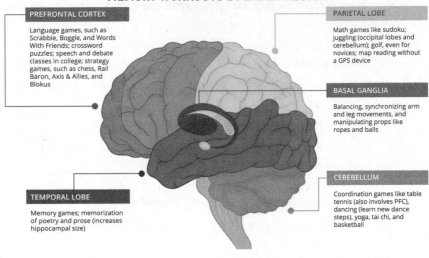

PREFRONTAL CORTEX

Language games, such as Scrabble, Boggle, and Words With Friends; crossword puzzles; speech and debate classes in college; strategy games, such as chess, Rail Baron, Axis & Allies, and Blokus

PARIETAL LOBE

Math games like sudoku; juggling (occipital lobes and cerebellum); golf, even for novices; map reading without a GPS device

BASAL GANGLIA

Balancing, synchronizing arm and leg movements, and manipulating props like ropes and balls

CEREBELLUM

Coordination games like table tennis (also involves PFC), dancing (learn new dance steps), yoga, tai chi, and basketball

TEMPORAL LOBE

Memory games; memorization of poetry and prose (increases hippocampal size)

BRIGHT MINDS TIP

The list of ways to stimulate your brain with new learning is endless. Just follow Marian Diamond's guidelines: Each activity should be challenging, new, and something you love.

Learning has a very real effect on neurons: It makes it easier for them to fire and to continue firing. There are approximately a thousand trillion synapses in the brain, and each one of them may wither and die if it is not actively firing. Like muscles that don't get used, idle nerve cells waste away. The brain has many different circuits connecting neurons in various parts of the brain. Any set of circuits that is not used grows weak.

Middle-aged people who go back to college, for example, often feel slow and stupid at first, and it takes a few semesters of mental exercise before they find academic studies easy again. Not only do they have to get back up to speed, the enzymatic activity in people's brain cells starts to decline as they get older. The cells become less efficient, so the 50-year-old's brain isn't quite as agile as an 18-year-old's. However, in some ways, younger people are at a disadvantage. The 50-year-old may actually do better in academic studies than his or her younger classmates because as one ages, the frontal lobes are better developed, which usually helps a person pay closer attention in class and ask better questions.

More developed frontal lobes allow you to take better advantage of new knowledge, know what to focus on, and relate that information to life experiences so it has more personal value. The 18-year-old may be able to memorize facts more easily, but his or her frontal lobes aren't as good at selecting *which* facts to memorize.

||||||||||||||||||||||||||||||||||||||||||||||||||||||||||||||||||||||||||||||||||||||||||||

10 More Ways to Exercise Your Brain to Boost Your Memory

Mental exercise is as important as diet and physical exercise for keeping both your body and brain strong. Here are activities that have been shown to make a difference.

1. **Dedicate yourself to new learning.** Devote just fifteen minutes a day to a new hobby, activity, or subject matter. Einstein once said that people who spend 15 minutes a day learning something new will become an expert within a year. As in school or business, commitment is critical if you want to reap the benefits.

2. **Be purposeful about cognitive training.** Community-dwelling seniors who took just a few weeks of cognitive training experienced significantly improved reasoning and speed of processing skills, as well as fewer difficulties with the activities of daily living 10 years later, compared with those who didn't get such training.[20] On our online portal Brain Fit Life (www.mybrainfitlife.com), we have cognitive brain training games for just this purpose.

3. **Take a class about something new and interesting.** Community colleges and online groups offer low-cost

courses on a wide variety of subjects. Challenge your brain to learn novel and interesting things by enrolling in a class that is unrelated to your work or daily life. Examples include square-dancing (great exercise), conversational Spanish, chess, tai chi, astronomy, or sculpture. Working with modeling clay or Play-Doh can help children or adults develop new neural connections, as well as agility and hand-brain coordination.

4. **Cross-train at work.** Learning someone else's job or even switching jobs for several weeks provides workers with better skills and brain function, and may offer the employer greater flexibility. In a grocery store, for example, employees can be taught to work as checkout clerks and to stock shelves, order products, and rotate among the produce, grocery, and dairy sections of the store.

5. **Limit television for kids and adults.** Adults who watched two or more hours of TV a day had a significantly higher risk of Alzheimer's disease. Watching TV is usually a "no brain" activity. To be fair, these studies did not specify if watching programs that teach you something, such as one of my shows on public television, had the same effect as situation comedies or sports.

6. **Alter daily routines to stimulate new parts of your brain.** Do the opposite of what feels natural to activate the other side of your brain and gain access to both hemispheres. When you write, dress, brush your teeth, set the table, shoot basketballs, play table tennis, or use your computer mouse, use your nondominant hand. These changes make your brain feel uncomfortable—in essence, breaking the patterned routine in your life and challenging your brain to make new connections.

7. **Travel to new and interesting places.** Exposing the brain to unique experiences, scents, sights, and people strengthens the brain. Using maps stimulates the brain in different ways and also exercises the parietal lobes, which are responsible for visual-spatial guidance.

8. **Develop friendships with smart people.** You become like the people you hang out with. You can trade ideas, get new perspectives, and generally stretch your mind if you are

surrounded by fascinating folks. Most of us know that to improve when playing any game, we have to play with people who are better than we are. The same principle holds true in pushing your brain to new heights. Spend time with people who challenge you.

9. **Use music to enhance your mind.** There is significant research suggesting that both learning to play music and listening to music, especially classical music, can enhance memory and mood. Classical music also enhances memory and cognitive function.[21] Listening to Mozart or Strauss for just 25 minutes, for example, has been shown to lower blood pressure and the stress hormone cortisol, while listening to ABBA has been shown to lower cortisol.[22] Listening to peaceful and joyful music lowered anxiety and depression.[23] Learning to play music helped to increase the size of the hippocampus.[24] Grab your guitar! Stevie Wonder once said, "Music, at its essence, is what gives us memories." Research shows that listening to happy or peaceful music leads to the recall of positive memories, while listening to frightening or sad music dredges up mostly negative memories.[25] Music matters.

10. **Treat learning problems.** Numerous studies show that better-educated people are at a lower risk of developing Alzheimer's disease and cognitive decline. Yet millions of children, teens, and adults struggle in school or with learning, despite having normal or even high intelligence. Often these difficulties stem from ADD or other learning issues. Recognizing and addressing these problems are essential to making "lifelong learning" a reality. You can take an online test to help you determine whether you have ADD at www.amenclinics.com.

‖‖

MEMORY STRATEGIES

Given all the information on rescuing your brain in this book, you may still be asking: *Are there specific exercises I can do to boost my memory?* Yes! BRIGHT MINDS is an example of a mnemonic, or a memory aid. It helps me immediately remember all 11 risk factors, so when I teach or talk about them on TV, I can sail through rather complicated material without any notes. It took my staff and me a while to come up with the mnemonic, but it was worth it.

I'd like to share three other memory magic tools that I've used with my patients and that I use myself to improve my ability to store and retain information. They are the types of tools that Jim Karol and other memory athletes use.

1. **Rhymes are a very popular tool for recalling rules or organization.** As children, most of us were taught certain popular rhymes to help us learn to spell, understand the time change each spring and fall, and familiarize ourselves with the number of days in each month of the year:

   - "*I* before *e* except after *c*"
   - "Spring ahead in spring; fall back in fall."
   - "Thirty days hath September, April, June, and November; all the rest have thirty-one, except February, which stands alone."

   Rhymes help connect into a metrical pattern those items that otherwise may seem totally unrelated. They help establish a definite informational progression because any mistake in the order of recall will destroy the rhyme. Following is an example of using a nursery rhyme ("One is a bun; two is a shoe," etc.) to help retain a sequence of facts:

   To use this mnemonic, choose 10 facts that you need to remember in a precise order and mentally picture an association between each one and its corresponding number's object. In less than a few minutes, you can easily memorize their order. Try this method with unrelated facts to observe its usefulness to you.

   As an example from my own life, here is a list of items I need to get at the store:

   1. Salmon
   2. Turkey
   3. Unsweetened almond milk
   4. Eggs
   5. Stevia
   6. Kale
   7. Sparkling water

8. Spinach, olive oil
9. Oranges
10. Coconut

It took me about two minutes to make the following associations:

1. One is a bun: I picture a salmon trying to jump out of the bun.
2. Two is a shoe: A turkey walks around in colorful high heels.
3. Three is a tree: An almond milk tree drips milk on the kids below, who are crying.
4. Four is a door: Someone has thrown eggs at the door, and I'm really mad about it.
5. Five is a hive: Bees are flying around a stevia plant.
6. Six are sticks: A kid at the fair holds organic kale on a stick, instead of cotton candy, and refuses to eat it.
7. Seven is heaven: I am handed a flute of champagne, but since it is heaven, it is really sparkling water.
8. Eight is a gate: Popeye stands outside my front gate, eating spinach with one hand and picking up Olive Oyl with the other.
9. Nine is a line: Oranges are lined up for miles in Orange County, where I live.
10. Ten is a hen: A clucking chicken runs around the yard dressed in a bikini with a coconut on its head.

Once I'm in the store, I run through these images in my head so I can remember the items I need to pick up—no written list needed. The more you do this exercise, the easier it becomes and the bigger your hippocampus may grow.

2. **Make words or phrases from the first letters of the words you need to remember—like BRIGHT MINDS.** When I have a series of facts to memorize, I immediately write down the first letter of each one to see if I can arrange them into an associative word or phrase. An example of this method:

On old Olympus' towering top, a Finn and German viewed a hop.

I learned this rhyme in medical school. Each first letter corresponds to the first letter of the twelve cranial nerves in their proper order: olfactory, optic, ocular, trochlear, trigeminal, abduceus, facial, acoustic, glossal pharyngeal, vagus, accessory, and hypoglossal.

BRASS is used by marksmen to remember the steps in firing a rifle: breathe, relax, aim, stabilize, and squeeze.

3. **Use places to remember specific things.** The Greek poet Simonides[26] was said to have left a banquet just before the roof collapsed and killed all those inside. Even though many bodies were unrecognizable, Simonides was able to identify them by their places at the table. The practical use of this technique involves visualizing what you want to remember in a certain location. Then when you go back to the location in your mind, the object or fact should come back to you. For example, when memorizing a speech that you have organized and outlined, choose the ideas or the major subdivisions and associate them in some way with the different rooms in your home. As you deliver the speech, imagine yourself walking from room to room discovering the associations you have made in the proper order.

In order to make this effective, use these two tips:

1. Make it active: Your brain does not think in still photographs, so the more action there is, the more details you can employ in a scene.
2. Make the picture as crazy and disproportionate as possible: It will be easier to remember the details as you recall the strange or unique things in the picture.

If you practice this technique, your associative powers will become limited only by the number of locations you can think of. I imagine walking in my front door, then the living room, dining room, kitchen, family room, and so on. You can associate literally hundreds of items and ideas with the insides of most homes.

USE YOUR MEMORY TO FEEL GREAT ANYTIME, ANYWHERE

Many people struggle with anxiety and depression because they have trouble forgetting their fears, their frustrations, and the negative events in their lives. Their undisciplined minds constantly go to places of anger, regret, and sadness. Recognizing these tendencies in others, I have developed a memory technique that relies on the power of associations and places to help you feel great anytime, anywhere. Using your memory will help you counteract the negative and accentuate the positive.

Begin by writing down your best 10 to 30 memories of all time (constantly update them as new memories come into your life). Then peg them to specific places in your home or another location. Here is an example from my own life.

As of this writing, 12 of my favorite memories are:

1. Marrying Tana and going on our honeymoon, which continues to this day
2. Being completely in love with our dog, Aslan, and cat, Miso
3. Helping my dad get well at the age of 87 and sharing his amazing story with the world
4. Having *Discover* magazine list our research on brain imaging as one of the top 100 stories in science for 2015
5. Eating dinner with my teenage daughter Breanne when she told me, "I kicked butt in a debate today, Dad"
6. Sitting at the dinner table playing strategy games with my son, Antony, when he was a child (he is now 40) and having him whip me
7. Having the world's most amazing, consistently loving mom
8. Standing at the stove with my grandpa when I was four years old
9. Being one of the chief architects with Pastor Rick Warren and Mark Hyman, MD, of *The Daniel Plan*, a program to make the world healthier through churches, done in thousands of congregations around the world
10. Watching my daughter Kaitlyn, now 30, perform in *Pocahontas* in second grade
11. Sitting with my then-two-year-old daughter Chloe, now 14, atop my shoulders at a Los Angeles Lakers game as she kissed my head and told me she loved me
12. Playing in the 1999 US Nationals Table Tennis Tournament

Walking through my home, here is how I peg these 12 memories to specific places using action and exaggeration.

1. At the front door—Carrying Tana across the threshold while she pleads for me not to drop her. (I almost dropped her when we practiced our wedding dance the night before we were married. We still laugh about it.)

2. In the foyer—Aslan and Miso are always there to greet me when I come home, looking for love. Well, Aslan is always there, wagging his tail; you never know about a cat.

3. In the living room to the right of the foyer—My 88-year-old dad is in his workout clothes, doing jumping jacks, getting ready to go to the gym to lift weights. He once did a six-minute plank, completely dominating me. I wimped out at three minutes but was so proud of him.

4. In the living room, where we put our Christmas tree—My friend and research collaborator Cyrus Raji, MD, gave me a framed copy of our *Discover* magazine honor, where our research was listed as one of the top 100 stories in science for 2015. We were listed at number 19. I also see a miniature Tesla car going around the room—Tesla was listed at number 18—being chased by a new vegan dinosaur species, listed at number 20.

5. In the dining room, next to the living room—At the table I see my daughter Breanne as a teenager (she is now 34 and the mother to two of my grandchildren). She winks at me and says, "I kicked butt in a debate today, Dad." In high school, she went from being shy to very confident, which made my heart soar.

6. In the dining room at the dinner table—I see my son, Antony, playing strategy games with me when he was a boy. He is very intense thinking about his next move. He is so smart; he started beating me at them early.

7. In the kitchen, which smells amazing—My mom is making a tantalizing salad with lemon, olive oil, fresh crushed garlic, avocados from my dad's ranch, grilled lamb, and asparagus. She's excited to hear about my day.

8. In the kitchen, at the stove—My four-year-old self is standing on a step stool, smiling, next to my grandfather, after whom I was named. He was my best friend when I was growing up. He has on his white apron, and we are preparing sugar-free chocolate-and-cashew-butter cups, a healthy, delicious version of the candy we used to make together. That way I can keep him with me longer.

9. In the kitchen, next to the sink—On the counter is a copy of *The Daniel Plan* and the accompanying cookbook. On top of the books, tens of thousands of tiny people are running around waving broccoli florets, symbolizing all the people who have undertaken our program.

10. In the family room, next to the kitchen—I see my then-seven-year-old daughter Kaitlyn in front of the TV performing in *Pocahontas*. She loved to perform, and being in front of the TV, blocking our view, never troubled her.

11. On the way upstairs—I see Chloe's room and imagine the zebra-hooded sweater she wore as she sat on my shoulders at the Lakers game, where she kissed my head and told me she loved me.

12. In my office upstairs—I see our Ping-Pong table, triggering the memory of the US Nationals, where I had a great time playing the game my mother taught me as a child.

Try this exercise on your own. Then anytime you feel sad or upset, walk through the house in your mind and trigger the positive memories, which in turn will trigger the release of positive chemicals in your brain to help you feel great.

 ## PICK ONE HEALTHY, MEMORY-SHARPENING HABIT TO START TODAY

1. **Dedicate yourself to new learning by devoting just 15 minutes a day to it.**

2. Grow your hippocampus: Break your routine and focus on learning things you love that are new and challenging.

3. **Do whole-brain workouts, including exercises to boost your prefrontal cortex (language and strategy games, prayer and meditation), temporal lobes (memory games and musical training), parietal lobes (math games, golf, and juggling), and cerebellum (coordination games, such as table tennis and dancing).**

4. Sign up for a course or conference on an unfamiliar topic that interests you.

5. Use your nondominant hand when brushing your teeth this week.

6. Cultivate friendships with smart people.

7. Listen to classical music and/or learn to play music.

8. Treat any learning problems as soon as possible.

9. Improve your recall with memory devices or mnemonics, especially rhymes and place anchors. Learn how to use them to your advantage.

10. Boost your mood anytime, anywhere, by writing down your top 10 to 30 memories and anchoring them to places in your home.

CHAPTER 18

MEMORY MEDICATIONS
WHEN AND WHAT TO CONSIDER

Medications almost always do it better if they're used in conjunction with other supports.
MEHMET OZ, MD

When it comes to addressing memory issues, there has been general disappointment with the medications currently available. None of them *cure* memory problems; they help only in the moment they are taken. Memory problems have too many causes for any silver bullet to do as much as was hoped. Yet pharmaceutical companies continue to spend billions of dollars with the hope of finding the next Prozac or Viagra. If we spent the same resources and scientific effort on prevention and lifestyle interventions, we would be much further ahead. But medications do have a place and can be worth a try. If your memory problems are not responding to simpler interventions, talk with your health-care professionals about medications. In this section, I'll review several of the most common medications and explain how we use them at Amen Clinics.

NAMENDA (MEMANTINE)

Namenda is approved for moderate to severe Alzheimer's disease. It has been shown to boost blood flow to the prefrontal cortex and, in some cases, delay the progression of the disease in its middle stages.

The drug modulates or partly blocks a receptor called N-methyl D-aspartate (NMDA), regulating the release of the neurotransmitter glutamate. This is important because excessive production of glutamate allows too much calcium to enter cells, which then turns on genes that are programmed to kill the neurons. (One take-home message: Don't overdo it with calcium supplements.)

Namenda sometimes produces substantial benefits in those with dementia. One of the more striking effects is the reduction in spasticity, which causes people to lose their balance, fall, or struggle to walk. Namenda can also help improve speech and fine motor skills, as well as reduce urinary incontinence. When Namenda is effective, the changes may be dramatic, easing the stress and burden on caregivers. Dosing usually starts at 5 mg a day for two weeks and is increased slowly to the maximum (typically 20 mg, although sometimes as much as 40 mg).

I've also seen this medication provide dramatic improvement in younger patients with mobility and speech issues. As a child, Ralph, a young man we saw at Amen Clinics, had a viral infection in his brain. Afterward, he struggled with his memory and learning. He also could no longer perform coordinated movements, speak clearly, or behave appropriately at work or in social settings. He had been fired several times because of his "poor attitude."

His SPECT scan showed almost no activity in the cerebellum. It also showed low activity in his prefrontal cortex (affecting judgment, impulse control, and concentration) and right temporal lobe (hampering his ability to read social cues), and increased activity in the anterior cingulate gyrus (often associated with trouble shifting attention, cognitive inflexibility, and oppositional and difficult behavior). After we treated him for three months with Namenda, his family reported that his coordination, speech, behavior, and job performance had all improved. A second SPECT scan looked much better as well.

**RALPH'S BRAIN SPECT SCANS (UNDERSIDE SURFACE VIEWS)
BEFORE AND AFTER TREATMENT WITH NAMENDA**

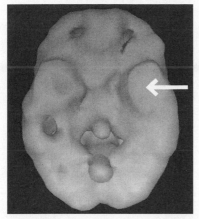 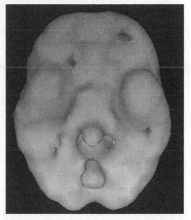

Before treatment: Decreased activity
in PFC, right temporal lobe

After treatment: Overall improved activity

THE CHOLINESTERASE INHIBITORS (EXELON, RAZADYNE, AND ARICEPT)

As we age, acetylcholine, the neurotransmitter most often associated with memory, declines. Improving the availability of acetylcholine in the brain has been shown to help sustain memory. One way to do this is to inhibit the enzymes that break it down. These medications are called acetylcholinesterase (AChE) inhibitors, or "cholinesterase" inhibitors, and tend to work by increasing blood flow in the prefrontal cortex and temporal lobes. Three are prescribed most often.

Important differences among the cholinesterase inhibitors may determine how effectively they work in people with significant memory issues. Because acetylcholine neurons are found throughout the cerebral cortex, increasing acetylcholine can strengthen many abilities. These medications reduce behavioral problems and, in the earlier stages of Alzheimer's disease, improve attention, short-term memory, comprehension, communication, and the ability to recognize people and objects.

Early treatment is critical, since people whose abilities are already severely impaired do not see significant gains. I have treated many patients with significant memory problems who had symptoms for less than six months, and in these patients, short-term memory has often improved.

Many patients seek help for existing problems; however, just as important is delaying or halting the progression of the disease process itself. Exelon, Razadyne, and Aricept differ most in how they seek to slow the disease.

1. **Exelon (rivastigmine).** All three of these drugs block AChE, but only Exelon blocks butyrylcholinesterase (BuChE), the other enzyme that breaks down acetylcholine.[1] About 80 percent of the cholinesterase is AChE and 20 percent is BuChE in people who are aging normally. However, as Alzheimer's disease (AD) progresses, the amount of AChE decreases and the amount of BuChE increases to the point where they are about equal. Both AChE and BuChE must be blocked to stall the progression of AD. At present, the only medication that does this is Exelon, which is why it is often my first choice, especially in the later stages of memory problems.

2. **Razadyne (galantamine).** Another option is Razadyne, which does not block BuChE and cannot raise the level of acetylcholine the way that Exelon can. However, Razadyne increases the levels of many different neurotransmitters, which generally increases brain activity.[2]

3. **Aricept (donepezil).** The first well-tolerated cholinesterase inhibitor produced in the United States, Aricept (donepezil) is now the most commonly prescribed of the cholinesterase inhibitors. (Though Cognex [tacrine] was the first cholinesterase inhibitor approved by the FDA, the medication produced many intolerable side effects and is no longer available in the United States.) Aricept is particularly effective in helping patients with mild AD, and patients report fewer side effects from it than from either Exelon or Razadyne. In addition, it needs to be given only once a day. Although its advantages make it attractive, particularly to busy physicians, it also has a couple of significant drawbacks that prevent it from being the first choice of many neurologists and psychiatrists.

   Because Aricept (like Razadyne) does not block BuChE, it is less effective at blocking the accumulation of beta-amyloid plaques. Aricept (like Exelon) does not bind to the nicotinic receptor, so it does not increase overall brain activity as effectively as Razadyne, and it may not block programmed cell death.

One of my colleagues has switched hundreds of memory-loss patients who were declining on Aricept to Exelon. About half of these patients noticeably improved on Exelon. In one research study, approximately 300 people with mild to moderate dementia who showed no benefit on Aricept were switched to Exelon and treated for six months. Of this group, half showed improvements in daily activities, behavior, and/or mental abilities on Exelon.[3]

Side effects of the cholinesterase inhibitors

About 10 to 20 percent of people who take these medications experience side effects. For instance, some people become aggressive, but that often occurs with improvement in mental abilities. Fortunately, any aggression usually resolves within two weeks, and in many cases, families prefer not to stop or decrease the medication because their loved one is functioning so much better.

The primary side effects of Exelon and Razadyne are nausea, vomiting, loss of appetite, dizziness, lightheadedness or fainting, generalized weakness, and muscle pain. These side effects are not related to the stomach or heart; rather, they result from increasing acetylcholine activity in the brain stem. Groups of brain-stem neurons control vomiting (to keep you from swallowing things that will kill you), breathing, heart rate, blood pressure, and metabolism. Acetylcholine slows the heart rate, which causes a drop in blood pressure. The fainting, lightheadedness, or dizziness that results is usually not life threatening and can be managed by reducing the dose of Exelon or Razadyne.

Aricept has similar side effects to Exelon and Razadyne, but they are less frequent. Aricept can also cause nightmares in some people who take it at bedtime. However, nightmares can usually be avoided by taking Aricept in the morning instead.

STIMULATING MEDICATIONS

Stimulant medications, such as Ritalin (methylphenidate) and Adderall (amphetamine salts), have been used to help enhance focus, memory, motivation, and learning. They are classically used to treat children who have attention deficit disorder (ADD)—also known as attention deficit hyperactivity disorder (ADHD)—but I have had good success using them with people of all ages. They work by enhancing dopamine production in the basal ganglia and can increase blood flow to the prefrontal cortex and temporal lobes. If you have had ADD/ADHD symptoms throughout your life (short attention span, distractibility, disorganization, restlessness, and impulse-control issues), these meds are worth considering.

Stimulants tend to help people who have low prefrontal cortex function after a traumatic brain injury, mold exposure, or infections.[4] Research also suggests they can reduce poor decision making and apathy in those with dementia.[5]

Because of the potential for addiction and side effects, Ritalin and Adderall are often not our first choices for patients with memory issues, but they should be considered if natural treatments are ineffective.

Provigil (modafinil) and Nuvigil (armodafinil) are commonly prescribed for narcolepsy. They also have been found to heighten alertness and boost higher-order cognitive functions in many studies.[6] In my experience, these medications can help with energy, focus, and memory. They have fewer side effects than Ritalin and Adderall but also tend to have a milder effect. One of my ADD patients who could not tolerate Ritalin or Adderall (he lost his appetite and his heart raced) was able to finish his doctorate on Provigil. He said it gave him sustained focus for six to eight hours.

Other medications, like selegiline (an antidepressant), reportedly have neurotrophic, or brain-enhancing, effects, but the research has been inconsistent.

I tell my patients that the issue should never be whether they are on or off medication, but rather what supports their best functioning. If medications can help, I encourage patients to think of them like eyeglasses, which we would never withhold from someone who could benefit from them.

CHAPTER 19

BRAIN-ENHANCEMENT THERAPIES
INNOVATIVE WAYS TO STRENGTHEN YOUR MEMORY

Although the world is full of suffering, it is also full of the overcoming of it.

HELEN KELLER

One of the most exciting lessons I've learned from looking at the brain is that there are many ways to strengthen it. Terry is one of my favorite examples. She shows that when one family member makes important lifestyle changes, others often follow suit.

Terry is the CEO of Amen Clinics. Before working with us, she was the CEO of AutoZone, Frederick's of Hollywood, and a number of other high-profile companies. My favorite story about Terry? She delivered one of her children while involved in a critical financial negotiation that rescued a billion-dollar company and 25,000 jobs. At 63, Terry is an older mom with kids ages 19 and 20 who still depend on her.

When her daughter was struggling in school, Terry brought her to Amen Clinics, and it transformed the girl's life.

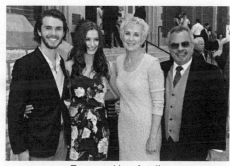

Terry and her family

That's when Terry fell in love with our mission. Curious about her own brain, Terry decided to get scanned. She had suffered eight concussions racing cars, had been electrocuted in an improperly wired elevator, and had been exposed to arsenic while being treated for tropical sprue when she was in the Peace Corps in Haiti.

Terry's brain looked damaged. The chronic work stress, insomnia, head injuries, and toxic exposure were visible on her scan, which revealed overall low blood flow, indicated by the holes and dents.

TERRY'S BRAIN SPECT SCANS

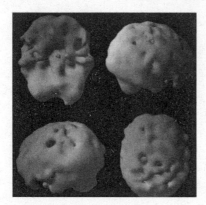 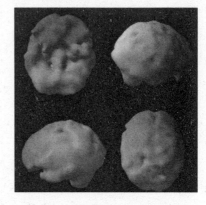

| Before treatment: severe decreases in blood flow | After treatment: significant overall improvement in activity and blood flow |

TERRY'S BRIGHT MINDS RISK FACTORS AND TREATMENT PLAN

BRIGHT MINDS	TERRY'S RISK FACTORS	INTERVENTIONS
Blood Flow	Low blood flow on SPECT	Exercise, diet, ginkgo biloba, and other supplements
Retirement/Aging	Early sixties	Continual new learning
Inflammation		
Genetics		
Head Trauma	Eight concussions, electrocution	Nutraceuticals and hyperbaric oxygen therapy
Toxins	Arsenic exposure	Support all the organs of detoxification

BRIGHT MINDS	TERRY'S RISK FACTORS	INTERVENTIONS
Mental Health	Chronic work stress from being a CEO	Stress management tools
Immunity/Infection Issues	Low vitamin D	Vitamin D3 supplements
Neurohormone Deficiencies		
Diabesity		
Sleep Issues	Chronic insomnia	Sleep hygiene, melatonin, magnesium, hypnosis strategies

The scan made Terry appropriately anxious about her brain. She had spent her life taking care of others; now it was time for her to take care of herself. Eleven months after she started on our program—which included our BRIGHT MINDS strategies, especially significant dietary changes, targeted supplements, 40 sessions in a hyperbaric oxygen chamber, and the sale of her Ducati motorcycle—Terry's scan looked much healthier and showed better activity overall. She became a more effective CEO for us as her focus and follow-through improved. Now, rather than becoming a burden to her children, she will likely be a positive force in their lives for decades to come.

It's worth repeating again and again: Your brain can be better, even if you've been bad to it, and with a better brain always comes a better life.

This chapter will discuss four innovative treatments to enhance your brain:

- Hyperbaric oxygen therapy (HBOT)
- Transcranial magnetic stimulation (TMS)
- Neurofeedback
- Audiovisual entrainment (AVE)

In addition, you'll learn which health issues each may help treat. Depending on your own risk factors, you may want to explore how one or more of these therapies might fit into your own Memory Rescue plan.

HYPERBARIC OXYGEN THERAPY: THE CHAMBER OF HEALING

I first became interested in hyperbaric oxygen therapy (HBOT) in the 1990s after listening to Michael Uszler, MD, a nuclear medicine physician, give a lecture on it at UCLA. Michael was one of the original pioneers in using brain SPECT imaging in the 1980s, and at this lecture he showed before-and-after SPECT scans of his patients who had undergone HBOT. They showed remarkable improvement in blood flow. As I started recommending this treatment, I saw the same improvement for many of our patients with low blood flow.

The body requires healthy oxygen levels in order to heal. HBOT uses the power of oxygen to create a regenerative environment inside the body, speeding up the healing process and reducing inflammation. During HBOT, a person lies down or sits in a chamber where the air pressure is 1.3 to 2 times greater than normal air pressure. This increased pressure allows the lungs to gather more oxygen. That means more oxygen gets into blood vessels and tissues, which can increase production of growth factors and stem cells, promoting healing.

Normally, only red blood cells carry oxygen throughout the body. With HBOT, oxygen dissolves into other bodily fluids, such as plasma, and can be carried to regions with low or damaged circulation. When someone is dealing with vascular problems, strokes, or nonhealing wounds, for example, adequate oxygen cannot reach damaged areas, so the body's natural healing ability is ineffective. When extra oxygen is able to reach these troubled areas, it speeds the healing process. Researchers have found that increased oxygen strengthens the ability of white blood cells to kill bacteria, reduces swelling, and allows new blood vessels to grow into damaged areas. HBOT is a simple, noninvasive, and painless treatment with minimal side effects.

In a study from Taiwan, HBOT reversed brain damage in patients who had significant neurological issues caused by carbon monoxide poisoning.[1] HBOT may be able to improve a person's quality of life when standard medicine is not working. Some research also suggests it may be helpful for several other conditions:

- head injuries[2]
- stroke[3]
- fibromyalgia[4]
- Lyme disease (as a helpful add-on treatment)[5]
- burns[6]

- diabetic ulcers and complications[7]
- wound healing[8]
- multiple sclerosis[9]
- inflammatory bowel disease[10]
- postsurgical healing[11]
- autism[12]
- cerebral palsy[13]

Improvement in soldiers

In 2011, Paul Harch, MD, and I, along with a number of colleagues, published a study on 16 soldiers who had experienced blast-induced traumatic brain injuries. They were studied with brain SPECT imaging and neuropsychological testing before and after 40 sessions of HBOT. Following treatment, our patients demonstrated significant improvement in their symptoms, full-scale IQ (a term for complete cognitive capacity; up 14.8 points), delayed and working memory scores, tests of impulsivity, mood, anxiety, and quality of life scores. Their SPECT scans showed remarkable overall improvement in blood flow.

COMPOSITE SCAN OF SOLDIERS' BRAINS BEFORE AND AFTER HBOT

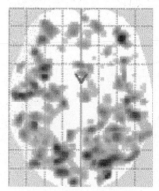

Increased blood flow after 40 sessions of HBOT indicated by dark areas on scan

Improvement in NFL and NHL players

Many of the NFL and NHL (National Hockey League) players treated at Amen Clinics also improved after undergoing HBOT treatments. Marvin Fleming, the first player in NFL history to play in five Super Bowls, is a good example. He played tight end for 12 years—first for the Green Bay Packers and then for the Miami Dolphins, including during the Dolphins' perfect season in 1972. When he first came to see us at age 67, his brain was in trouble. All our players undergo extensive cognitive testing, and Marvin's general cognitive testing was not good. But he made every healthy change we prescribed for him, including losing weight, eating right, taking supplements, and completing 40 sessions of HBOT. Two years later, he had lost 20 pounds, his brain looked dramatically younger (as did he), and his cognitive scores had improved by as much as 300 percent.

MARVIN'S "BEFORE" AND "AFTER" BRAIN SPECT SCANS

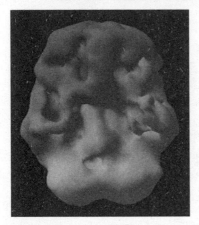 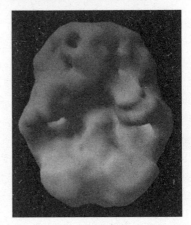

Damage to PFC and temporal lobes   Marked improvement

TRANSCRANIAL MAGNETIC STIMULATION: HEALING PULSES

A form of "brain stimulation," transcranial magnetic stimulation (TMS) is used to treat certain psychiatric and neurological disorders that have not improved through traditional approaches. TMS uses a noninvasive, highly focused, brief magnetic pulse to stimulate activity in the areas of the brain known to affect mood—without the troubling side effects people often experience from taking medication. While TMS has been approved by the FDA for the treatment of resistant depression, there is new evidence that it can enhance memory and potentially help improve a wide range of other brain-related issues, including

- anxiety[14]
- addiction[15]
- smoking cessation[16]
- post-traumatic stress disorder (PTSD)[17]

- obsessive-compulsive disorder (OCD)[18]
- cognitive problems, memory, and dementia[19]
- tinnitus (ringing in the ears)[20]
- stroke[21]

Electrical stimulation has been used for healing for centuries. The earliest known use occurred more than 2,000 years ago, when the Egyptians discovered that certain fish—including various electric rays—produced electrical impulses that could be used to treat pain and gout. These treatments were later practiced by the Greeks and Romans. In the 1780s Italian physician and physicist Luigi Galvani passed an electrical current through the spine of a frog, which resulted in the contraction of the frog's muscles. He discovered that nerves were not water pipes, as René Descartes thought, but electrical conductors carrying information within the nervous system. The young novelist Mary Shelley found inspiration from Galvani's research while writing her best-known work, *Frankenstein*. Roughly 50 years later, Michael Faraday's experiments in stimulating nerves and the brain laid the groundwork for the first use of transcranial magnetic stimulation in 1985. In 1997, TMS was approved for use in Canada, and in 2008 the FDA cleared it as a treatment for depression.

In a 2015 study, researchers from the University of São Paulo in Brazil studied the effect of TMS on memory in 34 elderly men and women with mild cognitive impairment (MCI), using 10 sessions of active TMS in one group and sham (or fake) treatment in the other to stimulate the left front side of the brain. Cognitive testing before and after TMS showed significant improvement of everyday memory in the treatment group as compared to the sham group. The researchers reported that their findings suggested that TMS might be effective as a treatment for MCI and "probably a tool to delay deterioration."[22]

TMS is a targeted treatment, and unlike medication, it has no systemic side effects (because it doesn't get into your bloodstream). It's noninvasive and usually well tolerated, although people with certain implants (particularly metal) may not be able to use it. Side effects are generally mild to moderate and may include headaches; scalp discomfort at the site of stimulation; tingling, spasms, or twitching of facial muscles; and lightheadedness. They improve shortly after an individual session and decrease over time with additional sessions. Serious side effects are rare but may include seizures and mania, particularly in people with bipolar disorder. Treatment sessions last about 40 minutes, and normal activities can be resumed immediately after each session. After a full course of treatment, which ranges from 16 to 30 sessions, a high percentage of patients report a significant reduction in symptoms and experience improvement in their quality of life.

Susan: lifted out of depression

Susan, 58, consulted Garrett Halweg, MD, a psychiatrist at Amen Clinics' Costa Mesa office, because of her severe depression. She succinctly explains the role of and benefits from TMS in her treatment plan:

> In January 2016, I received a devastating emotional shock. I was numb for several weeks but then started sinking into a deep depression. Amen Clinics had been recommended to me two years earlier to help one of my children with some emotional difficulties, and I was very impressed with how successful the treatment plan was. When I realized that I was sinking into depression, I called Dr. Halweg at the clinic. He placed me on one treatment for depression, then added a second and then a third. Each one helped, but I was still having difficulties. I was only getting about two hours of sleep per night. I had virtually no short-term memory and was struggling with long-term memory. I'd even lost my sense of direction. All I wanted to do was stay in bed all day with my door locked.
>
> I had to take a leave of absence from work and was just doing the minimum to care for my children. I thought my situation was completely hopeless and couldn't see how it could ever get better. After a few weeks, it was clear that I needed more help. At that time, Dr. Halweg performed a SPECT scan to determine the best course of treatment. He told me that my SPECT scan showed a high degree of post-traumatic stress disorder, where both anxiety and depression were cycling around and my brain couldn't shift out of those gears. He recommended TMS as a supplement to the antidepressants. I hoped and prayed that it would work. . . . By the fourth treatment, I started to see some improvement. My short-term memory had started to work a little bit. By the eighth treatment, my memory was much better, I regained my sense of direction, and I started sleeping better at night. By the twelfth treatment, I was actually beginning to feel tiny flickers of hope that maybe my situation could get better. At the end of my course of treatment, my memory was better than ever, I felt positive about my situation and my future, and I was able to return to work. Dr. Halweg stayed in close contact with me throughout my struggles, and I don't think I would have successfully made it

through without his help. I basically have my life back. I feel so good, I will actually sing along with the radio. And I'm able to manage the demands on a busy working mom. The TMS therapy is truly a life-changing experience.

SUSAN'S BRAIN SPECT SCAN BEFORE AND AFTER TMS

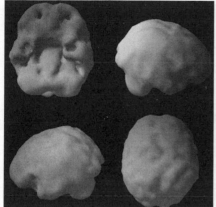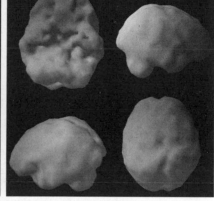

Low prefrontal and temporal lobe function   Improved prefrontal and temporal lobe function

NEUROFEEDBACK: YOU CAN CONTROL YOUR BRAIN WAVES

In 1987, I was the chief psychiatrist at Fort Irwin in the Mojave Desert. It was an isolated assignment, and I was looking for tools to help decrease the stress of soldiers who were training for challenging operations in a desert environment. There was a high incidence of depression, anxiety disorders, drug abuse, and domestic violence. I brought a treatment technique to the army post called biofeedback, which uses instruments to measure hand temperature, sweat gland activity, breathing, heart rate, muscle tension, and brain-wave patterns. The idea behind the treatment was that once people know their hand temperature or breathing patterns, for example, they could learn to change them with focused attention and mental exercises. They could learn to warm their hands, breathe with their bellies, decrease sweat gland activity, and so on; my goal was to use the technique to help the soldiers control their stress.

When I took the 10-day training in San Francisco to learn how to use biofeedback equipment that same year, it changed the trajectory of my career.

As I taught people that they could change their own physiology, I developed a consistent internal thought in dealing with my patients: *Teach them skills to manage their emotions and minds; don't just give them pills.*

Skills, not just pills.

The part of the training that completely blew my mind was neurofeedback, a specific form of biofeedback focused on the brain that is also called brain wave or EEG biofeedback. In the 1980s, the brain was still considered by many a "black box," but my professors were telling me and my classmates that we could look at brain wave signatures and teach people how to change them. It was a whole new world, which just a few years later led to my looking at the brain with SPECT scans. That series of lectures is where I first got the idea that would become the signature statement of my professional life:

You are not stuck with the brain you have; you can change it! You can change your brain *and* your life.

When I brought neurofeedback to Fort Irwin, I found it helped patients decrease their impulsivity and anxiety and improve their attention, learning, and mood. Now nearly 30 years later, more than 1,000 scientific studies show that neurofeedback can help a wide variety of mental-health and brain-related conditions, such as

- memory in healthy people[23]
- memory post-stroke[24]
- ADHD[25]
- obsessive-compulsive disorder[26]
- depression[27]
- traumatic brain injury[28]
- addiction[29]
- epilepsy[30]
- pain[31]
- balance in Parkinson's patients[32]

It can also help

- improve putting in golf[33]
- boost creativity in acting and business[34]

Here are the common brain-wave patterns (discussed in chapter 4), plus one more:

- *delta waves* (1–4 cycles per second)—very slow brain waves, seen mostly during sleep; high in traumatic brain injury and poor memory states
- *theta waves* (5–7 cycles per second)—slow brain waves, seen during creativity, daydreaming, and twilight states; higher in those with ADHD, impulsivity, poor memory, and brain fog states
- *alpha waves* (8–12 cycles per second)—brain waves seen during relaxed states
- *beta waves* (13–20 cycles per second)—fast brain waves seen during focused thinking and analytic states; higher in states of anxiety
- *high beta waves* (21–40 cycles per second)—fast brain waves seen during intense concentration or anxiety
- *gamma waves* (> 40 cycles per second)—very fast brain waves, often seen during meditation and creative states

A healthy brain will generate the wave frequency appropriate for any given situation. The basic neurofeedback technique uses behavioral reinforcement to help people change their brain-wave state accordingly. The more they can concentrate and produce fast beta brain waves, for example, the more rewards they can accrue. With Amen Clinics' neurofeedback equipment, a child or adult sits in front of a computer monitor with a biofeedback game. If he increases the beta activity or decreases the theta activity, the game continues. The game stops, however, when the player is unable to maintain the desired brain-wave state. People find the activity fun, and we gradually shape their brain-wave pattern to a healthier or more optimal one. This treatment technique is not an overnight cure. People often have to practice this form of biofeedback for 20 to 60 sessions to be able to recreate it on their own. But the results are worth it.

AUDIOVISUAL ENTRAINMENT: RHYTHMS OF SOUND AND LIGHT

Imagine sitting in a room at home with goggles and headphones on—strobe lights flicker through the goggles and pulses come through the headphones, both designed to stimulate your mind. Our minds "think" in states of brain-wave frequency. The changes in frequencies are based on brain activity. When the brain is stimulated with light and sound pulses (audiovisually), it begins to mimic or follow the same frequencies. This is called entrainment. In a sense, audiovisual entrainment (AVE) speaks to the mind in its own language—the language of rhythmic frequency—using a special machine that produces light and sound. The science of brain-wave entrainment, or the brain picking up the rhythm in the environment, is one of the fastest-growing technologies in brain enhancement.

A review of 20 clinical studies concluded that AVE was helpful for people suffering from cognitive functioning deficits, stress, anxiety, PMS, and behavioral problems.[35] It has also been found to improve overall brain activity[36] and help with several other issues:

- low brain blood flow[37]
- sleep[38]
- pain[39]
- stress reduction[40]
- migraines[41]
- depression[42]

Take Roger, age 62, a pastor who has Parkinson's disease. After having trouble sleeping for years, he came to Amen Clinics. From the first time he used audiovisual entrainment, he started sleeping better. Now he uses it multiple times a week to calm stress, balance his mood, and improve his focus.

Consider this: Everything in the universe vibrates and moves to certain rhythms. Striking one tuning fork near others of the same frequency will cause them to resonate also. Pendulum clocks hanging on the same wall, over time, will tick in synchrony. Crowds of people walking on a pedestrian bridge will unconsciously synchronize their steps if the bridge is slightly swaying. In concert halls, it is common for an audience's clapping to synchronize into rhythmic waves. Even the heartbeats and breathing patterns of couples sitting close to each other can match up. In hospitals, high-frequency oscillation ventilation machines are used to deliver stereo-speaker-like vibrations to help infants breathe. This phenomenon of vibration and synchronization is all around us and in the brain. The brain has its own vibrations. When masses of neurons fire in synchronized rhythmic oscillations, the small electrical vibrations emitted (brain waves) can change how we feel.

The idea of using rhythm and frequency to facilitate shifts in our brain is nothing new. From music to sunlight, sound and light have long played a central role in shaping our human consciousness. When we listen to music, certain songs can make us happy, sad, or irritated. Fast beats tend to speed up our brain waves. Slow beats tend to slow down our brain waves. Through the amazing use of AVE, we are able to stimulate the brain with rhythmic pulses of light and sounds at specific frequencies to purposefully guide the brain into different brain wave patterns.

I like AVE because it is so easy to use and cost-efficient, and you can use it in the comfort of your own home, on your own time. If you are looking for a clinically proven, pharmaceutical-free way to improve your life and want to learn more about how AVE can help, go to www.brainmdhealth.com/mind-alive.

This is an exciting time for brain-enhancement therapies, including the four discussed here. Outer space was once considered the new frontier. Now it is the space between your ears.

CHAPTER 20

MEMORY RESCUE MADE EASY
20 SHORT STORIES OF THE SEAHORSE TWINS, SCARLETT AND SAM

Even though *Memory Rescue* is based on a simple concept—that the best way to enhance your memory, decrease your risk of developing Alzheimer's disease, and rescue your memory from disaster is to prevent all the risk factors that steal your mind—it is backed by powerful neuroscience. In fact, that is why the book points you to more than 1,000 scientific references in the endnotes!

Yet none of the concepts is hard to grasp. To make it even easier, my team and I developed the mnemonic BRIGHT MINDS. Story can be another mnemonic tool to help you remember the book's takeaways—and stories can be shared with family members of any age. With that in mind, I came up with 20 short stories about Scarlett and Sam, the seahorse twins. Before I introduce you to them, I want you to answer a couple of questions about another type of horse. (At first, these questions might not seem to apply, but be patient and I'll connect the dots.)

If you had a million-dollar racehorse, would you ever feed it junk food?

Would you ever get it drunk or stoned?

Would you ever ignore it, abuse it, or keep it up all night?

Would you ever prevent it from exercising or allow it to breathe polluted air or drink polluted water if you could help it?

Of course not—unless you wanted to lose every race. Of course not, if you are a thoughtful, intelligent, caring person.

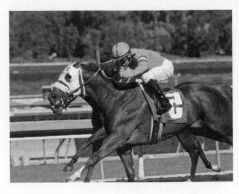

Yet aren't *you* worth more? Many people never treat themselves as well as they would treat a valuable thoroughbred, which is why they have trouble winning the races of their lives, whether at school, in work, in their relationships, or when it comes to their health.

As you learned in chapter 2, there is a special seahorse-shaped structure about the size of your thumb on the inside of your brain's temporal lobes. In fact, there are two of them. Most people don't even know they exist or consider their importance. One is called the hippocampus, the Greek word for seahorse; the pair are called the hippocampi.

Now, let's meet Scarlett and Sam, the hippocampi and the stars of this chapter (illustrated below). They are part of your emotional brain and help you feel happy or sad, and bonded to or disconnected from others. *They also are one of the main parts of your brain involved in memory.* They help you remember where you put your keys and whether you locked the door after you left the house. Your memories also make you who you are. They give you an identity, a family, and a sense of self-worth and purpose. They help you recognize those you love and those who love you. They enable you to remember important life lessons and learn from your mistakes.

Given how important the hippocampi are to your success in life, what is the best way for you to take care of Scarlett and Sam? The super-short stories below are designed to help you remember what makes your hippocampi weak, old, and frail, and how to reverse that trend to ensure they remain strong, vibrant, and healthy. Once again, I'm using the BRIGHT MINDS format you just learned as a framework.

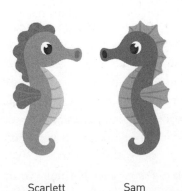

Scarlett   Sam

WHAT HURTS AND HELPS SCARLETT AND SAM?

<u>B</u> **Is for Blood Flow:** *Low blood flow is the number one predictor of Alzheimer's disease.*

1. Sam and Scarlett knew that the best way to ensure they got in regular workouts at the gym was to go first thing in the morning. As brother and sister, they could hold each other accountable. But then Sam got hooked on a late-night TV show. He convinced himself that he slept better after laughing along with the comedian host and his guests. Soon Sam was hitting the snooze button just about every morning. That was a problem—and not just because it was irritating Scarlett! Sam needed regular exercise to stay large and powerful. Once Sam realized that his late-night laugh fests were actually sapping his energy, he went back to walking, running, and lifting weights at the gym several times a week. He also made a point to engage regularly in coordination-building activities like dancing and table tennis. Before long, Sam felt younger and more energetic than he had in years.

2. One morning a vendor in the gym lobby was passing out free samples of energy drinks. Sam liked the taste and felt so good after drinking it that he picked up a case the next time he stopped at the grocery store. He started drinking a couple of cans in place of water after every workout. But soon his thinking became fuzzy, and he couldn't figure out why. Scarlett had been trying to kick her own caffeine habit, so she explained to Sam that she'd recently learned that caffeine (as well as nicotine) lowers blood flow to the brain, which meant the two of them would shrink if they consumed too much of it. They wouldn't be able to learn or remember as well as they once did either. That frightened them, so they replaced their caffeinated drinks with plenty of fresh, clean water and caffeine-free green tea, which is full of ingredients to keep their blood flow on track.

3. Scarlett went to her doctor, Dr. Amy G. Dala, and found out she had high blood pressure. At first, she didn't understand how serious it was and didn't do what her doctor asked of her. When Sam found out, he was very upset. "Don't you know that as blood pressure goes up, blood flow to the brain and to us goes down?" he asked. "You have to take this seriously!" Upon hearing the urgency in Sam's voice, Scarlett decided to exercise more and eat better (no more potato

chips and other salty snacks). Once she'd made these changes, she was able to get her blood pressure under control without taking medication.

R Is for Retirement/Aging: *When you stop learning, your brain starts dying.*

4. Scarlett and Sam had been working at the Seahorse Amusement Park for many years. They completed the same assignments—running the arcade, taking tickets, and fixing games—over and over. When they stopped learning and being interested in their work, they started to get smaller and weaker. When they weighed themselves and measured their height, they could see that boredom was making them waste away. They decided to look for new jobs at the park. Scarlett started to sing and act in the park's plays, and Sam took up the guitar so he could be in the band. As they learned new skills and took up challenging activities they felt passionate about, they started to grow bigger and stronger. They also felt happier.

5. After a family tragedy, Scarlett and Sam withdrew from their friends. They just didn't feel like being around other seahorses. But the more withdrawn they became, the more they noticed they had started to shrink. That really got their attention, and they started to volunteer at a local school, teaching seahorse children how to read. The sense of purpose and social connection helped them grow larger again.

6. As Scarlett and Sam got older, they slowed down. They stopped exercising, complained about their aches and pains, and stayed home more. Sam often told his children he was too old to exercise, too old to change his unhealthy eating habits, and too old to go dancing, which he had once loved. One day, his son, who was a seahorse physician, started to encourage his dad and aunt Scarlett to do more. He told them that seahorses shrink with age if they're not serious about taking care of themselves. Not wanting to be feeble and weak, and fearing that they could wind up being a burden on their grown children, they started taking better care of themselves. Now Sam and Scarlett regularly go dancing with their spouses.

I Is for Inflammation: *Inflammation comes from the Latin word for "setting a fire." It destroys your organs and shrinks your hippocampi.*

7. Sam struggled for many years with an upset stomach. He loved pizza but was sensitive to wheat and dairy. Whenever he had a slice, he paid for it with belly pain and the feeling of being bloated. As a child, Sam had many ear infections and his doctors gave him lots of antibiotics. Scarlett read that having many courses of childhood antibiotics and being sensitive to wheat and dairy were often associated with something called leaky gut, in which the lining of the intestinal tract becomes more permeable. This allows foreign invaders into the body, which causes inflammation. She encouraged Sam to stop eating pizza and other foods with wheat and dairy. She also recommended that he start taking a probiotic to help recolonize his gut with healthy bacteria. A month after making these changes, Sam felt much better, which helped him to remember to eat right.

8. Scarlett was a busy working seahorse and ate a lot of fast food filled with cheap oils, bread, potatoes, and sugar. She often complained of brain fog and joint pain. After Sam told Scarlett about a new test he'd read about called the Omega-3 Index, she went to her doctor and had the test. It turned out that her Omega-3 Index was very low. Once Scarlett changed her diet and added more omega-3-rich foods, such as shrimp (a seahorse's natural food), chia seeds, avocados, nuts, and seeds, her problems cleared up.

9 Sam's friend and coworker Seymour was a clownfish who was so busy that he never took care of his teeth. He had a nice smile anyway, so he didn't think it was that important. Over time, his gums started to bleed whenever he brushed his teeth. He wondered, though, why his favorite female clownfish never accepted his request for a date. Sam, who was fond of his fun-loving friend, finally told him he had bad breath. Then he added, "Don't you know that gum disease can cause inflammation in your body and damage your heart and brain?" Seymour got the message and started to floss every night and see his dentist regularly.

G Is for Genetics: *If memory problems run in your family, it is critical to be serious about brain health as soon as possible.*

10. Scarlett and Sam had a father and grandmother who both lost their memory as they got older. It was very hard on their family. Scarlett and Sam worried that maybe they would lose their memory too.

Instead of just being anxious about it, like their cousin Nervous Nancy, they decided to do everything they could to keep their memory strong as they aged, including exercising; learning new things; and eating delicious, healthy food.

H Is for Head Trauma: *Your brain is very soft, and it is housed in a very hard skull. The hippocampi sit on the inside of the temporal lobes, next to a sharp bony ridge, making them very susceptible to damage.*

11. Sam loved soccer. He had played as a young seahorse, and he even competed on weekends as an adult. He was particularly good at heading soccer balls, even though sometimes it left him feeling dazed and gave him headaches. Scarlett was worried about him. She had read that playing contact sports like football and soccer could cause long-term brain problems. At first Sam made fun of her, saying, "How can I have any fun? Do you want me to play badminton or Ping-Pong?" Because Scarlett loved her twin, she was courageous and said, "Who has more fun, Sam—the seahorse with a healthy brain or the one whose brain is damaged? You are smarter than you are acting. Seahorses who play racquet sports actually live longer than those who play any other sport. Get a Ping-Pong paddle and see if you can beat me. I doubt it!" Smart seahorses protect their brains.

T Is for Toxins: *Your brain cannot grow or heal in a toxic environment.*

12. Scarlett noticed that her skin was breaking out in rashes more often and that she had felt foggy-headed ever since an oil spill near their home. Her children had rashes, too, and they started to struggle in school. Sam, who lived a few miles away, was not having the same problems, so Scarlett took her children to live with his family. Over the next few weeks they felt better.

13. After the oil spill incident, Sam started to learn more about the effect of toxins on his brain. He read that the grooming products he used might contain toxins with funny-sounding names, such as phthalates and parabens. He was able to download a cool app for his smartphone that could scan the bar codes on his soap, deodorant, and toothpaste and provide ingredient information. He was horrified to learn that most of what he was using was not good for him. He told Scarlett, "What goes on your body goes in your body!" They both

used the app and got products for themselves and their families that were less harmful.

14. Scarlett's oldest son, Frisco, had always been a good student in school but often struggled with anxiety and nervousness. He started smoking marijuana at the suggestion of a friend, who told him it would cure his anxiety. After a few weeks, his grades started to drop, he became more forgetful, and he started to shrink. His mood changed, and he started fighting more with Scarlett. When she found out what Frisco was doing, Scarlett panicked and brought him to see Uncle Sam. Sam showed Frisco brain scans of seahorses who smoked marijuana from a study published in a medical journal. That frightened Frisco, who stopped smoking weed. Uncle Sam taught him to use meditation and exercise to calm his anxiety, which helped him regain his strength and vitality.

M Is for Mental Health: *The health of your mind is intertwined with the health of your brain and memory.*

15. When Scarlett's son Frisco started having problems with marijuana, she became very stressed out. She worried, developed tension headaches, had trouble sleeping, and became more withdrawn. The stress was making Scarlett smaller and weaker. Being a twin, Sam always knew when Scarlett was upset. He told her about the effect of stress on her brain and body. Not only did he teach her to meditate and exercise as he'd done with Frisco, he encouraged her to see a seahorse therapist to acquire skills to deal with stress. Once Scarlett began taking care of herself, she felt more relaxed and grew stronger.

16. One of the reasons Sam knew how to help Frisco and Scarlett was that he had gone through a period of depression many years earlier after losing his first wife to a hungry crab. It happened at a time when he was pregnant. (Female seahorses give males their eggs, and the males fertilize them and carry the developing baby seahorses. They can have up to 1,500 babies at a time.) Losing his wife and dealing with the stress of the pregnancy was very hard on Sam. He cried for weeks, had many negative thoughts and low energy, and wondered if life was worth living. Then he realized he had all the babies to nurture, and he went to see a therapist to get help. Using meditation, exercise, and healthy food, Sam began to feel better. He knew his wife would want him to be healthy for their babies.

I Is for Immunity/Infection Issues: *Protect your defenses so that they can protect you.*

17.　It was winter in the part of the sea that Scarlett and Sam called home. The water was very cold, and they hadn't seen light from the sun for weeks. They noticed they were more irritable with each other, got sick more often, and started to grow smaller and weaker. When they went to their seahorse physician, Dr. Amy G. Dala, she discovered they both had very low vitamin D levels. She explained that vitamin D is a very special nutrient we get from sun exposure; eating vitamin D–rich foods, such as cod liver oil and portobello mushrooms; or taking supplements. It helps keep bones strong and the immune system healthy, and it supports mood and memory. When vitamin D is low, seahorses get weaker and smaller. The doctor gave them a shot of vitamin D to give them a boost and some nutrients to take every day. Within a few weeks, they started to feel better.

N Is for Neurohormone Deficiencies: *Hormones keep your brain young and strong.*

18.　As Sam and Scarlett got older, they seemed to lose much of their energy and strength, even though they tried to eat right and exercise. Their skin became more wrinkled, and their recall of important information was not as good as it had been when they were younger. Dr. Dala checked their important numbers, which revealed that several of their hormones were low, including testosterone in both of them and estrogen in Scarlett. Boosting fiber and eliminating sugar helped, as did weight training and using special supplements and medication. Ensuring their hormones remained at healthy levels helped the seahorses regain their size and strength.

D Is for Diabesity: *As your weight and blood sugar go up, the size and function of your brain goes down.*

19.　While working at the Seahorse Amusement Park, both Scarlett and Sam ate too much of the tasty but very unhealthy food sold there, including corn dogs (with 29 ingredients), pizza, fries, sodas, and cotton candy. Even though the food made them feel good as they were eating it, they often felt sluggish later on. Over time they also noticed each other's bellies were getting bigger, while they were growing smaller and becoming weaker. Their blood sugar levels went up too. Dr. Dala told them that they were now obese, prediabetic seahorses, and if they wanted to live a long time with healthy brains, they had to change their ways. That got their attention. They began passing up the fast food and started bringing lunches to work. They reminded each other to be more thoughtful about what they put into their bodies. Their bellies stopped bulging, and they grew bigger and stronger.

S Is for Sleep Issues: *Your brain cleanses itself when you sleep. Poor sleep causes trash to build up, which can ruin your memory.*

20. Sam's new wife, Sophia, and Scarlett went out for green tea and blueberries together. Scarlett was so happy her brother had found someone new after he had lost his first wife. Sophia was a special seahorse, and Scarlett liked her very much, which was why she was concerned when Sophia told her she was not getting any sleep. Sam snored so loudly that he frequently woke Sophia up. She was worried because he seemed to stop breathing a lot. Scarlett recognized the symptoms of sleep apnea in her brother and talked to him about going to Dr. Dala for a sleep study. It turned out Sam had severe sleep apnea, and once it was treated, he slept much better, as did Sophia. Both of them became happier, healthier, stronger seahorses as a result.

See how easy it can be? Be sure to take care of your seahorses and your whole brain, because they run your life.

Postscript: As I was finishing this book, I had a brain MRI, both to test new quantification software we are using at Amen Clinics and to spot any potential trouble before it happens. The area of my temporal lobes where the hippocampi are housed was in the ninety-fifth percentile, meaning it was bigger than that of 95 percent of the population my age. Good news for Scarlett and Sam. I also had a test done to measure the length of my telomeres—the ends of chromosomes—that we discussed in chapter 6. I may be in my early sixties, but my telomere age is in the early forties. That made me smile.

Is getting healthy hard? I would argue that being sick is much harder. I know my brain and body were not this healthy when I had my first brain scan in 1991. But by living the message of this book, my brain and body are better, and yours can be too.

CHAPTER 21

HOW TO START YOUR PERSONAL MEMORY RESCUE PLAN

Be careful what you think, because your thoughts run your life. . . . Keep your
eyes focused on what is right, and look straight ahead to what is good.

PROVERBS 4:23, 25, NCV

Congratulations! You have taken the first giant step on the journey toward strengthening and rehabilitating your memory, bettering your brain, and improving your overall health and well-being. If you opened this book worried because your recall wasn't as sharp as it once was, I hope you are encouraged now that you have been introduced to dozens of ideas on how you can begin improving your memory *today*.

As I noted in the first few pages of *Memory Rescue*, having brain fog or trouble remembering things is not unusual, but you can do something about it. You are not stuck with the brain you currently have. Many patients have come to the Amen Clinics with memory-related health issues and gotten serious about bettering their brains. Their determination and efforts to overcome significant challenges have inspired me, and their successes make me optimistic about *your* ability to address individual health problems and rescue your memory.

The purpose of this chapter is to help you act on your new knowledge by putting together your personal Memory Rescue plan. The next steps are up to you. Taking them may be challenging as you let go of familiar behaviors, but don't let that stop you (we'll also help make the adoption of new habits as easy as possible; see step 4, page 341). Focus instead on the rewards that await you: a stronger memory and improved health.

Here are my recommendations as to what your next steps should be.

STEP 1: ASSESS YOUR PERSONAL RISK FACTORS

First, you need to know the reasons for your current memory problems. That means you need to determine how your body and your brain are functioning right now. Here are the assessments described early in the book that will provide you with this information:

☐ **A reliable cognitive test** (see page 30). A number of tests are available, but at Amen Clinics we use Brain Fit WebNeuro, which takes about 35 minutes to complete and provides an objective assessment of how your brain works in 17 specific areas. You can take it through our online Brain Fit Life program (www.mybrainfitlife.com). It produces a baseline score and, with retesting, a way to find out over time if your brain function is improving or deteriorating.

☐ **The BRIGHT MINDS risk factor assessment** (see page 48). This assessment provides you with two scores, one for your total number of BRIGHT MINDS risks and a second for your relative risks. Once you have those scores, enter them on pages 338–339.

☐ **Your important health numbers** (see page 52). These numbers (listed below) reveal the state of your health. Knowing which ones are too high or too low will help you identify which BRIGHT MINDS risks you need to address right away. If you don't know these numbers, now would be a good time to schedule an appointment with your health-care provider. I encourage you to work with an integrative medicine doctor, who will be knowledgeable about many of the tests, nutraceuticals, and additional therapies, such as neurofeedback, that are described in this book.

General Numbers to Know

☐ Body mass index (BMI; page 233)
☐ Waist-to-height ratio (WHtR; page 233)
☐ Blood pressure (page 68)

Blood Tests

- ☐ Complete blood count (CBC; page 69)
- ☐ General metabolic panel (kidney and liver function; page 157)
- ☐ Lipid panel (page 69)
- ☐ Fasting blood sugar (page 87)
- ☐ Hemoglobin A1c (HbA1c; page 87)
- ☐ Fasting insulin (page 234)
- ☐ Homocysteine (page 102)
- ☐ C-reactive protein (CRP; page 101)
- ☐ Ferritin level (measure of iron store; page 88)
- ☐ Thyroid panel (page 217)
- ☐ Testosterone level (page 135)
- ☐ DHEA level (page 87)
- ☐ Vitamin D (pages 194 and 197)
- ☐ Folate (page 102)
- ☐ Vitamin B12 level (page 102)
- ☐ Plasma zinc (page 157)
- ☐ Serum copper
- ☐ Magnesium (page 238)
- ☐ Omega-3 Index (pages 102–103)
- ☐ *APOE* gene type (page 115)

STEP 2: DECIDE WHICH BRIGHT MINDS RISK FACTOR(S) TO ADDRESS FIRST

Once you have assessed the health of your brain and the rest of your body, you are ready to decide which BRIGHT MINDS risk factor(s) to focus on first. Chapters 5 through 15 explain all the risk factors and how each one is linked to memory issues. Each of these chapters includes a "checkup" of tests that will reveal problems related to that risk factor; a "prescription" of strategies, nutraceuticals, and foods (to avoid or add) designed to help you eliminate that particular risk factor; and a list of healthy habits to adopt. The Memory Rescue Diet, in chapter 16, includes healthy foods for each risk factor; I recommend that *anyone* who has memory problems adopt a healthier diet based on the principles of this plan. As I noted earlier, proper nutrition is one of the key strategies for enduring good health. Chapters 17 through 19 contain overviews of brain workouts and mnemonic devices; memory medications; and tools to strengthen your memory, from hyperbaric oxygen therapy (HBOT) to audiovisual entrainment (AVE).

Whether you have one or multiple risk factors, a good way to keep track of them and the remedies you have selected to address them is to fill out the chart entitled "Your BRIGHT MINDS Risk Factors and Interventions" on pages 338–339. For example, for blood flow you might enter "high blood pressure & elevated total cholesterol/1-7-18" under "Known Risk Factors/ Dates Evaluated" and under "Interventions," list "aerobic exercise 3x/week, weight loss, daily prayer." Once you begin working to eliminate a risk factor, be sure to get follow-up testing after 12 or more weeks to track your progress. (For a look at how charts like this one have been filled out, page through the book to see the many "BRIGHT MINDS Risk Factors and Interventions" charts of patients we have treated at Amen Clinics; two examples are the charts of Jim, a successful businessman, on pages 60–61, and champion surfer Shawn Dollar, on page 122.)

You also might want to jot down your healthy actions/activities in a daily journal or calendar and review them at the end of each day or week. Doing so will help you stay on top of your interventions, monitor their effectiveness, and see your progress more clearly. Research has shown that using a journal in this way will help you reach your goals.

If you prefer to concentrate on becoming healthier overall—or you simply want to take action while you await the date of a health exam or the arrival of test results—here is a quick-start checklist of actions that will reduce your risk in every BRIGHT MINDS category:

Blood flow
- ✓ Avoid anything that hurts your vascular health, such as caffeine or nicotine
- ✓ Drink more water
- ✓ Engage in regular exercise; racquet sports are particularly beneficial

Retirement and aging
- ✓ Spend 15 minutes a day learning something new (musical training, dancing, a new language)
- ✓ Volunteer
- ✓ Try a daily 12- to 16-hour fast

Inflammation
- ✓ Floss your teeth daily and care for your gums
- ✓ Eliminate trans fats
- ✓ Add omega-3s and probiotic foods or supplements to your diet

Genetics

- ✓ If dementia runs in your family, be serious about brain health starting now, and get early screening for memory issues
- ✓ Get tested for the ApoE4 gene
- ✓ Eat organic blueberries

Head trauma

- ✓ Do not text while walking or driving
- ✓ Be careful going up and down stairs; hold the handrail
- ✓ Always wear a seat belt when you drive or ride in a vehicle

Toxins

- ✓ Limit alcohol to two glasses a week
- ✓ Scan all your personal products with an app like Think Dirty
- ✓ Eat cruciferous vegetables for their detoxifying ability

Mental health

- ✓ Write down three things you are grateful for every day
- ✓ Take a walk in nature
- ✓ Pray to release your worries and to rejoice over the good things around you

Immunity/infection issues

- ✓ Start an elimination diet for a month to see if you have food allergies
- ✓ Watch comedies to boost your immunity
- ✓ Optimize your vitamin D level

Neurohormone deficiencies

- ✓ Eat more fiber
- ✓ Lift weights to boost testosterone
- ✓ Avoid hormone disruptors, such as BPA, phthalates, parabens, and pesticides

Diabesity

- ✓ Know your BMI (body mass index); if it's over 25, lose weight
- ✓ Start the Memory Rescue Diet
- ✓ Don't drink your calories

Sleep issues

- ✓ If you snore, get assessed for sleep apnea
- ✓ Turn off your electronic gadgets an hour before bed
- ✓ Listen to audio created to help with sleep

YOUR BRIGHT MINDS RISK FACTORS AND INTERVENTIONS

BRIGHT MINDS	KNOWN RISK FACTORS/ DATE(S) EVALUATED	INTERVENTIONS	PROGRESS REPORT/ DATE(S) EVALUATED
Blood Flow			
Retirement/ Aging			
Inflammation			
Genetics			
Head Trauma			
Toxins			

BRIGHT MINDS	KNOWN RISK FACTORS/ DATE(S) EVALUATED	INTERVENTIONS	PROGRESS REPORT/ DATE(S) EVALUATED
Mental Health			
Immunity/ Infection Issues			
Neurohormone Deficiencies			
Diabesity			
Sleep Issues			

YOUR BRIGHT MINDS RISK FACTORS AND INTERVENTIONS

_____Your total number of risk factors

_____Your relative risk score

STEP 3: JUMP-START YOUR MEMORY RESCUE

Everyone needs to take basic supplements daily for good brain and body health, including a 100 percent multivitamin/mineral complex daily with extra vitamins B6 and B12, folate, and vitamin D3, plus omega-3 fatty acids EPA and DHA. Beyond these basics, I recommend taking targeted nutraceuticals (which I define as supplements with medicinal properties), based on your specific BRIGHT MINDS needs.

I am aware, however, that if you have numerous risk factors, the number of recommended nutraceuticals can quickly add up, along with the cost, which usually is not covered by health insurance. For these reasons, and to address those readers who might ask, "Dr. Amen, which of these nutraceuticals are the *best ones* to help me get my memory back?" my team developed the chart below. (Presiding over the chart are Sam and Scarlett from chapter 20, the seahorse twins who "embody" the hippocampi, the gateway brain structures for memory. The key provides the full name of each nutraceutical.)

The nutraceuticals are divided into three categories, based on the amount of quality scientific research supporting each one. The categories are "best proven," "moderately proven," and "promising." So if for any reason you need to limit the nutraceuticals you take for brain fog and memory problems,

BRIGHT MINDS MEMORY NUTRACEUTICALS

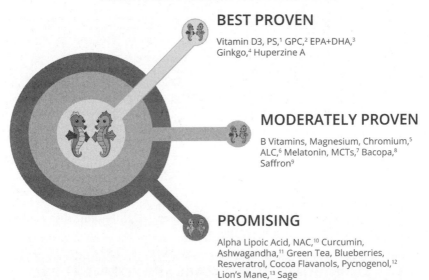

BEST PROVEN

Vitamin D3, PS,[1] GPC,[2] EPA+DHA,[3]
Ginkgo,[4] Huperzine A

MODERATELY PROVEN

B Vitamins, Magnesium, Chromium,[5]
ALC,[6] Melatonin, MCTs,[7] Bacopa,[8]
Saffron[9]

PROMISING

Alpha Lipoic Acid, NAC,[10] Curcumin,
Ashwagandha,[11] Green Tea, Blueberries,
Resveratrol, Cocoa Flavanols, Pycnogenol,[12]
Lion's Mane,[13] Sage

---

[1]PS = phosphatidylserine, [2]GPC = glycerophosphocholine, [3]EPA+DHA = eicosapentaenoic acid plus docosahexaenoic acid omega-3 fatty acids, [4]Ginkgo = *Ginkgo biloba* standardized extract, [5]Chromium = chromium as picolinate, [6]ALC = acetyl-L-carnitine, [7]MCTs = medium chain triglycerides, [8]Bacopa = *Bacopa monnieri* Synapsa™ standardized extract, [9]Saffron = *Crocus sativus* standardized extract, [10]NAC = N-acetylcysteine, [11]Ashwagandha = *Withania somnifera* Sensoril® standardized extract, [12]Pycnogenol = *Pinus maritima* standardized extract, [13]Lion's mane = *Hericium erinaceus* standardized extract

choose first from among the six that are the "best proven" (which already include two from the basic supplement list), next from the "moderately proven" group, and lastly from the "promising" ones. Finally, as I noted, I highly recommend that you work with an integrative medicine doctor who can help you decide which nutraceuticals to take based on your needs and any medications you are currently taking. Nutraceuticals, while generally safer than prescription medications, are not without risks, and there can be harmful consequences, such as reducing the effectiveness of a prescription drug due to an interaction with a nutraceutical.

STEP 4: HOW TO INITIATE CHANGE— AND MAKE IT STICK

Making big changes can be daunting, and depending on your personal risk factors, you may discover you need to alter your lifestyle in a number of ways. If you find that you feel not only motivated by the challenge but also a bit apprehensive, it may help to acknowledge that this is a sizable undertaking that will take time, energy, and determination.[1] That awareness can help you plot a strategy that works for you.

Everyone knows that the best intentions can easily go awry when obstacles arise. You set a goal to exercise three times a week, and it rains on two of the days you had earmarked to go outdoors for a walk. Temptation in the form of strawberry rhubarb pie—your favorite!—overwhelms your resolve to give up sweets. An ongoing work project interferes with your plans to get at least seven hours of sleep every night. Life happens, and you have to figure out a way to adapt and make headway toward your goals.

Here is a quick refresher of suggestions introduced in chapter 4 (see page 51), along with additional science-backed tips, that can help you maintain your resolve:

Plan first, and be specific. Reaching a goal is easier when you think about the what, when, where, and how of it before you put a plan into action. If you have been sedentary and want to start exercising, for example, you might decide to walk (what) around your neighborhood (where) for 15 minutes a day right after breakfast (when). As a reminder, when you get dressed in the morning, you will put on your walking shoes (how). Plotting out strategies in this way contributes to the likelihood of success.

Begin with small, measurable steps. They will build your confidence in your ability to reach your goals. Do you want to eat healthier? In the first week, you might choose three "foods to avoid" and three "foods to consider adding" from the lists for your specific risk factor in chapter 16 (see page 278). During the week, note down every time you avoid or add one of those foods, and at the end of the week, congratulate yourself on having met your goal.

Write it down. Committing goals to paper (or the computer) reaffirms your determination to make changes. Post them where you will see them and be reminded (and motivated) to stick with your plan.

Make it routine. Repeating the same action or behavior over and over again in the same context until it becomes automatic (i.e., a habit) is one way to stay on track. (The classic example is strapping on a seat belt whenever you get into a car.) A big side benefit is that once the action is automatic, it becomes second nature—you don't have to think about doing it and your brain is free to focus on something else. Your routines might include adding berries whenever you have yogurt for breakfast, flossing right after you brush your teeth, and holding the handrail whenever you descend a set of stairs. Be patient: Research shows that it may take 10 weeks for an action to become automatic.[2]

Enlist family and/or friends. Share your intentions with one or more people who will support you, help you through any rough patches, and celebrate your successes. Be sure to call on them when your motivation flags or you backslide and find yourself tempted to quit.

Keep a journal (or use an app). Writing down the actions you plan to take and checking them off when you have accomplished them will help you achieve your goals. Consider using an app, like the Momentum Habit Tracker (free; iOS), to help you stay focused.

Mark it in your calendar. Incorporating change into your life usually requires making space for it, whether "it" is shopping in a new store for healthier foods or remembering to take your nutraceuticals every day. Enter commitments into your calendar, and program alerts on your smartphone as reminders. Keep your family apprised of your commitments so that they can make any necessary accommodations and support you.

When tempted, say "I don't," not "I can't." Self-talk is an important part of staying the course. When you are confronted with a temptation, such as a glazed doughnut, research suggests that passing up the treat by saying "I don't eat doughnuts" is a better response than saying "I can't have doughnuts." The first is an empowering statement of self-control; the second implies lack of choice and being constrained by forces outside yourself. Learning to say "I don't" is more likely to result in long-term success.[3]

Embrace your victories *and* your mess-ups. Keep looking back at what you have accomplished to build your motivation to move forward; that's more helpful than looking ahead at what still has to be done. And when you step off the path, forgive yourself and recommit to your goals as quickly as you can. Overcoming your risk factors and rescuing your memory rely on the accretion of small changes that you stick with over the long haul.

Lifestyle changes are at the heart of the BRIGHT MINDS Memory Rescue plan. The reasons are twofold. First, prescription drugs have been ineffective at preventing Alzheimer's disease and other dementias. And second, well-designed scientific studies, including my own, have shown that lifestyle interventions do work. Just one example is the two-year FINGER study, which found that a combination of healthy diet, physical activity, cognitive training, and social activities successfully prevented cognitive decline in 1,260 at-risk individuals.[4] Similar studies are under way, and I suspect that when they are concluded, they, too, will support the idea that a healthy lifestyle can preserve memory and keep Alzheimer's and other dementias at bay.

Don't wait. Begin today, right now, to follow the BRIGHT MINDS path to memory rescue.

About Daniel G. Amen, MD

The *Washington Post* has called Dr. Daniel G. Amen the most popular psychiatrist in America, and Sharecare, a digital health company designed to help people manage their health in one place, named him the web's most influential expert and advocate on mental health.

Dr. Amen is a physician, double board–certified psychiatrist, 10-time *New York Times* bestselling author, and international speaker. He is the founder of Amen Clinics in Costa Mesa and San Francisco, California; Bellevue, Washington; Reston, Virginia; Atlanta; New York; and Chicago. Amen Clinics have one of the highest published success rates treating complex psychiatric issues, and they have built the world's largest database of functional brain scans, totaling more than 135,000 scans on patients from 111 countries.

Dr. Amen is the lead researcher on the world's largest brain imaging and rehabilitation study of professional football players. His research has not only demonstrated high levels of brain damage in players, it has also shown the possibility of significant recovery for many with the principles that underlie his work.

Together with Pastor Rick Warren and Mark Hyman, MD, Dr. Amen is also one of the chief architects of Saddleback Church's Daniel Plan, a program to get the world healthy through religious organizations.

Dr. Amen is the author or coauthor of more than 70 professional articles, seven book chapters, and more than 30 books, including the #1 New York Times bestsellers *The Daniel Plan* and *Change Your Brain, Change Your Life*; as well as *Magnificent Mind at Any Age*; *Change Your Brain, Change Your Body*;

Use Your Brain to Change Your Age; *Healing ADD*; *The Brain Warrior's Way*; and *The Brain Warrior's Way Cookbook*.

Dr. Amen's published scientific articles have appeared in the prestigious journals *Brain Imaging and Behavior*, Nature's *Molecular Psychiatry*, *PLOS ONE*, Nature's *Translational Psychiatry*, Nature's *Obesity*, the *Journal of Neuropsychiatry and Clinical Neurosciences*, *Minerva Psichiatrica*, *Journal of Neurotrauma*, the *American Journal of Psychiatry*, *Nuclear Medicine Communications*, *Neurological Research*, *Journal of the American Academy of Child & Adolescent Psychiatry*, *Primary Psychiatry*, *Military Medicine*, and *General Hospital Psychiatry*. His research on post-traumatic stress disorder and traumatic brain injury was recognized by *Discover* magazine in its Year in Science issue as one of the "100 Top Stories of 2015."

Dr. Amen has written, produced, and hosted 12 popular shows about the brain on public television. He has appeared in movies, including *After the Last Round* and *The Crash Reel*, and in Emmy Award–winning television shows, such as *The Truth about Drinking* and *The Dr. Oz Show*. He was a consultant on the movie *Concussion*, starring Will Smith. He has also spoken for the National Security Agency (NSA), the National Science Foundation (NSF), Harvard's Learning & the Brain Conference, the Department of the Interior, the National Council of Juvenile and Family Court Judges, and the Supreme Courts of Delaware, Ohio, and Wyoming. Dr. Amen's work has been featured in *Newsweek*, *Time* magazine, the *Huffington Post*, the BBC, the *Guardian*, *Parade* magazine, the *New York Times*, the *New York Times Magazine*, the *Washington Post*, *Los Angeles Times*, *Men's Health*, and *Cosmopolitan*.

Dr. Amen is married to Tana. He is the father of four children and grandfather to Elias, Emmy, Liam, and Louie. He is also an avid table tennis player.

Gratitude and Appreciation

So many people have been involved in the process of creating the Memory Rescue program and this book. I am grateful to them all, especially the tens of thousands of patients and families who have come to Amen Clinics and allowed us to help them on their healing journey.

I am grateful to the amazing staff at Amen Clinics, who work hard every day serving our patients. Thanks to our creative team, including CJ Ramos and Shabnam Agahi, for creating many of the illustrations in the book. Special appreciation to Jenny Cook, who helped me craft the book to make it easily accessible to our readers. I hope you agree. I also thank our fearless leader, CEO Terry Weber, and my colleagues Dr. Parris Kidd, Dr. Rob Johnson, Lorenzo Sevilla, and Natalie Buchoz, who also read every word in this book to be sure it makes sense.

I am grateful to Jan Long Harris at Tyndale, who saw the potential for this book to help many people, and my editor, Kim Miller, who helped make this book the best it can be.

I remain grateful to my friends and colleagues at public television stations across the country, including my mentors and friends Alan Foster, BaBette Davidson, Alicia Steele, Kurt Mendelsohn, Greg Sherwood, Camille Dixon, Stacey Wiggins, Maura Phinney, Henry Brodersen, Jerry Liwanag, Suzanne Fiske, Claire O'Connor-Solomon, and countless others. Public television is a treasure, and we are grateful to be able to partner with stations to bring our message of hope and healing to millions of people.

Of course, I am grateful to my amazing wife, Tana, who is my partner in all I do, and to my family, who have tolerated my obsession with making brains better, especially my children, Antony, Breanne, Kaitlyn, and Chloe; grandchildren; and parents, Mary Meeks (Tana's mom) and Louis and Dorie Amen.

Resources

AMEN CLINICS

www.amenclinics.com

Amen Clinics, Inc., (ACI) was established in 1989 by Daniel G. Amen, MD. We specialize in innovative diagnosis and treatment planning for a wide variety of behavioral, learning, emotional, cognitive, and weight issues for children, teenagers, and adults. ACI has an international reputation for evaluating brain-behavior problems, such as ADD/ADHD, depression, anxiety, school failure, traumatic brain injury and concussions, obsessive-compulsive disorders, aggressiveness, marital conflict, cognitive decline, brain toxicity from drugs or alcohol, and obesity. In addition, we work with patients to optimize brain function and decrease the risk for Alzheimer's disease and other age-related issues.

One of the primary diagnostic tools used at ACI is brain SPECT imaging. ACI has the world's largest database of brain scans for emotional, cognitive, and behavioral problems. We welcome referrals from physicians, psychologists, social workers, marriage and family therapists, drug and alcohol counselors, and individual patients and families.

Our toll-free number is (888) 288-9834.

Amen Clinics Los Angeles
5363 Balboa Blvd., Suite 100
Encino, CA 91316

Amen Clinics Orange County,
California
3150 Bristol St., Suite 400
Costa Mesa, CA 92626

Amen Clinics Northern California
350 N Wiget Ln.
Walnut Creek, CA 94598

Amen Clinics New York
16 East 40th St., 9th Floor
New York, NY 10016

Amen Clinics Northwest
616 120th Ave. NE, Suite C100
Bellevue, WA 98005

Amen Clinics Atlanta
5901-C Peachtree Dunwoody Rd.
NE, Suite 65
Atlanta, GA 30328

Amen Clinics Washington, DC
10701 Parkridge Blvd., Suite 110
Reston, VA 20191

Amen Clinics Chicago
2333 Waukegan Rd., Suite 150
Bannockburn, IL 60015

Amenclinics.com is an educational, interactive website geared toward mental health and medical professionals, educators, students, and the public. It offers a wealth of information and resources to help you learn about optimizing your brain. The site contains more than 300 color brain SPECT images, thousands of scientific abstracts on brain SPECT imaging for psychiatry, a free brain health assessment, and much more.

BRAIN FIT LIFE

www.mybrainfitlife.com

Based on Dr. Amen's 35 years as a clinical psychiatrist, he and his wife, Tana, have developed a sophisticated online community to help you feel smarter, happier, and younger. It includes

- Detailed questionnaires to help you know your brain type and a personalized program targeted to your own needs
- WebNeuro, a sophisticated neuropsychological test that assesses your brain
- Fun brain games and tools to boost your motivation
- Exclusive, award-winning, 24-7 brain gym membership
- Physical exercises and tutorials led by Tana
- Hundreds of Tana's delicious, brain-healthy recipes
- Exercises to kill the ANTs (automatic negative thoughts)
- Meditation and hypnosis audios for sleep, anxiety relief, overcoming weight issues, pain management, and peak performance

- Amazing brain-enhancing music from Grammy Award winner Barry Goldstein
- Online forum for questions and answers, and a community of support
- Access to monthly live coaching calls with Daniel and Tana

BRAINMD HEALTH

www.brainmdhealth.com

For the highest-quality brain health supplements, courses, books, and information products

Notes

THE PROBLEM . . . THE PROMISE . . . THE PROGRAM

1. Christopher A. Taylor et al., "Deaths from Alzheimer's Disease—United States, 1999–2014," *Centers for Disease Control and Prevention Morbidity and Mortality Weekly Report* 66, no. 20 (May 26, 2017), https://www.cdc.gov/mmwr/volumes/66/wr/pdfs /mm6620a1.pdf.

2. R. Brookmeyer et al., "Forecasting the Global Burden of Alzheimer's Disease," *Alzheimer's Dementia* 3, no. 3 (July 2007): 186–91.

PREFACE

1. Kevin McSpadden, "You Now Have a Shorter Attention Span Than a Goldfish," *Time*, May 14, 2015, http://time.com/3858309/attention-spans-goldfish/.

CHAPTER 1: A BREAKTHROUGH APPROACH TO MEMORY ISSUES, AGING, AND ALZHEIMER'S

1. Cleusa P. Ferri et al., "Global Prevalence of Dementia: A Delphi Consensus Study," *Lancet* 366, no. 9503 (December 17, 2005): 2112–17, doi: 10.1016/S0140-6736(05)67889-0.

2. "Who Has the Better Memory, Men or Women?" *ScienceDaily*, November 9, 2016, https://www.sciencedaily.com/releases/2016/11/161109112447.htm.

3. Miia Kivipelto and Krister Håkansson, "A Rare Success against Alzheimer's," *Scientific American*, April 2017, 32–34.

4. Ibid.

5. Brian Krans, "Dementia Drugs Ineffective at Slowing Mental Decline," *Healthline News*, September 17, 2013, http://www.healthline.com/health-news/mental -cognitive-enhancement-medications-dont-slow-mental-decline-091713#1.

6. Eric Rieman et al., "Brain Imaging and Fluid Biomarker Analysis in Young Adults at Genetic Risk for Autosomal Dominant Alzheimer's Disease in the Presenilin 1 E280A Kindred: A Case-Control Study," *Lancet Neurology* 11, no. 12 (December 2012): 1048–56; Yakeel T. Quiroz et al., "Brain Imaging and Blood Biomarker Abnormalities in Children with Autosomal-Dominant Alzheimer's Disease: A Cross-Sectional Study," *JAMA Neurology* 72, no. 8 (August 2015): 912–19, doi: 10.1001/jamaneurol.2015.1099; Camilla Ferrari et al., "Imaging and Cognitive Reserve Studies Predict Dementia in Presymptomatic Alzheimer's Disease Subjects," *Neurodegenerative Diseases* 13 (August 2014): 157–59, doi: 10.1159/000353690; Victor L. Villemagne et al., "Amyloid β Deposition, Neurodegeneration, and Cognitive Decline in Sporadic Alzheimer's Disease: A Prospective Cohort Study," *Lancet Neurology* 12, no. 4 (April 2013): 357–67, doi: 10.1016 /S1474-4422(13)70044-9.

7. S. Gauthier et al., "Mild Cognitive Impairment," *Lancet* 367, no. 9518 (April 15, 2006): 1262–70; F. Jessen et al., "AD Dementia Risk in Late MCI, in Early MCI, and in Subjective Memory Impairment," *Alzheimers & Dementia* 10, no. 1 (January 2014): 76–83; A. J. Mitchell et al., "Risk of Dementia and Mild Cognitive Impairment in Older People with Subjective Memory Complaints: Meta-Analysis," *Acta Psychiatrica Scandinavica* 130, no. 6 (December 2014): 439–51.

8. Yasser Iturria-Medina et al., "Early Role of Vascular Dysregulation on Late-Onset Alzheimer's Disease Based on Multifactorial Data-Driven Analysis," *Nature Communications* 7 (June 21, 2016), article number 11934, doi: 10.1038/ncomms11934.

CHAPTER 2: HOW THE BRAIN WORKS

1. Frederico A. Azevedo et al., "Equal Numbers of Neuronal and Nonneuronal Cells Make the Human Brain an Isometrically Scaled-Up Primate Brain," *Journal of Comparative Neurology* 513, no. 5 (April 10, 2009): 532–41, doi: 10.1002/cne.21974.

2. Elizabeth D. Kirby et al., "Adult Hippocampal Neural Stem and Progenitor Cells Regulate the Neurogenic Niche by Secreting VEGF," *Proceedings of the National Academy of Sciences of the United States of America* 112, no. 13 (March 31, 2015), 4128–33, doi: 10.1073/pnas .1422448112; C. Rolando and V. Taylor, "Neural Stem Cell of the Hippocampus: Development, Physiology Regulation, and Dysfunction in Disease," *Current Topics in Developmental Biology* 107 (2014): 183–206, doi: 10.1016/B978-0-12-416022-4.00007-X.

3. Majid Fotuhi, "Can You Grow Your Hippocampus? Yes. Here's How, and Why It Matters," SharpBrains.com, November 4, 2015, http://sharpbrains.com/blog/2015/11/04/can-you -grow-your-hippocampus-yes-heres-how-and-why-it-matters/.

CHAPTER 3: WHAT TROUBLE LOOKS LIKE

1. Cyndy B. Cordell et al., "Alzheimer's Association Recommendations for Operationalizing the Detection of Cognitive Impairment during the Medicare Annual Wellness Visit in a Primary Care Setting," *Alzheimers & Dementia* 9, no. 2 (2013): 141–50; Soo Borson et al., "Improving Identification of Cognitive Impairment in Primary Care," *Internal Journal of Geriatric Psychiatry* 21, no. 4 (2006): 349–55.

2. American Academy of Neurology, "Low Scores on Memory and Thinking Tests May Signal Alzheimer's 18 Years Prior to Disease," *ScienceDaily*, June 25, 2015, http://www.sciencedaily.com/releases/2015/06/150625143929.htm.

3. Tara Bahrampour, "PET Scans Show Many Alzheimer's Patients May Not Actually Have the Disease," *Washington Post*, July 19, 2017, https://www.washingtonpost .com/national/health-science/brain-scans-show-many-alzheimers-patients-may -not-actually-have-the-disease/2017/07/18/52013620-6bf2-11e7-9c15-177740635e83 _story.html?utm_term=.9f465231f5e5.

CHAPTER 4: THE BRIGHT MINDS APPROACH TO RESCUING YOUR MEMORY

1. Sebastian Köhler et al., "Depression, Vascular Factors, and Risk of Dementia in Primary Care: A Retrospective Cohort Study," *Journal of the American Geriatrics Society* 63, no. 4 (April 2015): 692–98, doi: 10.1111/jgs.13357.

2. B. N. Justin, M. Turek, and A. M. Hakim, "Heart Disease as a Risk Factor for Dementia," *Clinical Epidemiology* 5 (April 26, 2013): 135–45, doi: 10.2147/CLEP.S30621.

3. Köhler et al., "Depression, Vascular Factors, and Risk of Dementia," 692–98; Emanuelle Duron and Olivier Hanon, "Vascular Risk Factors, Cognitive Decline, and Dementia," *Vascular Health and Risk Management* 4, no. 2 (2008): 363–81.

4. Sean P. Kennelly, Brian A. Lawlor, and Rose A. Kenny, "Blood Pressure and the Risk for Dementia: A Double Edged Sword," *Ageing Research Reviews* 8, no. 2 (April 2009): 61–70, doi: 10.1016/j.arr.2008.11.001.

5. Chun-Ming Yang et al., "Increased Risk of Dementia in Patients with Erectile Dysfunction: A Population-Based, Propensity Score-Matched, Longitudinal Follow-Up Study," *Medicine (Baltimore)* 94, no. 24 (June 2015): e990.

6. Jenni Kulmala et al., "Association between Mid- to Late Life Physical Fitness and Dementia: Evidence from the CAIDE Study," *Journal of Internal Medicine* 276, no. 3 (September 2014): 296–307; Kay Deckers et al., "Target Risk Factors for Dementia Prevention: A Systematic Review and Delphi Consensus Study on the Evidence from Observational Studies," *International Journal of Geriatric Psychiatry* 30, no. 3 (November 2014): 234–46, doi: 10.1002/gps.4245; Robert P. Friedland et al., "Patients with Alzheimer's Disease Have Reduced Activities in Midlife Compared with Healthy Control-Group Members," *Proceedings of the National Academy of Sciences of the United States of America* 98, no. 6 (March 13, 2001): 3440–45, doi: 10.1073/pnas.061002998.

7. "Preventing Alzheimer's Disease: What Do We Know?," National Institute on Aging, last updated February 1, 2016, https://www.nia.nih.gov/alzheimers/publication/preventing -alzheimers-disease/risk-factors-alzheimers-disease; Alzheimer's Association, "2014 Alzheimer's Disease Facts and Figures," *Alzheimer's & Dementia* 10, no. 2 (March 2014): 347–92; L. E. Hebert et al., "Change in Risk of Alzheimer Disease over Time," *Neurology* 75, no. 9 (August 31, 2010): 736–91, doi: 10.1212/WNL.0b013e3181f0754f.

8. John Gever, "Link Seen in Age at Retirement and Risk of Alzheimer's," *MedPage Today*, July 15, 2013, http://www.medpagetoday.com/MeetingCoverage/AAIC/40474; Heather A. Lindstrom et al., "The Relationships between Television Viewing in Midlife and the Development of Alzheimer's Disease in a Case-Control Study," *Brain and Cognition* 58, no. 2 (July 2005): 157–65.

9. Dennis Thompson, "These Kinds of Jobs May Help Protect Your Brain from Alzheimer's," *HealthDay*, July 25, 2016, http://www.cbsnews.com/news/jobs-protect-brain -dementia-alzheimers.

10. "Loneliness and Alzheimer's," Rush University Medical Center, https://www.rush.edu /health-wellness/discover-health/loneliness-and-alzheimers.

11. José Antonio Gil-Montoya et al., "Oral Hygiene in the Elderly with Different Degrees of Cognitive Impairment and Dementia," *Journal of the American Geriatrics Society* 65, no. 3 (March 2017): 642–47, doi: 10.1111/jgs.14697/full.

12. Deckers et al., "Target Risk Factors for Dementia Prevention," 234–46.

13. Antonio Cherubini et al., "Low Plasma N-3 Fatty Acids and Dementia in Older Persons: The InCHIANTI Study," *Journals of Gerontology, Series A: Biological Sciences and Medical Sciences* 62, no. 10 (October 2007): 1120–26.

14. Robert C. Green et al., "Risk of Dementia among White and African American Relatives of Patients with Alzheimer Disease," *Journal of the American Medical Association* 287, no. 3 (2002): 329–36, doi: 10.1001/jama.287.3.329; Richard Mayeux et al., "Risk of Dementia in First-Degree Relatives of Patients with Alzheimer's Disease and Related Disorders," *Archives of Neurology* 48, no. 3 (March 1991): 269–73, doi: 10.1001/archneur.1991 .00530150037014.

15. Lindsay A. Farrer et al., "Effects of Age, Sex, and Ethnicity on the Association between

Apolipoprotein E Genotype and Alzheimer Disease: A Meta-Analysis," *Journal of the American Medical Association* 278, no. 16 (October 1997): 1349–56, doi: 10.1001/jama.278.16.1349.

16. Tanya C. Lye and Edwin A. Shores, "Traumatic Brain Injury as a Risk Factor for Alzheimer's Disease: A Review," *Neuropsychology Review* 10, no. 2 (July 2000): 115–29, doi: 10.1023/A:1009068804787; Brenda L. Plassman et al., "Documented Head Injury in Early Adulthood and Risk of Alzheimer's Disease and Other Dementias," *Neurology* 55, no. 8 (October 24, 2000): 1158–66, doi: 10.1212/WNL.55.8.1158; Raquel C. Gardner and Kristine Yaffe, "Traumatic Brain Injury May Increase Risk of Young Onset Dementia," *Annals of Neurology* 75, no. 3 (March 2014): 339–41, doi: 10.1002/ana.24121.

17. Douglas H. Smith, Victoria E. Johnson, and William Stewart, "Chronic Neuropathologies of Single and Repetitive TBI: Substrates of Dementia?," *Nature Reviews: Neurology* 9, no. 4 (April 2013): 211–21; K. M. Guskiewicz, "Association between Recurrent Concussion and Late-Life Cognitive Impairment in Retired Professional Football Players," *Neurosurgery* 57, no. 4 (October 2005): 719–26.

18. Rosebud O. Roberts et al., "Association between Olfactory Dysfunction and Amnestic Mild Cognitive Impairment and Alzheimer Disease Dementia," *Journal of the American Medical Association Neurology* 73, no. 1 (January 2016): 93–101, doi: 10.1001/jamaneurol.2015.2952.

19. Deckers et al., "Target Risk Factors for Dementia Prevention," 234–46; Guochao Zhong, "Smoking Is Associated with an Increased Risk of Dementia: A Meta-Analysis of Prospective Cohort Studies with Investigation of Potential Effect Modifiers," *PLOS One* 10, no. 3 (March 12, 2015): e0118333, doi: 10.1371/journal.pone.0126169.

20. Suzanne L. Tyes, "Alcohol Use and the Risk of Developing Alzheimer's Disease," National Institute on Alcohol Abuse and Alcoholism, https://pubs.niaaa.nih.gov/publications/arh25-4/299-306.htm; Juan Deng, "A 2-Year Follow-Up Study of Alcohol Consumption and Risk of Dementia," *Clinical Neurology and Neurosurgery* 108 (2006): 378–83.

21. Jin-Hua Chen et al., "Dementia Risk in Irradiated Patients with Head and Neck Cancer," *Medicine (Baltimore)* 94, no. 45 (November 2015): e1983, doi: 10.1097/MD.0000000000001983.

22. Jeanne S. Mandelblatt et al., "Long-Term Trajectories of Self-Reported Cognitive Function in a Cohort of Older Survivors of Breast Cancer: CALGB 369901 (Alliance)," *Cancer* 122, no. 22 (July 22, 2016): doi: 10.1002/cncr.30208.

23. Xianglin L. Du, Yi Cai, and Elaine Symanski, "Association between Chemotherapy and Cognitive Impairments in a Large Cohort of Patients with Colorectal Cancer," *International Journal of Oncology* 42, no. 6 (June 2013): 2123–33, doi: 10.3892/ijo.2013.

24. Anushruti Ashok et al., "Exposure to As-, Cd-, and Pb-Mixture Induces Aβ, Amyloidogenic APP Processing and Cognitive Impairments via Oxidative Stress-Dependent Neuroinflammation in Young Rats," *Toxicological Sciences* 143, no. 1 (January 2015): 64–80.

25. L. D. Empting, "Neurologic and Neuropsychiatric Syndrome Features of Mold and Mycotoxin Exposure," *Toxicology and Industrial Health* 25, nos. 9–10 (October 23, 2009): 577–81, doi: 10.1177/0748233709348393.

26. Deckers et al., "Target Risk Factors for Dementia Prevention," 234–46.

27. TsungYang Wang et al., "Risk for Developing Dementia among Patients with Posttraumatic Stress Disorder: A Nationwide Longitudinal Study," *Journal of Affective Disorders* 205 (November 15, 2016): 306–10, doi: 10.1016/j.jad.2016.08.013.

28. Osvaldo P. Almeida et al., "Risk of Dementia and Death in Community-Dwelling Older Men with Bipolar Disorder," *British Journal of Psychiatry* 209, no. 2 (August 2016): 121–26, doi: 10.1192/bjp.bp.115.180059; M. H. Chen et al., "Risk of Subsequent Dementia among Patients with Bipolar Disorder or Major Depression: A Nationwide Longitudinal Study in Taiwan," *Journal of the American Medical Directors Association* 16, no. 6 (June 1, 2015): 504–8.

29. Renate R. Zilkens et al., "Severe Psychiatric Disorders in Mid-Life and Risk of Dementia in

Late-Life (Age 65–84 Years): A Population Based Case-Control Study," *Current Alzheimer Research* 11, no. 7 (2014): 681–93, doi: 10.2174/1567205011666140812115004.

30. Yang et al., "Increased Risk of Dementia in Patients with Erectile Dysfunction: A Population-Based, Propensity Score-Matched, Longitudinal Follow-Up Study," e990.

31. Shireen Sindi et al., "Midlife Work-Related Stress Increases Dementia Risk in Later Life: The CAIDE 30-Year Study," *Journals of Gerontology, Series B: Psychological Sciences and Social Sciences* (April 8, 2016): gbw043, doi: 10.1016/j.jalz.2014.05.1408; Antonio Terracciano et al., "Personality and Resilience to Alzheimer's Disease Neuropathology: A Prospective Autopsy Study," *Neurobiology of Aging* 34, no. 4 (April 2013): 1045–50, doi: 10.1016/j.neurobiolaging.2012.08.008; Lena Johansson et al., "Midlife Psychological Distress Associated with Late-Life Brain Atrophy and White Matter Lesions: A 32-Year Population Study of Women," *Psychosomatic Medicine* 74, no. 2 (February–March 2012): 120–25, doi: 10.1097/PSY.0b013e318246eb10.

32. Richard C. Chou et al., "Treatment for Rheumatoid Arthritis and Risk of Alzheimer's Disease: A Nested Case-Control Analysis," *CNS Drugs* 30, no. 11 (November 2016): 1111–20, doi: 10.1007/s40263-016-0374-z.

33. Yu-Ru Lin et al., "Increased Risk of Dementia in Patients with Systemic Lupus Erythematosus: A Nationwide Population-Based Cohort Study," *Arthritis Care & Research* 68, no. 12 (December 2016): 1774–79, doi: 10.1002/acr.22914.

34. Dennis Thompson, "Immune Disorders Such as MS, Psoriasis May Be Tied to Dementia Risk," *HealthDay*, March 1, 2017, https://consumer.healthday.com/diseases-and -conditions-information-37/immune-disorder-news-404/immune-disorders-such -as-ms-psoriasis-may-be-tied-to-dementia-risk-720235.html.

35. Katrina Abuabara et al., "Cause-Specific Mortality in Patients with Severe Psoriasis: A Population-Based Cohort Study in the U.K.," *British Journal of Dermatology* 163, no. 3 (September 2010): 586–92, doi: 10.1111/j.1365-2133.2010.09941.x.

36. Yi-Hao Peng et al., "Adult Asthma Increases Dementia Risk: A Nationwide Cohort Study," *Journal of Epidemiology and Community Health* 69, no. 2 (February 2015): 123–28, doi: 10.1136/jech-2014-204445; M. Rusanen et al., "Chronic Obstructive Pulmonary Disease and Asthma and the Risk of Mild Cognitive Impairment and Dementia: A Population Based CAIDE Study," *Current Alzheimer Research* 10, no. 5 (June 2013): 549–55.

37. Frederic Blanc et al., "Lyme Neuroborreliosis and Dementia," *Journal of Alzheimer's Disease* 41, no. 4 (April 2014): 1087–93, doi: 10.3233/JAD-130446; Judith Miklossy et al., "Borrelia Burgdorferi Persists in the Brain in Chronic Lyme Neuroborreliosis and May Be Associated with Alzheimer Disease," *Journal of Alzheimer's Disease* 6, no. 6 (December 2004): 639–49.

38. Timo E. Strandberg et al., "Impact of Viral and Bacterial Burden on Cognitive Impairment in Elderly Persons with Cardiovascular Diseases," *Stroke* 34, no. 9 (September 2003): 2126–31, doi: 10.1161/01.STR.0000086754.32238.DA.

39. Anthony T. Dugbartey, "Neurocognitive Aspects of Hypothyroidism," *Archives of Internal Medicine* 158, no. 13 (July 13, 1998): 1413–18, doi:10.1001/archinte.158.13.1413.

40. Stephen C. Waring et al., "Postmenopausal Estrogen Replacement Therapy and Risk of AD: A Population-Based Study," *Neurology* 52, no. 5 (March 1999): 965–70, doi: 10.1212 /WNL.52.5.965.

41. Leung-Wing Chu et al., "Bioavailable Testosterone Predicts a Lower Risk of Alzheimer's Disease in Older Men," *Journal of Alzheimer's Disease* 21, no. 4 (September 10, 2010): 1335–45, doi: 10.3233/JAD-2010-100027.

42. American Academy of Neurology, "Removing Ovaries before Menopause Can Lead to Memory and Movement Problems," *ScienceDaily*, August 30, 2007, www.sciencedaily .com/releases/2007/08/070829162824.htm.

43. Kevin T. Nead et al., "Association between Androgen Deprivation Therapy and Risk of Dementia," *Journal of the American Medical Association Oncology* 3, no. 1 (January 1, 2017): 49–55, doi: 10.1001/jamaoncol.2016.3662.

44. Duron and Hanon, "Vascular Risk Factors, Cognitive Decline, and Dementia," 363–81.

45. Rachel A. Whitmer, "The Epidemiology of Adiposity and Dementia," *Current Alzheimer Research* 4, no. 2 (April 2007): 117–22; Duron and Hanon, "Vascular Risk Factors, Cognitive Decline, and Dementia," 363–81.

46. José A. Luchsinger et al., "Measures of Adiposity and Dementia Risk in Elderly Persons," *Archives of Neurology* 64, no. 3 (March 2007): 392–98.

47. Pin-Liang Chen et al., "Risk of Dementia in Patients with Insomnia and Long-Term Use of Hypnotics: A Population-Based Retrospective Cohort Study," *PLOS One* 7, no. 11 (2012): e49113, doi: 10.1371/journal.pone.0049113.

48. Kristine Yaffe et al., "Sleep-Disordered Breathing, Hypoxia, and Risk of Mild Cognitive Impairment and Dementia in Older Women," *Journal of the American Medical Association* 306, no. 6 (August 10, 2011): 613–19, doi: 10.1001/jama.2011.1115; W. P. Chang et al., "Sleep Apnea and the Risk of Dementia: A Population-Based 5-Year Follow-Up Study in Taiwan," *PLOS One* 8, no. 10 (October 24, 2013): e78655, doi: 10.1371/journal.pone .0078655.

49. Miia Kivipelto et al., "Risk Score for the Prediction of Dementia Risk in 20 Years among Middle Aged People: A Longitudinal, Population-Based Study," *Lancet Neurology* 5, no. 9 (September 2006): 735–41.

50. Mark Hyman, *The UltraMind Solution: Fix Your Broken Brain by Healing Your Body First* (New York: Scribner, 2009), 114.

51. Daniel G. Amen et al., "Reversing Brain Damage in Former NFL Players: Implications for Traumatic Brain Injury and Substance Abuse Rehabilitation," *Journal of Psychoactive Drugs* 43, no. 1 (January–March 2011): 1–5; Daniel G. Amen et al., "Effects of Brain-Directed Nutrients on Cerebral Blood Flow and Neuropsychological Testing: A Randomized, Double-Blind, Placebo-Controlled, Crossover Trial," *Advances in Mind-Body Medicine* 27, no. 2 (Spring 2013): 24–33.

52. Antoine Pariente et al., "The Benzodiazepine-Dementia Disorders Link: Current State of Knowledge," *CNS Drugs* 30, no. 1 (January 2016): 1–7, doi: 10.1007/s40263-015 -0305-4; Heidi Taipale et al., "Use of Benzodiazepines and Related Drugs Is Associated with a Risk of Stroke among Persons with Alzheimer's Disease," *International Clinical Psychopharmacology* 32, no. 3 (May 2017): 135–41, doi: 10.1097/YIC.0000000000000161.

CHAPTER 5: <u>B</u> IS FOR BLOOD FLOW

1. Y. Iturria-Medina et al., "Early Role of Vascular Dysregulation on Late-Onset Alzheimer's Disease Based on Multifactorial Data-Driven Analysis," *Nature Communications* 7 (June 21, 2016): 11934; Marije R. Benedictus et al., "Lower Cerebral Blood Flow Is Associated with Faster Cognitive Decline in Alzheimer's Disease," *European Radiology* 27, no. 3 (March 2017): 1169–75.

2. K. A. Tsvetanov et al., "The Effect of Ageing on fMRI: Correction for the Confounding Effects of Vascular Reactivity Evaluated by Joint fMRI and MEG in 335 Adults," *Human Brain Mapping* 36, no. 6 (June 2015): 2248–69.

3. H. A. Feldman et al., "Impotence and Its Medical and Psychosocial Correlates: Results of the Massachusetts Male Aging Study," *Journal of Urology* 151, no. 1 (January 1994): 54–61.

4. David Perlmutter, *Brain Maker: The Power of Gut Microbes to Heal and Protect Your Brain— for Life* (New York: Little, Brown and Company, 2015).

5. V. Berislav et al., "Blood-Brain Barrier Breakdown in the Aging Human Hippocampus," *Neuron* 85, no. 2 (January 21, 2015): 296–302.

6. O. Kosunen et al., "Relation of Coronary Atherosclerosis and Apolipoprotein E Genotypes in Alzheimer Patients," *Stroke* 26, no. 5 (May 1995): 743–48.

7. F. C. Goldstein et al., "The Relationship between Cognitive Functioning and the JNC-8 Guidelines for Hypertension in Older Adults," *Journals of Gerontology: Series A, Biological Sciences and Medical Sciences* 72, no. 1 (January 2017): 121–26.

8. "High Blood Pressure," Centers for Disease Control and Prevention, http://www.cdc .gov/bloodpressure/facts.htm.

9. F. van Kooten et al., "The Dutch Vascular Factors in Dementia Study: Rationale and Design," *Journal of Neurology* 245, no. 1 (January 1998): 32–39.

10. Joshua O. Cerasuolo et al., "Population-Based Stroke and Dementia Incidence Trends: Age and Sex Variations," *Alzheimer's & Dementia* (March 28, 2017): doi: 10.1016/j .jalz.2017.02.010.

11. Shai Efrati et al., "Hyperbaric Oxygen Induces Late Neuroplasticity in Post Stroke Patients—Randomized, Prospective Trial," *PLOS One* 8, no. 1 (2013): e53716.

12. D. Laurin et al., "Physical Activity and Risk of Cognitive Impairment and Dementia in Elderly Persons," *Archives of Neurology* 58, no. 3 (March 2001): 498–504.

13. Stephanie Studenski et al., "Gait Speed and Survival in Older Adults," *Journal of the American Medical Association* 305, no. 1 (January 5, 2011): 50–58.

14. M. L. Callisaya et al., "Longitudinal Relationships between Cognitive Decline and Gait Slowing: The Tasmanian Study of Cognition and Gait," *Journals of Gerontology: Series A, Biological Sciences and Medical Sciences* 70, no. 10 (October 2015): 1226–32; L. H. Kuller et al., "Risk of Dementia and Death in the Long-Term Follow-Up of the Pittsburgh Cardiovascular Health Study-Cognition Study," *Alzheimer's & Dementia* 12, no. 2 (February 2016): 170–83.

15. C. W. Cotman and N. C. Berchtold, "Exercise: A Behavioral Intervention to Enhance Brain Health and Plasticity," *Trends in Neurosciences* 25, no. 6 (June 2002): 295–301; William D. S. Killgore, Elizabeth A. Olson, and Mareen Weber, "Physical Exercise Habits Correlate with Gray Matter Volume of the Hippocampus in Healthy Adult Humans," *Scientific Reports* 3 (December 12, 2013): 3457.

16. K. M. Gerecke et al., "Exercise Protects against Chronic Restraint Stress-Induced Oxidative Stress in the Cortex and Hippocampus," *Brain Research* 1509 (May 6, 2013): 66–78.

17. V. R. Varma et al., "Low-Intensity Daily Walking Activity Is Associated with Hippocampal Volume in Older Adults," *Hippocampus* 25, no. 5 (May 2015): 605–15.

18. L. F. ten Brinke et al., "Aerobic Exercise Increases Hippocampal Volume in Older Women with Probable Mild Cognitive Impairment: A 6-Month Randomised Controlled Trial," *British Journal of Sports Medicine* 49, no. 4 (February 2015): 248–54; C. Rosano et al., "Hippocampal Response to a 24-Month Physical Activity Intervention in Sedentary Older Adults," *American Journal of Geriatric Psychiatry* 25, no. 3 (March 2017): 209–17; M. M. Kleemeyer et al., "Changes in Fitness Are Associated with Changes in Hippocampal Microstructure and Hippocampal Volume among Older Adults," *NeuroImage* 131 (May 1, 2016): 155–61; F. G. Pajonk et al., "Hippocampal Plasticity in Response to Exercise in Schizophrenia," *Archives of General Psychiatry* 67, no. 2 (February 2010): 133–43.

19. P. A. Adlard et al., "Voluntary Exercise Decreases Amyloid Load in a Transgenic Model of Alzheimer's Disease," *Journal of Neuroscience* 25, no. 17 (April 27, 2005): 4217–21.

20. "Physical Activity May Leave the Brain More Open to Change," *ScienceDaily*, December 7, 2015, http://www.sciencedaily.com/releases/2015/12/151207131508.htm; Giles Sheldrick, "Exercise Keeps Dementia at Bay: Running and Walking 'Significantly' Boosts Brain Power," *Sunday Express*, May 24, 2017, http://www.express.co.uk/life-style/health/795908 /Dementia-running-walking-support-health-medical-lifestyle-swimming-tennis; Laird Harrison, "Aerobic Exercise Reverses Alzheimer's Symptoms," *Medscape*, June 2, 2017, http://www.medscape.com/viewarticle/881057.

21. C. Lenfant et al., "Seventh Report of the Joint National Committee on the Prevention, Detection, Evaluation, and Treatment of High Blood Pressure (JNC 7): Resetting the Hypertension Sails," *Hypertension* 41, no. 6 (June 2001): 1178–79.

22. P. K. Elias et al., "Serum Cholesterol and Cognitive Performance in the Framingham Heart Study," *Psychosomatic Medicine* 67, no. 1 (January–February 2005): 24–30.

23. M. M. Mielke et al., "High Total Cholesterol Levels in Late Life Associated with a Reduced Risk of Dementia," *Neurology* 64, no. 10 (May 24, 2005): 1689–95; A. W. Weverling-Rijnsburger et al., "Total Cholesterol and Risk of Mortality in the Oldest Old," *Lancet* 350, no. 9085 (October 18, 1997): 1119–23.

24. M. Leandri et al., "Balance Features in Alzheimer's Disease and Amnestic Mild Cognitive Impairment," *Journal of Alzheimer's Disease* 16, no. 1 (2009): 113–20; O. Beauchet et al., "Poor Gait Performance and Prediction of Dementia: Results from a Meta-Analysis," *Journal of the American Medical Directors Association* 17, no. 6 (June 1, 2016): 482–90.

25. G. Faraco et al., "Water Deprivation Induces Neurovascular and Cognitive Dysfunction through Vasopressin-Induced Oxidative Stress," *Journal of Cerebral Blood Flow and Metabolism* 34, no. 5 (May 2014): 852–60.

26. A. Newberg et al., "Cerebral Blood Flow during Meditative Prayer: Preliminary Findings and Methodological Issues," *Perceptual and Motor Skills* 97, no. 2 (October 2003): 625–30.

27. M. Lehmann et al., "Vitamin B12-B6-Folate Treatment Improves Blood-Brain Barrier Function in Patients with Hyperhomocysteinaemia and Mild Cognitive Impairment," *Dementia and Geriatric Cognitive Disorders* 16, no. 3 (2003): 145–50.

28. S. Won et al., "Vitamin D Prevents Hypoxia/Reoxygenation-Induced Blood-Brain Barrier Disruption via Vitamin D Receptor-Mediated NF-kB Signaling Pathways," *PLOS One* 10, no. 3 (March 27, 2015): e0122821.

29. B. N. Ames and J. Liu, "Delaying the Mitochondrial Decay of Aging with Acetylcarnitine," *Annals of the New York Academy of Sciences* 1033 (November 2004): 108–16.

30. G. Schreibelt et al., "Lipoic Acid Affects Cellular Migration into the Central Nervous System and Stabilizes Blood-Brain Barrier Integrity," *Journal of Immunology* 177, no. 4 (August 15, 2006): 2630–37.

31. S. K. Tayebati, F. Amenta, and D. Tomassoni, "Cerebrovascular and Blood-Brain Barrier Morphology in Spontaneously Hypertensive Rats: Effect of Treatment with Choline Alphoscerate," *CNS and Neurological Disorders Drug Targets* 14, no. 3 (2015): 421–29.

32. Y. F. Wang et al., "Curcumin Ameliorates the Permeability of the Blood-Brain Barrier during Hypoxia by Upregulating Heme Oxygenase-1 Expression in Brain Microvascular Endothelial Cells," *Journal of Molecular Neuroscience* 41, no. 2 (October 2013): 344–51.

33. H. Wei et al., "Resveratrol Attenuates the Blood-Brain Barrier Dysfunction by Regulation of the MMP-9/TIMP-1 Balance after Cerebral Ischemia Reperfusion in Rats," *Journal of Molecular Neuroscience* 55, no. 4 (April 2015): 872–79.

34. K. L. Russell et al., "Fish Oil Improves Motor Function, Limits Blood-Brain Barrier Disruption, and Reduces Mmp9 Gene Expression in a Rat Model of Juvenile Traumatic Brain Injury," *Prostaglandins, Leukotreines, and Essential Fatty Acids* 90, no. 1 (January 2014): 5–11.

35. J. E. James, "Critical Review of Dietary Caffeine and Blood Pressure: A Relationship That Should Be Taken More Seriously," *Psychosomatic Medicine* 66, no. 1 (January–February 2004): 63–71.

36. C. Borghi and A. F. Cicero, "Nutraceuticals with a Clinically Detectable Blood Pressure-Lowering Effect: A Review of Available Randomized Clinical Trials and Their Meta-analyses," *British Journal of Clinical Pharmacology* 83, no. 1 (January 2017): 163–71.

37. Matthew H. Robinson et al., "Enhanced Protein Translation Underlies Improved Metabolic and Physical Adaptations to Different Exercise Training Modes in Young and Old Humans," *Cell Metabolism* 25, no. 3 (March 7, 2017): 581–92.

38. Callisaya et al., "Longitudinal Relationships between Cognitive Decline and Gait Slowing: The Tasmanian Study of Cognition and Gait," 1226–32.

39. J. C. Davis et al., "An Economic Evaluation of Resistance Training and Aerobic Training versus Balance and Toning Exercises in Older Adults with Mild Cognitive Impairment," *PLOS One* 8, no. 5 (May 14, 2013): e63031.

40. Y. Mavros et al., "Mediation of Cognitive Function Improvements by Strength Gains after Resistance Training in Older Adults with Mild Cognitive Impairment: Outcomes of the Study of Mental and Resistance Training," *Journal of the American Geriatrics Society* 65, no. 3 (March 2017): 550–59.

41. Pekka Oja et al., "Associations of Specific Types of Sports and Exercise with All-Cause and Cardiovascular-Disease Mortality: A Cohort Study of 80 306 British Adults," *British Journal of Sports Medicine* (November 28, 2016), doi: 10.1136/bjsports-2016-096822.

42. Bog Ja Jeoung, "Relationships of Exercise with Frailty, Depression, and Cognitive Function in Older Women," *Journal of Exercise and Rehabilitation* 10, no. 5 (October 31, 2014): 291–94.

43. A. E. Den Heijer et al., "Sweat It Out? The Effects of Physical Exercise on Cognition and Behavior in Children and Adults with ADHD: A Systematic Literature Review," *Journal of Neural Transmission (Vienna)* 124, suppl. 1 (February 2017): 3–26.

44. R. F. Santos et al., "Cognitive Performance, SPECT, and Blood Viscosity in Elderly Non-demented People Using Ginkgo Biloba," *Pharmacopsychiatry* 36, no. 4 (July 2003): 127–33; J. A. Mix and W. D. Crews Jr., "A Double-Blind, Placebo-Controlled, Randomized Trial of Ginkgo Biloba Extract EGb 761 in a Sample of Cognitively Intact Older Adults: Neuropsychological Findings," *Human Psychopharmacology* 17, no. 6 (August 2002): 267–77; A. Mashayekh et al., "Effects of Ginkgo Biloba on Cerebral Blood Flow Assessed by Quantitative MR Perfusion Imaging: A Pilot Study," *Neuroradiology* 3, no. 3 (March 2011): 185–91; F. Eckmann, "Cerebral Insufficiency—Treatment with Ginkgo-Biloba Extract. Time of Onset of Effect in a Double-Blind Study with 60 Inpatients," *Fortschritte der Medizin* 108, no. 29 (October 10, 1990): 557–60; H. Herrschaft et al., "Ginkgo Biloba Extract EGb 761® in Dementia with Neuropsychiatric Features: A Randomised, Placebo-Controlled Trial to Confirm the Efficacy and Safety of a Daily Dose of 240 mg," *Journal of Psychiatric Research* 46, no. 6 (June 2012): 716–23.

45. D. J. Lamport et al., "The Effect of Flavanol-Rich Cocoa on Cerebral Perfusion in Healthy Older Adults during Conscious Resting State: A Placebo Controlled, Crossover, Acute Trial," *Psychopharmacology (Berlin)* 232, no. 14 (September 2015): 3227–34; D. T. Field, C. M. Williams, and L. T. Butler, "Consumption of Cocoa Flavanols Results in an Acute Improvement in Visual and Cognitive Functions," *Physiology and Behavior* 103, nos. 3–4 (June 1, 2011): 255–60; S. T. Francis et al., "The Effect of Flavanol-Rich Cocoa on the fMRI Response to a Cognitive Task in Healthy Young People," *Journal of Cardiovascular Pharmacology* 47, suppl. 2 (2006): S215–20; F. A. Sorond et al., "Neurovascular Coupling, Cerebral White Matter Integrity, and Response to Cocoa in Older People," *Neurology* 81, no. 10 (September 3, 2013): 904–9.

46. K. Ried et al., "Effect of Cocoa on Blood Pressure," *Cochrane Database of Systematic Reviews*, no. 8 (August 15, 2012): CD008893; Karin Ried et al., "Does Chocolate Reduce Blood Pressure? A Meta-analysis," *BMC Medicine* 8, no. 39 (June 28, 2010).

47. G. Desideri et al., "Benefits in Cognitive Function, Blood Pressure, and Insulin Resistance through Cocoa Flavanol Consumption in Elderly Subjects with Mild Cognitive Impairment: The Cocoa, Cognition, and Aging (CoCoA) Study," *Hypertension* 60, no. 3 (September 2012): 794–801; Daniela Mastroiacovo et al., "Cocoa Flavanol Consumption Improves Cognitive Function, Blood Pressure Control, and Metabolic Profile in Elderly Subjects: The Cocoa, Cognition, and Aging (CoCoA) Study—A Randomized Controlled Trial," *American Journal of Clinical Nutrition* 101, no. 3 (March 2015): 538–48.

48. D. Grassi et al., "Flavanol-Rich Chocolate Acutely Improves Arterial Function and Working Memory Performance Counteracting the Effects of Sleep Deprivation in Healthy Individuals," *Journal of Hypertension* 34, no. 7 (July 2016): 1298–308.

49. Mandy Oaklander, "5 Surprising Ways to Help Your Memory," *Time* (June 10, 2015), http://time.com/3915030/boost-memory-exercise/; P. A. Jackson et al., "DHA-Rich Oil Modulates the Cerebral Haemodynamic Response to Cognitive Tasks in Healthy Young Adults: A Near IR Spectroscopy Pilot Study," *British Journal of Nutrition* 107, no. 8 (April 2012): 1093–98; T. J. Song et al., "Low Levels of Plasma Omega 3-Polyunsaturated Fatty Acids Are Associated with Cerebral Small Vessel Diseases in Acute Ischemic Stroke Patients," *Nutrition Research* 35, no. 5 (May 2015): 368–74; Daniel G. Amen et al., "Quantitative Erythrocyte Omega-3 EPA Plus DHA Levels Are Related to Higher Regional Cerebral Blood Flow on Brain SPECT," *Journal of Alzheimer's Disease* 58, no. 4 (May 2017): 1189–99, doi: 10.3233/JAD-17028.

50. F. Jernerén et al., "Brain Atrophy in Cognitively Impaired Elderly: The Importance of Long-Chain ω-3 Fatty Acids and B Vitamin Status in a Randomized Controlled Trial," *American Journal of Clinical Nutrition* 102, no. 1 (July 2015): 215–21.

51. E. L. Boespflug et al., "Fish Oil Supplementation Increases Event-Related Posterior Cingulate Activation in Older Adults with Subjective Memory Impairment," *Journal of Nutrition, Health, and Aging* 20, no. 2 (February 2016): 161–69.

52. A. V. Witte et al., "Long-Chain Omega-3 Fatty Acids Improve Brain Function and Structure in Older Adults," *Cerebral Cortex* 24, no. 11 (November 2014): 3059–68.

53. N. Hamazaki-Fujita et al., "Polyunsaturated Fatty Acids and Blood Circulation in the Forebrain during a Mental Arithmetic Task," *Brain Research* 1397 (June 23, 2011): 38–45.

54. "Omega-3 Fatty Acids," website of the University of Maryland Medical Center, http://umm .edu/health/medical/altmed/supplement/omega3-fatty-acids.

55. E. L. Wightman et al., "Epigallocatechin Gallate, Cerebral Blood Flow Parameters, Cognitive Performance and Mood in Healthy Humans: A Double-Blind, Placebo-Controlled, Crossover Investigation," *Human Psychopharmacology* 27, no. 2 (March 2012): 177–86.

56. X. Peng et al., "Effect of Green Tea Consumption on Blood Pressure: A Meta-analysis of 13 Randomized Controlled Trials," *Scientific Reports* 4 (September 2014): 6251.

57. Li Shen et al., "Tea Consumption and Risk of Stroke: A Dose-Response Meta-analysis of Prospective Studies," *Journal of Zhejiang University: Science B* 13, no. 8 (August 2012): 652–62.

58. X. X. Zheng et al., "Green Tea Intake Lowers Fasting Serum Total and LDL Cholesterol in Adults: A Meta-analysis of 14 Randomized Controlled Trials," *American Journal of Clinical Nutrition* 94, no. 2 (August 2011): 601–10.

59. X. X. Zheng et al., "Effects of Green Tea Catechins with or without Caffeine on Glycemic Control in Adults: A Meta-analysis of Randomized Controlled Trials," *American Journal of Clinical Nutrition* 97, no. 4 (April 2013): 750–62.

60. Q. Zhang et al., "Effect of Green Tea on Reward Learning in Healthy Individuals: A Randomized, Double-Blind, Placebo-Controlled Pilot Study," *Nutrition Journal* 12 (June 18, 2013): 84.

61. Q. P. Ma et al., "Meta-Analysis of the Association between Tea Intake and the Risk of Cognitive Disorders," *PLOS One* 11, no. 11 (November 8, 2016): e0165861; L. Feng et al., "Tea Consumption Reduces the Incidence of Neurocognitive Disorders: Findings from the Singapore Longitudinal Aging Study," *Journal of Nutrition, Health & Aging* 20, no. 10 (2016): 1002, doi: 10.1007/s12603-016-0687-0.

62. S. Iravani and B. Zolfaghari, "Pharmaceutical and Nutraceutical Effects of Pinus Pinaster Bark Extract," *Research in Pharmaceutical Sciences* 6, no. 1 (January 2011): 1–11.

63. R. Luzzi et al., "Pycnogenol Supplementation Improves Cognitive Function, Attention, and Mental Performance in Students," *Panminerva Medica*, 53, no. 3, suppl. 1 (September 2011): 75–82; J. Ryan et al., "An Examination of the Effects of the Antioxidant Pycnogenol on Cognitive Performance, Serum Lipid Profile, Endocrinological and Oxidative Stress Biomarkers in an Elderly Population," *Journal of Psychopharmacology* 22, no. 5 (July 2008): 553–62.

64. D. C. Kennedy et al., "Effects of Resveratrol on Cerebral Blood Flow Variables and Cognitive Performance in Humans: A Double-Blind, Placebo-Controlled, Crossover Investigation," *American Journal of Clinical Nutrition* 91, no. 6 (June 2010): 1590–97; R. H. Wong, D. Raederstorff, and P. R. Howe, "Acute Resveratrol Consumption Improves Neurovascular Coupling Capacity in Adults with Type 2 Diabetes Mellitus," *Nutrients* 8, no. 7 (July 12, 2016): pii: E425.

65. R. M. Thushara et al., "Cardiovascular Benefits of Probiotics: A Review of Experimental and Clinical Studies," *Food and Function* 7, no. 2 (February 2016): 632–42.

66. Heike Wersching, Hannah Gardener, and Ralph L. Sacco, "Sugar-Sweetened and Artificially-Sweetened Beverages in Relation to Stroke and Dementia," *Stroke* 48 (2017): 1129–31, doi: 10.1161/STROKEAHA.117.017198.

67. Matthew P. Pase et al., "Sugar- and Artificially Sweetened Beverages and the Risks of Incident Stroke and Dementia: A Prospective Cohort Study," *Stroke* (April 20, 2017): [Epub ahead of print].

68. Mustafa Chopan and Benjamin Littenberg, "The Association of Hot Red Chili Pepper Consumption and Mortality: A Large Population-Based Cohort Study." *PLOS One* 12, no. 1 (2017): e0169876.

69. L. C. Tapsell et al., "Health Benefits of Herbs and Spices: The Past, the Present, the Future," *Medical Journal of Australia* 185, suppl. 4 (August 21, 2006): S4–24.

70. S. Rastogi, M. M. Pandey, and A. Rawat, "Spices: Therapeutic Potential in Cardiovascular Health," *Current Pharmaceutical Design* (October 21, 2016): [Epub ahead of print].

71. Ibid.

72. Pasupuleti Visweswara Rao and Siew Hua Gan, "Cinnamon: A Multifaceted Medicinal Plant," *Evidence-Based Complementary and Alternative Medicine* (2014): article ID 642942.

73. T. D. Presley et al., "Acute Effect of a High Nitrate Diet on Brain Perfusion in Older Adults," *Nitric Oxide* 24, no. 1 (January 1, 2011): 34–42; E. L. Wightman et al., "Dietary Nitrate Modulates Cerebral Blood Flow Parameters and Cognitive Performance in Humans: A Double-Blind, Placebo-Controlled, Crossover Investigation," *Physiology and Behavior* 149 (October 1, 2015): 149–58; Diego dos Santos Baião et al., "Beetroot Juice Increase Nitric Oxide Metabolites in Both Men and Women Regardless of Body Mass," *International Journal of Food Sciences and Nutrition* 67, no. 1 (2016): 40–46.

74. A. Aleixandre and M. Miguel, "Dietary Fiber and Blood Pressure Control," *Food and Function* 7, no. 4 (April 2016): 1864–71.

75. P. Surampudi et al., "Lipid Lowering with Soluble Dietary Fiber," *Current Atherosclerosis Reports* 18, no. 12 (December 2016): 75.

76. L. Stojanovska et al., "Maca Reduces Blood Pressure and Depression, in a Pilot Study in Postmenopausal Women," *Climacteric* 18, no. 1 (February 2015): 69–78.

CHAPTER 6: R IS FOR RETIREMENT AND AGING

1. Maureen Salamon, "Delaying Retirement May Help Stave Off Alzheimer's," WebMD (July 15, 2013), http://www.webmd.com/alzheimers/news/20130715/putting-off-retirement -may-help-stave-off-alzheimers#1.

2. Dave Asprey, *Head Strong: The Bulletproof Plan to Activate Untapped Brain Energy to Work Smarter and Think Faster—in Just Two Weeks* (New York: Harper Wave, 2017), 19.

3. C. Porter et al., "Mitochondrial Respiratory Capacity and Coupling Control Decline with Age in Human Skeletal Muscle," *American Journal of Physiology: Endocrinology and Metabolism* 309, no. 3 (August 1, 2015): E224–32.

4. Dominic J. Hare et al., "Is Early-Life Iron Exposure Critical in Neurodegeneration?" *Nature Reviews Neurology* 11, no. 9 (September 2015): 536–44; A. C. Leskovjan et al., "Increased Brain Iron Coincides with Early Plaque Formation in a Mouse Model of Alzheimer's Disease," *NeuroImage* 55, no. 1 (March 1, 2011): 32–38.

5. R. M. Cawthon et al., "Association between Telomere Length in Blood and Mortality in People Aged 60 Years or Older," *Lancet* 361, no. 9355 (February 1, 2003): 393–95.

6. J. Zhang et al., "Ageing and the Telomere Connection: An Intimate Relationship with Inflammation," *Ageing Research Reviews* 25 (January 2016): 55–69.

7. C. C. Meltzer et al., "Serotonin in Aging, Late-Life Depression, and Alzheimer's Disease: The Emerging Role of Functional Imaging," *Neuropsychopharmacology* 18, no. 6 (June 1998): 407–30.

8. Scott E. Hemby, John Q. Trojanowski, and Stephen D. Ginsberg, "Neuron-Specific Age-Related Decreases in Dopamine Receptor Subtype mRNAs," *Journal of Comparative Neurology* 465, no. 2 (February 3, 2003): 176–83; Jean-Claude Dreher et al., "Age-Related Changes in Midbrain Dopaminergic Regulation of the Human Reward System," *Proceedings of the National Academy of Sciences of the United States of America* 105, no. 39 (September 30, 2008): 15106–11.

9. Thomas H. McNeill and Michael Jakowec, "Neurotransmitters—Gaba and Glutamate," http://medicine.jrank.org/pages/1225/Neurotransmitters-GABA-glutamate.html.

10. J. L. Muir, "Acetylcholine, Aging, and Alzheimer's Disease," *Pharmacology, Biochemistry, and Behavior* 56, no. 4 (April 1997): 687–96.

11. T. J. Holwerda et al., "Feelings of Loneliness, but Not Social Isolation, Predict Dementia Onset: Results from the Amsterdam Study of the Elderly (AMSTEL)," *Journal of Neurology, Neurosurgery, and Psychiatry* 85, no. 2 (February 2014), doi: 10.1136/jnnp-2012-302755.

12. Bryan D. James et al., "Late-Life Social Activity and Cognitive Decline in Old Age," *Journal of the International Neuropsychological Society* 17, no. 6 (November 2011): 998–1005, doi: 10.1017/S1355617711000531.

13. "Loneliness on the Rise: One in Eight People Have No Close Friends to Turn To," *Express* (March 1, 2017), http://www.express.co.uk/news/uk/773002/One-in-eight-people-faced -with-loneliness.

14. P. Sebastiani et al., "Biomarker Signatures of Aging," *Aging Cell* 16, no. 2 (Epub January 6, 2017): doi: 10.1111/acel.12557.

15. Joseph Mercola, "Iron: This Life-Saving Mineral Found to Actually Increase Senility in Many," *Mercola*, July 19, 2012, http://articles.mercola.com/sites/articles/archive/2012/07 /19/excess-iron-leads-to-alzheimers.aspx#_edn1.

16. "Telomere Testing," SpectraCell Laboratories, https://www.spectracell.com/clinicians /products/telomere-testing/.

17. "The Tall Tail of Telomeres," *Mark's Daily Apple*, May 30, 2012, http://www.marksdailyapple .com/the-tall-tail-of-telomeres/; Yasumichi Arai et al., "Inflammation, but Not Telomere Length, Predicts Successful Ageing at Extreme Old Age: A Longitudinal Study of Semi- Supercentenarians," *EBioMedicine* 2, no. 10 (July 29, 2015): 1549–58.

18. S. Kamhieh-Milz et al., "Regular Blood Donation May Help in the Management of Hypertension: An Observational Study on 292 Blood Donors," *Transfusion* 56, no. 3 (March 2016): 637–44.

19. S. Samman et al., "Green Tea or Rosemary Extract Added to Foods Reduces Nonheme- Iron Absorption," *American Journal of Clinical Nutrition* 73, no. 3 (March 2001): 607–12.

20. Y. Jiao et al., "Iron Chelation in the Biological Activity of Curcumin," *Free Radical Biology and Medicine* 40, no. 7 (April 1, 2006): 1152–60.

21. Lindsay Lyon, "How 5 Longevity Researchers Stave Off Aging," *U.S. News & World Report*, December 23, 2009, http://health.usnews.com/health-news/family-health/slideshows /how-5-longevity-researchers-stave-off-aging.

22. Alan Mozes, "DNA 'Telomere' Length Tied to Aging, Death Risk," *HealthDay*, November 8, 2012, https://consumer.healthday.com/senior-citizen-information-31/misc-aging -news-10/dna-telomere-length-tied-to-aging-death-risk-670426.html.

23. Ibid.

24. N. Shivappa et al., "Association between the Dietary Inflammatory Index (DII) and Telomere Length and C-Reactive Protein from the National Health and Nutrition Examination Survey—1999–2002," *Molecular Nutrition and Food Research* 61, no. 4 (April 2016); J. Y. Wong et al., "The Relationship between Inflammatory Biomarkers and Telomere Length in an Occupational Prospective Cohort Study," *PLOS One* 9, no. 1 (January 27, 2014): e87348.

25. J. B. Richards et al., "Homocysteine Levels and Leukocyte Telomere Length," *Atherosclerosis* 200, no. 2 (October 2008): 271–77; see comment in PubMed Commons below G. Rane et al., "Association between Leukocyte Telomere Length and Plasma Homocysteine in a Singapore Chinese Population," *Rejuvenation Research* 18, no. 3 (June 2015): 203–10.

26. M. A. Babizhayev, K. S. Vishnyakova, and Y. E. Yegorov, "Oxidative Damage Impact on Aging and Age-Related Diseases: Drug Targeting of Telomere Attrition and Dynamic Telomerase Activity Flirting with Imidazole-Containing Dipeptides," *Recent Patents on Drug Delivery and Formulation* 8, no. 3 (2014): 163–92.

27. J. Shen et al., "Telomere Length, Oxidative Damage, Antioxidants and Breast Cancer Risk," *International Journal of Cancer* 124, no. 7 (April 1, 2009): 1637–43.

28. Aric A. Prather et al., "Tired Telomeres: Poor Global Sleep Quality, Perceived Stress, and Telomere Length in Immune Cell Subsets in Obese Men and Women," *Brain, Behavior, and Immunity* 47 (July 2015): 155–62.

29. Ibid; Stacy Lu, "How Chronic Stress Is Harming Our DNA," *Monitor on Psychology* 45, no. 9 (October 2014): 18, http://www.apa.org/monitor/2014/10/chronic-stress.aspx.

30. Q. Shen et al., "Association of Leukocyte Telomere Length with Type 2 Diabetes in Mainland Chinese Populations," *Journal of Clinical Endocrinology and Metabolism* 97, no. 4 (April 2012): 1371–74.

31. L. Rode et al., "Increased Body Mass Index, Elevated C-Reactive Protein, and Short Telomere Length," *Journal of Clinical Endocrinology and Metabolism* 99, no. 4 (September 2014): E1671–75.

32. J. H. Kim et al., "Habitual Physical Exercise Has Beneficial Effects on Telomere Length in Postmenopausal Women," *Menopause* 19, no. 10 (October 2012): 1109–15; Per Sjögren et al., "Stand Up for Health—Avoiding Sedentary Behaviour Might Lengthen Your Telomeres: Secondary Outcomes from a Physical Activity RCT in Older People," *British Journal of Sports Medicine* 48 (September 3, 2014): 1407–9.

33. D. Ornish et al., "Increased Telomerase Activity and Comprehensive Lifestyle Changes: A Pilot Study," *Lancet Oncology* 9, no. 11 (November 2008): 1048–57.

34. N. Adler et al., "Educational Attainment and Late Life Telomere Length in the Health, Aging and Body Composition Study," *Brain, Behavior, and Immunology* 47, no. 1 (January 2013): 15–21.

35. Linda E. Carlson et al., "Mindfulness-Based Cancer Recovery and Supportive-Expressive Therapy Maintain Telomere Length Relative to Controls in Distressed Breast Cancer Survivors," *Cancer* 121, no. 3 (February 1, 2015): 476–84.

36. J. K. Kiecolt-Glaser et al., "Omega-3 Fatty Acids, Oxidative Stress, and Leukocyte Telomere Length: A Randomized Controlled Trial," *Brain, Behavior, and Immunology* 28 (February 2013): 16–24; A. Barden et al., "n-3 Fatty Acid Supplementation and Leukocyte Telomere Length in Patients with Chronic Kidney Disease," *Nutrients* 8, no. 3 (March 19, 2016): 175.

37. L. Salvador et al., "A Natural Product Telomerase Activator Lengthens Telomeres in Humans: A Randomized, Double Blind, and Placebo Controlled Study," *Rejuvenation Research* 19, no. 6 (December 2016): 478–84.

38. J. B. Richards et al., "Higher Serum Vitamin D Concentrations Are Associated with Longer Leukocyte Telomere Length in Women," *American Journal of Clinical Nutrition* 86, no. 5 (November 2007): 1420–25; Mohsen Mazidi, Erin D. Michos, and Maciej Banach, "The Association of Telomere Length and Serum 25-Hydroxyvitamin D Levels in US Adults: The National Health and Nutrition Examination Survey," *Archives of Medical Science* 13, no. 1 (February 1, 2017): 61–65.

39. Ornish et al., "Increased Telomerase Activity," 1048–57.

40. Q. Xu et al., "Multivitamin Use and Telomere Length in Women," *American Journal of Clinical Nutrition* 89, no. 6 (June 2009): 1857–63.

41. Sonja Hilbrand et al., "Caregiving within and beyond the Family Is Associated with Lower Mortality for the Caregiver: A Prospective Study," *Evolution and Human Behavior* 39, no. 3 (2016): doi: 10.1016/j.evolhumbehav.2016.11.010.

42. Hayley Wright, Rebecca A. Jenks, and Nele Demeyere, "Frequent Sexual Activity Predicts Specific Cognitive Abilities in Older Adults," *The Journals of Gerontology: Series B* (June 21, 2017): doi: 10.1093/geronb/gbx065.

43. F. Amenta et al., "The ASCOMALVA (Association between the Cholinesterase Inhibitor Donepezil and the Cholinergic Precursor Choline Alphoscerate in Alzheimer's Disease) Trial: Interim Results after Two Years of Treatment," *Journal of Alzheimer's Disease* 42, suppl. 3 (2014): S281–88; A. Carotenuto et al., "The Effect of the Association between Donepezil and Choline Alphoscerate on Behavioral Disturbances in Alzheimer's Disease: Interim Results of the ASCOMALVA Trial," *Journal of Alzheimer's Disease* 56, no. 2 (2017): 805–15; R. Rea et al., "Apathy Treatment in Alzheimer's Disease: Interim Results of the

ASCOMALVA Trial," *Journal of Alzheimer's Disease* 48, no. 2 (2015): 377–83; T. Kawamura et al., "Glycerophosphocholine Enhances Growth Hormone Secretion and Fat Oxidation in Young Adults," *Nutrition* 28, nos. 11–12 (November–December 2012): 1122–26; G. Strifler et al., "Targeting Mitochondrial Dysfunction with L-Alpha Glycerylphosphorylcholine," *PLOS One* 11, no. 11 (November 18, 2016): e0166682.

44. Parris M. Kidd, "Phosphatidylserine, Membrane Nutrient for Memory: A Clinical and Mechanistic Assessment," *Alternative Medicine Review* 1, no. 2 (1996): 70–84.

45. T. H. Crook et al., "Effects of Phosphatidylserine in Age-Associated Memory Impairment," *Neurology* 41 (1991): 644–49.

46. Adriana Cristofano et al., "Serum Levels of Acyl-Carnitines along the Continuum from Normal to Alzheimer's Dementia," *PLOS One* 11, no. 5 (2016): e0155694.

47. S. A. Montgomery, L. J. Thal, and R. Amrein, "Meta-Analysis of Double Blind Randomized Controlled Clinical Trials of Acetyl-L-carnitine versus Placebo in the Treatment of Mild Cognitive Impairment and Mild Alzheimer's Disease," *International Clinical Psychopharmacology* 18, no. 2 (March 2003): 61–71.

48. S. Kasperczyk et al., "The Administration of N-acetylcysteine Reduces Oxidative Stress and Regulates Glutathione Metabolism in the Blood Cells of Workers Exposed to Lead," *Clinical Toxicology (Philadelphia)* 51, no. 6 (July 2013): 480–86.

49. G. S. Kelly, "Clinical Applications of N-acetylcysteine," *Alternative Medicine Review: A Journal of Clinical Therapeutic* 3, no. 2 (April 1998): 114–27.

50. Olive Dean, Frank Giorlando, and Michael Berk, "N-acetylcysteine in Psychiatry: Current Therapeutic Evidence and Potential Mechanisms of Action," *Journal of Psychiatry and Neuroscience* 36, no. 2 (March 2011): 78–86.

51. J. C. Adair, J. E. Knoefel, and N. Morgan, "Controlled Trial of N-acetylcysteine for Patients with Probable Alzheimer's Disease," *Neurology* 57, no. 8 (October 23, 2001): 1515–17; W. R. Shankle et al., "CerefolinNAC Therapy of Hyperhomocysteinemia Delays Cortical and White Matter Atrophy in Alzheimer's Disease and Cerebrovascular Disease," *Journal of Alzheimer's Disease* 54, no. 3 (October 4, 2016): 1073–84.

52. Y. Ashani, J. O. Peggins, and B. P. Doctor, "Mechanism of Inhibition of Cholinesterases by Huperzine A," *Biochemical and Biophysical Research Communications* 18, no. 2 (April 30, 1992): 719–26.

53. B. S. Wang et al., "Efficacy and Safety of Natural Acetylcholinesterase Inhibitor Huperzine A in the Treatment of Alzheimer's Disease: An Updated Meta-analysis," *Journal of Neural Transmission* 116, no. 4 (April 2009): 457–65.

54. H. S. Ved et al., "Huperzine A, a Potential Therapeutic Agent for Dementia, Reduces Neuronal Cell Death Caused by Glutamate," *Neuroreport* 8, no. 4 (March 3, 1997): 963–68; A. A. Skolnick, "Old Chinese Herbal Medicine Used for Fever Yields Possible New Alzheimer Disease Therapy," *Journal of the American Medical Association* 277, no. 10 (March 12, 1997): 776.

55. Seyedeh Zeinab Mousavi and Seyedeh Zahra Bathale, "Historical Uses of Saffron: Identifying Potential New Avenues for Modern Research," *Avicenna Journal of Phytomedicine* 1, no. 2 (September 2011): 57–66.

56. H. A. Hausenblas et al., "Saffron (Crocus Sativus L.) and Major Depressive Disorder: A Meta-analysis of Randomized Clinical Trials," *Journal of Integrative Medicine* 11, no. 6 (November 2013): 377–83.

57. M. Agha-Hosseini et al., "Crocus Sativus L. (Saffron) in the Treatment of Premenstrual Syndrome: A Double-Blind, Randomised and Placebo-Controlled Trial," *British Journal of Obstetrics and Gynaecology* 115, no. 4 (March 2008): 515–19.

58. L. Kashani et al., "Saffron for Treatment of Fluoxetine-Induced Sexual Dysfunction in Women: Randomized Double-Blind Placebo-Controlled Study," *Human Psychopharmacology* 28, no. 1 (January 2013): 54–60; A. Modabbernia et al., "Effect of Saffron on Fluoxetine-Induced Sexual Impairment in Men: Randomized Double-Blind Placebo-Controlled Trial," *Psychopharmacology (Berlin)* 223, no. 4 (October 2012): 381–88.

59. M. A. Papandreou et al., "Inhibitory Activity on Amyloid-beta Aggregation and Antioxidant

Properties of Crocus Sativus Stigmas Extract and Its Crocin Constituents," *Journal of Agricultural and Food Chemistry* 54, no. 23 (November 15, 2006): 8762–68.

60. S. Soeda et al., "Neuroprotective Activities of Saffron and Crocin," *Advances in Neurobiology* 12 (2016): 275–92.

61. M. Tsolaki et al., "Efficacy and Safety of Crocus Sativus L. in Patients with Mild Cognitive Impairment: One Year Single-Blind Randomized, with Parallel Groups, Clinical Trial," *Journal of Alzheimer's Disease* 54, no. 1 (July 27, 2016): 129–33.

62. S. Akhondzadeh et al., "A 22-Week, Multicenter, Randomized, Double-Blind Controlled Trial of Crocus Sativus in the Treatment of Mild-to-Moderate Alzheimer's Disease," *Psychopharmacology (Berlin)* 207, no. 4 (January 2010): 637–43; S. Akhondzadeh et al., "Saffron in the Treatment of Patients with Mild to Moderate Alzheimer's Disease: A 16-Week, Randomized and Placebo-Controlled Trial," *Journal of Clinical Pharmacy and Therapeutics* 35, no. 5 (October 2010): 581–88.

63. M. Farokhnia et al., "Comparing the Efficacy and Safety of Crocus Sativus L. with Memantine in Patients with Moderate to Severe Alzheimer's Disease: A Double-Blind Randomized Clinical Trial," *Human Psychopharmacology* 29, no. 4 (July 2014): 351–59.

64. Esmaeal Tamaddonfard et al., "Crocin Improved Learning and Memory Impairments in Streptozotocin-Induced Diabetic Rats," *Iranian Journal of Basic Medical Sciences* 16, no. 1 (January 2013): 91–100.

65. G. D. Geromichalos et al., "Saffron as a Source of Novel Acetylcholinesterase Inhibitors: Molecular Docking and In Vitro Enzymatic Studies," *Journal of Agricultural and Food Chemistry* 60, no. 24 (June 20, 2012): 6131–38.

66. Sabrina Morelli et al., "Neuronal Membrane Bioreactor as a Tool for Testing Crocin Neuroprotective Effect in Alzheimer's Disease," *Chemical Engineering Journal* 305 (January 2016): doi: 10.1016/j.cej.2016.01.035.

67. M. Rashedinia et al., "Protective Effect of Crocin on Acrolein-Induced Tau Phosphorylation in the Rat Brain," *Acta Neurobiologiae Experimentalis* 75, no. 2 (2015): 208–19.

68. Steven Roodenrys et al., "Chronic Effects of Brahmi (Bacopa Monnieri) on Human Memory," *Neuropsychopharmacology* 27, no. 2 (2002): 279–81, doi:10.1016/S0893-133X(01)00419-5; C. Stough et al., "Examining the Cognitive Effects of a Special Extract of Bacopa Monniera: A Review of Ten Years of Research at Swinburne University," *Journal of Pharmacy and Pharmaceutical Science* 16, no. 2 (2013): 254–58.

69. N. R. Tildesley et al., "Salvia Lavandulaefolia (Spanish Sage) Enhances Memory in Healthy, Young Volunteers," *Pharmacology, Biochemistry, and Behavior* 75, no. 3 (June 2003): 669–74; A. B. Scholey et al., "An Extract of Salvia (Sage) with Anticholinesterase Properties Improves Memory and Attention in Healthy Older Volunteers," *Psychopharmacology (Berlin)* 198, no. 1 (May 2008): 127–39; D. O. Kennedy et al., "Monoterpenoid Extract of Sage (Salvia Lavandulaefolia) with Cholinesterase Inhibiting Properties Improves Cognitive Performance and Mood in Healthy Adults," *Journal of Psychopharmacology* 25, no. 8 (August 2011): 1088–100.

70. Rao and Gan, "Cinnamon: A Multifaceted Medicinal Plant," article ID 642942, doi: http://dx.doi.org/10.1155/2014/642942; Anjali Ganjre et al., "Anti-carcinogenic and Anti-bacterial Properties of Selected Spices: Implications in Oral Health," *Clinical Nutrition Research* 4, no. 4 (October 2015): 209–15.

71. C. Poly et al., "The Relation of Dietary Choline to Cognitive Performance and White-Matter Hyperintensity in the Framingham Offspring Cohort," *American Journal of Clinical Nutrition* 94, no. 6 (December 2011): 1584–91.

72. M. Herdener et al., "Musical Training Induces Functional Plasticity in Human Hippocampus," *Journal of Neuroscience* 30, no. 4 (January 27, 2010): 1377–84; B. R. Zendel, K. A. Willoughby, and J. F. Rovet, "Neuroplastic Effects of Music Lessons on Hippocampal Volume in Children with Congenital Hypothyroidism," *Neuroreport* 24, no. 17 (December 4, 2013): 947–50; M. S. Oechslin et al., "Hippocampal Volume Predicts Fluid Intelligence in Musically Trained People," *Hippocampus* 23, no. 7 (July 2013): 552–58.

CHAPTER 7: I IS FOR INFLAMMATION

1. A. C. Logan and M. Katzman, "Major Depressive Disorder: Probiotics May Be an Adjuvant Therapy," *Medical Hypotheses* 64, no. 3 (2005): 533–38, doi: 10.1016/j.mehy.2004.08.019.

2. Y. Wang et al., "Effects of Alcohol on Intestinal Epithelial Barrier Permeability and Expression of Tight Junction–Associated Proteins," *Molecular Medicine Reports* 9, no. 6 (2014): 2352–56.

3. L. Möhle et al., "Ly6C(hi) Monocytes Provide a Link between Antibiotic-Induced Changes in Gut Microbiota and Adult Hippocampal Neurogenesis," *Cell Reports* 15, no. 9 (May 31, 2016): 1945–56, doi: 10.1016/j.celrep.2016.04.074.

4. "Smoking, High Blood Pressure and Being Overweight Top Three Preventable Causes of Death in the U.S.," Harvard School of Public Health website, April 27, 2009, https://www.hsph.harvard.edu/news/press-releases/smoking-high-blood-pressure -overweight-preventable-causes-death-us/.

5. T. A. Mori and L. J. Beilin, "Omega-3 Fatty Acids and Inflammation," *Current Atherosclerosis Reports* 6, no. 6 (November 2004): 461–67; D. Moertl et al., "Dose-Dependent Effects of Omega-3-Polyunsaturated Fatty Acids on Systolic Left Ventricular Function, Endothelial Function, and Markers of Inflammation in Chronic Heart Failure of Nonischemic Origin: A Double-Blind, Placebo-Controlled, 3-Arm Study," *American Heart Journal* 161, no. 5 (May 2011): 915.e1–9, doi: 10.1016/j.ahj.2011.02.011; J. G. Devassy et al., "Omega-3 Polyunsaturated Fatty Acids and Oxylipins in Neuroinflammation and Management of Alzheimer Disease," *Advances in Nutrition* 7, no. 5 (September 15, 2016): 905–16, doi: 10.3945/an.116.012187.

6. C. von Schacky, "The Omega-3 Index as a Risk Factor for Cardiovascular Diseases," *Prostaglandins & Other Lipid Mediators* 96, nos. 1–4 (November 2011): 94–98, doi: 10.1016/j.prostaglandins.2011.06.008; S. P. Whelton et al., "Meta-Analysis of Observational Studies on Fish Intake and Coronary Heart Disease," *American Journal of Cardiology* 93, no. 9 (May 1, 2004): 1119–23, doi: 10.1016/j.amjcard.2004.01.038.

7. E. Messamore et al., "Polyunsaturated Fatty Acids and Recurrent Mood Disorders: Phenomenology, Mechanisms, and Clinical Application," *Progress in Lipid Research* 66 (April 2017): 1–13, doi: 10.1016/j.plipres.2017.01.001; J. Sarris, D. Mischoulon, and J. Schweitzer, "Omega-3 for Bipolar Disorder: Meta-Analyses of Use in Mania and Bipolar Depression," *Journal of Clinical Psychiatry* 73, no. 1 (January 2012): 81–86, doi: 10.4088 /JCP.10r06710; R. J. Mocking et al., "Meta-Analysis and Meta-Regression of Omega-3 Polyunsaturated Fatty Acid Supplementation for Major Depressive Disorder," *Translational Psychiatry* 6 (March 15, 2016): e756, doi: 10.1038/tp.2016.2.

8. J. R. Hibbeln and R. V. Gow, "The Potential for Military Diets to Reduce Depression, Suicide, and Impulsive Aggression: A Review of Current Evidence for Omega-3 and Omega-6 Fatty Acids," *Military Medicine* 179, suppl. 11 (November 2014): 117–28, doi: 10.7205/MILMED-D-14-00153; M. Huan et al., "Suicide Attempt and n-3 Fatty Acid Levels in Red Blood Cells: A Case Control Study in China," *Biological Psychiatry* 56, no. 7 (October 1, 2004): 490–96, doi: 10.1016/j.biopsych.2004.06.028; M. E. Sublette et al., "Omega-3 Polyunsaturated Essential Fatty Acid Status as a Predictor of Future Suicide Risk," *American Journal of Psychiatry* 163, no. 6 (June 2006): 1100–1102, doi: 10.1176 /ajp.2006.163.6.1100; M. D. Lewis et al., "Suicide Deaths of Active-Duty US Military and omega-3 Fatty-Acid Status: A Case-Control Comparison," *Journal of Clinical Psychiatry* 72, no. 12 (December 2011): 1585–90, doi: 10.4088/JCP.11m06879.

9. C. M. Milte et al., "Increased Erythrocyte Eicosapentaenoic Acid and Docosahexaenoic Acid Are Associated with Improved Attention and Behavior in Children with ADHD in a Randomized Controlled Three-Way Crossover Trial," *Journal of Attention Disorders* 19, no. 11 (November 2015): 954–64, doi: 10.1177/1087054713510562; M. H. Bloch and A. Qawasmi, "Omega-3 Fatty Acid Supplementation for the Treatment of Children with Attention-Deficit/Hyperactivity Disorder Symptomatology: Systematic Review and Meta-Analysis," *Journal of the American Academy of Child and Adolescent Psychiatry* 50, no. 10 (October 2011): 991–1000, doi: 10.1016/j.jaac.2011.06.008.

10. Y. Zhang et al., "Intakes of Fish and Polyunsaturated Fatty Acids and Mild-to-Severe

Cognitive Impairment Risks: A Dose-Response Meta-Analysis of 21 Cohort Studies," *American Journal of Clinical Nutrition* 103, no. 2 (February 2016): 330–40, doi: 10.3945 /ajcn.115.124081; T. A. D'Ascoli et al., "Association between Serum Long-Chain Omega-3 Polyunsaturated Fatty Acids and Cognitive Performance in Elderly Men and Women: The Kuopio Ischaemic Heart Disease Risk Factor Study," *European Journal of Clinical Nutrition* 70, no. 8 (August 2016): 970–75, doi: 10.1038/ejcn.2016.59.

11. C. Couet et al., "Effect of Dietary Fish Oil on Body Fat Mass and Basal Fat Oxidation in Healthy Adults," *International Journal of Obesity and Related Metabolic Disorders* 21, no. 8 (August 1997): 637–43; J. D. Buckley and P. R. Howe, "Anti-Obesity Effects of Long-Chain Omega-3 Polyunsaturated Fatty Acids," *Obesity Reviews* 10, no. 6 (November 2009): 648–59, doi: 10.1111/j.1467-789X.2009.00584.x.

12. K. Lukaschek et al., "Cognitive Impairment Is Associated with a Low Omega-3 Index in the Elderly: Results from the KORA-Age Study," *Dementia and Geriatric Cognitive Disorders* 42, nos. 3–4 (2016): 236–45, doi: 10.1159/000448805.

13. A. D. Smith et al., "Homocysteine-Lowering by B Vitamins Slows the Rate of Accelerated Brain Atrophy in Mild Cognitive Impairment: A Randomized Controlled Trial," *PLOS One* 5, no. 9 (September 8, 2010): e12244, doi: 10.1371/journal.pone.0012244.

14. G. Douaud et al., "Preventing Alzheimer's Disease-Related Gray Matter Atrophy by B-Vitamin Treatment," *Proceedings of the National Academy of Sciences of the United States of America* 110, no. 23 (June 4, 2013): 9523–28, doi: 10.1073/pnas.1301816110.

15. Mandy Oaklander, "5 Surprising Ways to Help Your Memory," *Time,* June 10, 2015, http://time.com/3915030/boost-memory-exercise/; P. A. Jackson et al., "DHA-Rich Oil Modulates the Cerebral Haemodynamic Response to Cognitive Tasks in Healthy Young Adults: A Near IR Spectroscopy Pilot Study," *British Journal of Nutrition* 107, no. 8 (April 2012): 1093–98, doi: 10.1017/S0007114511004041; T. J. Song et al., "Low Levels of Plasma Omega 3-Polyunsaturated Fatty Acids Are Associated with Cerebral Small Vessel Diseases in Acute Ischemic Stroke Patients," *Nutrition Research* 35, no. 5 (May 2015): 368–74, doi: 10.1016/j.nutres.2015.04.008.

16. F. Jernerén et al., "Brain Atrophy in Cognitively Impaired Elderly: The Importance of Long-Chain ω-3 Fatty Acids and B Vitamin Status in a Randomized Controlled Trial," *American Journal of Clinical Nutrition* 102, no. 1 (July 2015): 215–21, doi: 10.3945/ajcn.114.103283.

17. E. L. Boespflug et al., "Fish Oil Supplementation Increases Event-Related Posterior Cingulate Activation in Older Adults with Subjective Memory Impairment," *Journal of Nutrition, Health & Aging* 20, no. 2 (February 2016): 161–69, doi: 10.1007/s12603-015 -0609-6.

18. A. V. Witte et al., "Long-Chain Omega-3 Fatty Acids Improve Brain Function and Structure in Older Adults," *Cerebral Cortex* 24, no. 11 (November 2014): 3059–68, doi: 10.1093 /cercor/bht163.

19. Marta K. Zamroziewicz et al., "Determinants of Fluid Intelligence in Healthy Aging: Omega-3 Polyunsaturated Fatty Acid Status and Frontoparietal Cortex Structure," *Nutritional Neuroscience* 11 (published online May 11, 2017): 1–10, http://dx.doi.org/10 .1080/1028415X.2017.1324357; N. Hamazaki-Fujita et al., "Polyunsaturated Fatty Acids and Blood Circulation in the Forebrain during a Mental Arithmetic Task," *Brain Research* 1397 (June 23, 2011): 38–45, doi: 10.1016/j.brainres.2011.04.044.

20. "Omega-3 Fatty Acids," University of Maryland Medical Center website, accessed June 2, 2017, http://umm.edu/health/medical/altmed/supplement/omega3-fatty-acids.

21. J. K. Kiecolt-Glaser et al., "Omega-3 Supplementation Lowers Inflammation and Anxiety in Medical Students: A Randomized Controlled Trial," *Brain, Behavior, and Immunity* 25, no. 8 (November 2011): 1725–34, doi: 10.1016/j.bbi.2011.07.229.

22. J. A. Gil-Montoya et al., "Is Periodontitis a Risk Factor for Cognitive Impairment and Dementia? A Case-Control Study," *Journal of Periodontology* 86, no. 2 (February 2015): 244–53, doi: 10.1902/jop.2014.140340; J. Luo et al., "Association between Tooth Loss and Cognitive Function among 3063 Chinese Older Adults: A Community-Based Study," *PLOS One* 10, no. 3 (March 24, 2015): e0120986, doi: 10.1371/journal.pone.0120986.

23. S. Ghosh, S. Banerjee, and P. C. Sil, "The Beneficial Role of Curcumin on Inflammation, Diabetes and Neurodegenerative Disease: A Recent Update," *Food and Chemical Toxicology* 83 (September 2015): 111–24, doi: 10.1016/j.fct.2015.05.022.

24. Z. Asemi et al., "Effects of Daily Consumption of Probiotic Yoghurt on Inflammatory Factors in Pregnant Women: A Randomized Controlled Trial," *Pakistan Journal of Biological Sciences* 14, no. 8 (April 15, 2011): 476–82; L. Valentini et al., "Impact of Personalized Diet and Probiotic Supplementation on Inflammation, Nutritional Parameters and Intestinal Microbiota - The 'RISTOMED Project': Randomized Controlled Trial in Healthy Older People," *Clinical Nutrition* 34, no. 4 (August 2015): 593–602, doi: 10.1016/j.clnu.2014.09.023; S. K. Hegazy and M. M. El-Bedewy, "Effect of Probiotics on Pro-Inflammatory Cytokines and NF-kappaB Activation in Ulcerative Colitis," *World Journal of Gastroenterology* 16, no. 33 (September 7, 2010): 4145–51; E. J. Giamarellos-Bourboulis et al., "Pro- and Synbiotics to Control Inflammation and Infection in Patients with Multiple Injuries," *Journal of Trauma* 67, no. 4 (October 2009): 815–21, doi: 10.1097/TA.0b013e31819d979e; D. Viramontes-Hörner et al., "Effect of a Symbiotic Gel (Lactobacillus Acidophilus + Bifidobacterium Lactis + Inulin) on Presence and Severity of Gastrointestinal Symptoms in Hemodialysis Patients," *Journal of Renal Nutrition* 25, no. 3 (May 2015): 284–91, doi: 10.1053/j.jrn.2014.09.008; J. Villar-García et al., "Effect of Probiotics (Saccharomyces Boulardii) on Microbial Translocation and Inflammation in HIV-Treated Patients: A Double-Blind, Randomized, Placebo-Controlled Trial," *Journal of Acquired Immune Deficiency Syndromes* 68, no. 3 (March 1, 2015): 256–63, doi: 10.1097/QAI.0000000000000468; A. Toiviainen et al., "Impact of Orally Administered Lozenges with Lactobacillus Rhamnosus GG and Bifidobacterium Animalis Subsp. Lactis BB-12 on the Number of Salivary Mutans Streptococci, Amount of Plaque, Gingival Inflammation and the Oral Microbiome in Healthy Adults," *Clinical Oral Investigations* 19, no. 1 (January 2015): 77–83, doi: 10.1007/s00784-014-1221-6; S. J. Spaiser et al., "Lactobacillus Gasseri KS-13, Bifidobacterium Bifidum G9-1, and Bifidobacterium Longum MM-2 Ingestion Induces a Less Inflammatory Cytokine Profile and a Potentially Beneficial Shift in Gut Microbiota in Older Adults: A Randomized, Double-Blind, Placebo-Controlled, Crossover Study," *Journal of the American College of Nutrition* 34, no. 6 (2015): 459–69, doi: 10.1080/07315724.2014.983249; A. K. Szkaradkiewicz et al., "Effect of Oral Administration Involving a Probiotic Strain of *Lactobacillus Reuteri* on Pro-Inflammatory Cytokine Response in Patients with Chronic Periodontitis," *Archivum Immunologiae Therapiae Experimentalis* 62, no. 6 (December 2014): 495–500, doi: 10.1007/s00005-014-0277-y; Z. H. Liu et al., "The Effects of Perioperative Probiotic Treatment on Serum Zonulin Concentration and Subsequent Postoperative Infectious Complications after Colorectal Cancer Surgery: A Double-Center and Double-Blind Randomized Clinical Trial," *American Journal of Clinical Nutrition* 97, no. 1 (January 2013): 117–26, doi: 10.3945/ajcn.112.040949.

25. H. Rajkumar et al., "Effect of Probiotic Lactobacillus Salivarius UBL S22 and Prebiotic Fructo-Oligosaccharide on Serum Lipids, Inflammatory Markers, Insulin Sensitivity, and Gut Bacteria in Healthy Young Volunteers: A Randomized Controlled Single-Blind Pilot Study," *Journal of Cardiovascular Pharmacology and Therapeutics* 20, no. 3 (May 2015): 289–98, doi: 10.1177/1074248414555004.

26. T. P. Ng et al., "Curry Consumption and Cognitive Function in the Elderly," *American Journal of Epidemiology* 164, no. 9 (November 1, 2006): 898–906, doi: 10.1093/aje/kwj267; A. Ganjre et al., "Anti-Carcinogenic and Anti-Bacterial Properties of Selected Spices: Implications in Oral Health," *Clinical Nutrition Research* 4, no. 4 (October 2015): 209–15, doi: 10.7762/cnr.2015.4.4.209.

27. Ganjre et al., "Anti-Carcinogenic and Anti-Bacterial Properties of Selected Spices: Implications in Oral Health," 209–15.

28. Rao and Gan, "Cinnamon: A Multifaceted Medicinal Plant," article ID 642942.

29. Ganjre et al., "Anti-Carcinogenic and Anti-Bacterial Properties of Selected Spices: Implications in Oral Health," 209–15.

30. H. R. Schumacher et al., "Randomized Double-Blind Crossover Study of the Efficacy of a Tart Cherry Juice Blend in Treatment of Osteoarthritis (OA) of the Knee," *Osteoarthritis and Cartilage* 21, no. 8 (August 2013): 1035–41, doi: 10.1016/j.joca.2013.05.009;

G. Howatson et al., "Influence of Tart Cherry Juice on Indices of Recovery Following Marathon Running," *Scandinavian Journal of Medicine & Science in Sports* 20, no. 6 (December 2010): 843–52, doi: 10.1111/j.1600-0838.2009.01005.x.

CHAPTER 8: G IS FOR GENETICS

1. J. Jankovic, "Parkinson's Disease: Clinical Features and Diagnosis," *Journal of Neurology, Neurosurgery, and Psychiatry* 79, no. 4 (April 2008): 368–76, doi: 10.1136/jnnp.2007.131045; N. Caballol, M. J. Marti, and E. Tolosa, "Cognitive Dysfunction and Dementia in Parkinson Disease," *Movement Disorders* 22, suppl. 17 (September 2007): S358–66, doi: 10.1002/mds.21677.

2. Allison Abbott and Elie Dolgin, "Failed Alzheimer's Trial Does Not Kill Leading Theory of Disease," *Nature* 540, no. 7631 (November 23, 2016), http://www.nature.com/news/failed-alzheimer-s-trial-does-not-kill-leading-theory-of-disease-1.21045.

3. R. M. Corbo and R. Scacchi, "Apolipoprotein E (APOE) Allele Distribution in the World. Is APOE*4 a 'Thrifty' Allele?," *Annals of Human Genetics* 63, part 4 (July 1999): 301–10.

4. I. Lonskaya et al., "Tau Deletion Impairs Intracellular β-amyloid-42 Clearance and Leads to More Extracellular Plaque Deposition in Gene Transfer Models," *Molecular Neurodegeneration* 9 (November 10, 2014): 46, doi: 10.1186/1750-1326-9-46.

5. A. C. McKee et al., "The Spectrum of Disease in Chronic Traumatic Encephalopathy," *Brain* 136, part 1 (January 2013): 43–64, doi: 10.1093/brain/aws307.

6. J. R. Prasanthi et al., "Deferiprone Reduces Amyloid-β and Tau Phosphorylation Levels but Not Reactive Oxygen Species Generation in Hippocampus of Rabbits Fed a Cholesterol-Enriched Diet," *Journal of Alzheimer's Disease* 30, no. 1 (2012): 167–82, doi: 10.3233/JAD-2012-111346.

7. D. J. Selkoe, "Alzheimer's Disease: Genotypes, Phenotypes, and Treatment," *Science* 275, no. 5300 (1997): 630–31.

8. D. M. Michaelson, "APOE ε4: The Most Prevalent Yet Understudied Risk Factor for Alzheimer's Disease," *Alzheimer's & Dementia* 10, no. 6 (November 2014): 861–68, doi: 10.1016/j.jalz.2014.06.015; S. Schilling et al., "APOE Genotype and MRI Markers of Cerebrovascular Disease: Systematic Review and Meta-Analysis," *Neurology* 81, no. 3 (July 2013): 292–300, doi: 10.1212/WNL.0b013e31829bfda4.

9. M. Thambisertty et al., "APOE Epsilon4 Genotype and Longitudinal Changes in Cerebral Blood Flow in Normal Aging," *Archives of Neurology* 67, no. 1 (January 2010): 93–98, doi: 10.1001/archneurol.2009.913.

10. T. D. Bird, "Clinical Genetics of Familial Alzheimer's Disease," in *Alzheimer Disease*, ed. R. D. Terry et al. (Philadelphia: Lippincott Williams & Wilkins, 1999), 57–67.

11. M. E. Pembrey et al., "Sex-Specific, Male-Line Transgenerational Responses in Humans," *European Journal of Human Genetics* 14, no. 2 (February 2006): 159–66, doi: 10.1038/sj.ejhg.5201538.

12. D. Zhou and Y. X. Pan, "Pathophysiological Basis for Compromised Health beyond Generations: Role of Maternal High-Fat Diet and Low-Grade Chronic Inflammation," *Journal of Nutritional Biochemistry* 26, no. 1 (January 2015): 1–8, doi: 10.1016/j.jnutbio.2014.06.011.

13. S. Karsli-Ceppioglu et al., "Epigenetic Mechanisms of Breast Cancer: An Update of the Current Knowledge," *Epigenomics* 6, no. 6 (2014): 651–64, doi: 10.2217/epi.14.59; M. Ngollo et al., "Epigenetic Modifications in Prostate Cancer," *Epigenomics* 6, no. 4 (2014): 415–26, doi: 10.2217/epi.14.34; M. J. Dauncey, "Nutrition, the Brain and Cognitive Decline: Insights from Epigenetics," *European Journal of Clinical Nutrition* 68, no. 11 (November 2014): 1179–85, doi: 10.1038/ejcn.2014.173; M. Devall, J. Mill, and K. Lunnon, "The Mitochondrial Epigenome: A Role in Alzheimer's Disease?," *Epigenomics* 6, no. 6 (2014): 665–75, doi: 10.2217/epi.14.50; O. Babenko, I. Kovalchuk, and G. A. Metz, "Stress-Induced Perinatal and Transgenerational Epigenetic Programming of Brain Development and Mental Health," *Neuroscience and Biobehavioral Reviews* 48 (January 2015): 70–91, doi: 10.1016/j.neubiorev.2014.11.013; M. Debnath, G. Venkatasubramanian, and M. Berk, "Fetal

Programming of Schizophrenia: Select Mechanisms," *Neuroscience and Biobehavioral Reviews* 49 (February 2015): 90–104, doi: 10.1016/j.neubiorev.2014.12.003; C. Lesseur, A. G. Paquette, and C. J. Marsit, "Epigenetic Regulation of Infant Neurobehavioral Outcomes," *Medical Epigenetics* 2, no. 2 (May 2014): 71–79, doi: 10.1159.000361026; M. A. Reddy, E. Zhang, and R. Natarajan, "Epigenetic Mechanisms in Diabetic Complications and Metabolic Memory," *Diabetologia* 58, no. 3 (March 2015): 443–55, doi: 10.1007/s00125 -014-3462-y; W. Yuan et al., "An Integrated Epigenomic Analysis for Type 2 Diabetes Susceptibility Loci in Monozygotic Twins," *Nature Communications* 5 (December 12, 2014): 5719, doi: 10.1038/ncomms6719.

14. T. A. Ahles et al., "The Relationship of APOE Genotype to Neuropsychological Performance in Long-Term Cancer Survivors Treated with Standard Dose Chemotherapy," *Psycho-oncology* 12, no. 6 (September 2003): 612–19, doi: 10.1002 /pon.742; D. W. Lawrence et al., "The Role of Apolipoprotein E Episilon (ε)-4 Allele on Outcome Following Traumatic Brain Injury: A Systematic Review," *Brain Injury* 29, no. 9 (2015): 1018–31, doi: 10.3109/02699052.2015.1005131.

15. Emilie Reas, "Exercise Counteracts Genetic Risk for Alzheimer's," *Scientific American*, November 1, 2014, https://www.scientificamerican.com/article/exercise-counteracts -genetic-risk-for-alzheimer-s/.

16. C. Liu et al., "Apolipoprotein E and Alzheimer Disease: Risk, Mechanisms, and Therapy," *Nature Reviews Neurology* 9 (February 2013): 106–18, doi: 10.1038/nrneurol.2012.263.

17. J. A. Joseph et al., "Blueberry Supplementation Enhances Signaling and Prevents Behavioral Deficits in an Alzheimer Disease Model," *Nutritional Neuroscience* 6, no. 3 (June 2003): 153–62, doi: 10.1080/1028415031000111282; Y. Zhu et al., "Blueberry Opposes Beta-Amyloid Peptide-Induced Microglial Activation via Inhibition of p44/42 Mitogen-Activation Protein Kinase," *Rejuvenation Research* 11, no. 5 (October 2008): 891–901, doi: 10.1089/rej.2008.0757.

18. T. C. Huang et al., "Resveratrol Protects Rats from Aβ-Induced Neurotoxicity by the Reduction of iNOS Expression and Lipid Peroxidation," *PLOS One* 6, no. 12 (2011): e29102, doi: 10.1371/journal.pone.0029102; H. Capiralla et al., "Resveratrol Mitigates Lipopolysaccharide- and Aβ-Mediated Microglial Inflammation by Inhibiting the TLR4/ NF-kappaB/STAT Signaling Cascade," *Journal of Neurochemistry* 120, no. 3 (February 2012): 461–72, doi: 10.1111/j.1471-4159.2011.07594.x.

19. S. Sinha et al., "Comparison of Three Amyloid Assembly Inhibitors: The Sugar Scyllo-Inositol, the Polyphenol Epigallocatechin Gallate, and the Molecular Tweezer CLR01," *ACS Chemical Neuroscience* 3, no. 6 (June 20, 2012): 451–58, doi: 10.1021/cn200133x; J. M. Lopez del Amo et al., "Structural Properties of EGCG-Induced, Nontoxic Alzheimer's Disease Aβ Oligomers," *Journal of Molecular Biology* 421, nos. 4–5 (August 24, 2012): 517–24, doi: 10.1016/j.jmb.2012.01.013.

20. H. M. Abdul et al., "Acetyl-L-Carnitine-Induced Up-Regulation of Heat Shock Proteins Protects Cortical Neurons against Amyloid-Beta Peptide 1-42-Mediated Oxidative Stress and Neurotoxicity: Implications for Alzheimer's Disease," *Journal of Neuro-science Research* 84, no. 2 (August 1, 2006): 398–408, doi: 10.1002/jnr.20877; G. Traina, G. Federighi, and M. Brunelli, "Up-Regulation of Kinesin Light-Chain 1 Gene Expression by Acetyl-L-Carnitine: Therapeutic Possibility in Alzheimer's Disease," *Neurochemistry International* 53, nos. 6–8 (December 2008): 244–47, doi: 10.1016/j.neuint.2008.08.001; P. Zhou et al., "Acetyl-L-Carnitine Attenuates Homocysteine-Induced Alzheimer-Like Histopathological and Behavioral Abnormalities," *Rejuvenation Research* 14, no. 6 (December 2011): 669–79, doi: 10.1089/rej.2011.1195.

21. S. Mishra and K. Palanivelu, "The Effect of Curcumin (Turmeric) on Alzheimer's Disease: An Overview," *Annals of Indian Academy of Neurology* 11, no. 1 (January–March 2008): 13–19, doi: 10.4103/0972-2327.40220; L. N. Zhao et al., "The Effect of Curcumin on the Stability of Amyloid Beta Dimers," *Journal of Physical Chemistry B* 116, no. 25 (June 28, 2012): 7428–35, doi: 10.1021/jp3034209; R. A. DiSilvestro et al., "Diverse Effects of a Low Dose Supplement of Lipidated Curcumin in Healthy Middle Aged People," *Nutrition Journal* 11 (September 26, 2012): 79, doi: 10.1186/1475-2891-11-79.

22. S. R. Rainey-Smith et al., "Curcumin and Cognition: A Randomised, Placebo-Controlled, Double-Blind Study of Community-Dwelling Older Adults," *The British Journal of Nutrition* 115, no. 12 (June 2016): 2106–13, doi: 10.1017/S0007114516001203.

23. B. Jayaprakasam, K. Pradmanabhan, and M. G. Nair, "Withanamides in Withania Somnifera Fruit Protect PC-12 Cells from Beta-Amyloid Responsible for Alzheimer's Disease," *Phytotherapy Research* 24, no. 6 (June 2010): 859–63, doi: 10.1002/ptr.3033; K. R. Kurapati et al., "β-Amyloid1-42, HIV-1Ba-L (Clade B) Infection and Drugs of Abuse Induced Degeneration in Human Neuronal Cells and Protective Effects of Ashwagandha (Withania somnifera) and Its Constituent Withanolide A," *PLOS One* 9, no. 11 (November 21, 2014): e112818, doi: https://doi.org/10.1371/journal.pone.0112818.

24. L. Yang et al., "Ginsenoside Rg3 Promotes Beta-Amyloid Peptide Degradation by Enhancing Gene Expression of Neprilysin," *Journal of Pharmacy and Pharmacology* 61, no. 3 (March 2009): 375–80, doi: 10.1211/jpp/61.03.0013; L. M. Chen et al., "Ginsenoside Rg1 Attenuates β-Amyloid Generation via Suppressing PPARγ-Regulated BACE1 Activity in N2a-APP695 Cells," *European Journal of Pharmacology* 675, nos. 1–3 (January 30, 2012): 15–21, doi: 10.1016/j.ejphar.2011.11.039.

25. Y. H. Hsiao et al., "Amelioration of Social Isolation-Triggered Onset of Early Alzheimer's Disease-Related Cognitive Deficit by N-Acetylcysteine in a Transgenic Mouse Model," *Neurobiology of Disease* 45, no. 3 (March 2012): 1111–20, doi: 10.1016/j.nbd.2011.12.031.

26. J. C. Adair, J. E. Knoefel, and N. Morgan, "Controlled Trial of N-Acetylcysteine for Patients with Probable Alzheimer's Disease," *Neurology* 57, no. 8 (October 23, 2001): 1515–17.

27. X. Yang et al., "Coenzyme Q10 Reduces Beta-Amyloid Plaque in an APP/PS1 Transgenic Mouse Model of Alzheimer's Disease," *Journal of Molecular Neuroscience* 41, no. 1 (May 2010): 110–13, doi: 10.1007/s12031-009-9297-1; M. Dumont et al., "Coenzyme Q10 Decreases Amyloid Pathology and Improves Behavior in a Transgenic Mouse Model of Alzheimer's Disease," *Journal of Alzheimer's Disease* 27, no. 1 (2011): 211–23, doi: 10.3233/JAD-2011-110209.

28. J. Yu et al., "Magnesium Modulates Amyloid-Beta Protein Precursor Trafficking and Processing," *Journal of Alzheimer's Disease* 20, no. 4 (2010): 1091–106, doi: 10.3233/JAD-2010-091444.

29. L. Flicker et al., "B-Vitamins Reduce Plasma Levels of Beta Amyloid," *Neurobiology of Aging* 29, no. 2 (February 2008): 303–5, doi: 10.1016/j.neurobiolaging.2006.10.007.

30. M. T. Mizwicki et al., "Genomic and Nongenomic Signaling Induced by 1α,25(OH)2-Vitamin D3 Promotes the Recovery of Amyloid-β Phagocytosis by Alzheimer's Disease Macrophages," *Journal of Alzheimer's Disease* 29, no. 1 (2012): 51–62, doi: 10.3233/JAD-2012-110560; A. Masoumi et al., "1alpha,25-dihydroxyvitamin D3 Interacts with Curcuminoids to Stimulate Amyloid-Beta Clearance by Macrophages of Alzheimer's Disease Patients," *Journal of Alzheimer's Disease* 17, no. 3 (2009): 703–17, doi: 10.3233/JAD-2009-1080.

31. C. Annweiler et al., "Vitamin D Insufficiency and Mild Cognitive Impairment: Cross-Sectional Association," *European Journal of Neurology* 19, no. 7 (July 2012): 1023–29, doi: 10.1111/j.1468-1331.2012.03675.x.

32. H. Yassine et al., "Association of Docosahexaenoic Acid Supplementation with Alzheimer Disease Stage in Apolipoprotein E ε4 Carriers: A Review," *JAMA Neurology* 74, no. 3 (March 1, 2017): 339–47, doi: 10.1001/jamaneurol.2016.4899.

33. Y. Kashiwaya et al., "A Ketone Ester Diet Exhibits Anxiolytic and Cognition-Sparing Properties, and Lessens Amyloid and Tau Pathologies in a Mouse Model of Alzheimer's Disease," *Neurobiology of Aging* 4, no. 6 (June 2013): 1530–39, doi: 10.1016/j.neurobiolaging.2012.11.023.

CHAPTER 9: H IS FOR HEAD TRAUMA

1. K. Dams-O'Connor et al., "Risk for Late-Life Re-Injury, Dementia and Death among Individuals with Traumatic Brain Injury: A Population-Based Study," *Journal of Neurology,*

Neurosurgery, and Psychiatry 84, no. 2 (February 2013): 177–82, doi: 10.1136/jnnp-2012 -303938.

2. B. D. Jordan et al., "Apolipoprotein E Epsilon4 Associated with Chronic Traumatic Brain Injury in Boxing," *JAMA* 278, no. 2 (July 9, 1997): 136–40; K. C. Kutner et al., "Lower Cognitive Performance of Older Football Players Possessing Apolipoprotein E Epsilon4," *Neurosurgery* 47, no. 3 (September 2000): 651–57.

3. Visit this link to watch a video of a newly autopsied brain, so you can see how soft it really is: https://m.youtube.com/watch?v=jHxyP-nUhUY. The video features Suzanne Stensaas, PhD, professor of neurobiology and anatomy at the University of Utah, and is produced by the University of Utah Neuroscience Initiative.

4. "DoD Worldwide Numbers for TBI," Defense and Veterans Brain Injury Center website, accessed May 19, 2017, http://dvbic.dcoe.mil/dod-worldwide-numbers-tbi.

5. "Fighting in Ice Hockey," *Wikipedia*, last modified May 3, 2017, https://en.wikipedia .org/wiki/Fighting_in_ice_hockey.

6. Z. M. Weil, J. D. Corrigan, and K. Karelina, "Alcohol Abuse after Traumatic Brain Injury: Experimental and Clinical Evidence," *Neuroscience and Biobehavioral Reviews* 62 (March 2016): 89–99, doi: 10.1016/j.neubiorev.2016.01.005; M. R. Hibbard et al., "Axis I Psychopathology in Individuals with Traumatic Brain Injury," *Journal of Head Trauma Rehabilitation* 13, no. 4 (August 1998): 24–39; A. L. Zaninotto et al., "Updates and Current Perspectives of Psychiatric Assessments after Traumatic Brain Injury: A Systematic Review," *Frontiers in Psychiatry* 7 (June 14, 2016): 95, doi: 10.3389/fpsyt.2016.00095; J. E. Max, "Neuropsychiatry of Pediatric Traumatic Brain Injury," *Psychiatric Clinics of North America* 37, no. 1 (March 2014): 125–40, doi: 10.1016/j.psc.2013.11.003; J. R. Sullivan and C. A. Riccio, "Language Functioning and Deficits Following Pediatric Traumatic Brain Injury," *Applied Neuropsychology* 17, no. 2 (April 2010): 93–98, doi: 10.1080/09084281003708852; Vanessa X. Barrat et al., "School Mobility, Dropout, and Graduation Rates across Student Disability Categories in Utah," National Center for Education Evaluation and Regional Assistance, November 2014, http://files.eric.ed.gov /fulltext/ED548546.pdf; S. Fazel et al., "Risk of Violent Crime in Individuals with Epilepsy and Traumatic Brain Injury: A 35-Year Swedish Population Study," *PLOS Medicine* 8, no. 12 (December 2011): e1001150, doi: 10.1371/journal.pmed.1001150; M. A. Nowrangi, K. B. Kortte, and V. A. Rao, "A Perspectives Approach to Suicide after Traumatic Brain Injury: Case and Review," *Psychosomatics* 55, no. 5 (September–October 2014): 430–37, doi: https://doi.org/10.1016/j.psym.2013.11.006; J. P. Cuthbert et al., "Unemployment in the United States after Traumatic Brain Injury for Working-Age Individuals: Prevalence and Associated Factors 2 Years Postinjury," *Journal of Head Trauma Rehabilitation* 30, no. 3 (May–June 2015): 160–74, doi: 10.1097/HTR.0000000000000090; K. E. McIsaac et al., "Association between Traumatic Brain Injury and Incarceration: A Population-Based Cohort Study," *CMAJ Open* 4, no. 4 (December 6, 2016): E746–E753, doi: 10.9778 /cmajo.20160072; J. Topolovec-Vranic et al., "Traumatic Brain Injury among People Who Are Homeless: A Systematic Review," *BMC Public Health* 12 (December 8, 2012): 1059, doi: 10.1186/1471-2458-12-1059.

7. S. W. Hwang et al., "The Effect of Traumatic Brain Injury on the Health of Homeless People," *CMAJ* 178, no. 8 (October 7, 2008): 779–84, doi: 10.1503/cmaj.080341.

8. D. G. Amen et al., "Impact of Playing American Professional Football on Long-Term Brain Function," *Journal of Neuropsychiatry and Clinical Neurosciences* 23, no. 1 (Winter 2011), doi: 10.1176/appi.neuropsych.23.1.98.

9. Nate Scott, "Researchers Find Evidence of CTE in 96% of Deceased NFL Players They Tested," *For the Win* (*USA Today* Sports website), September 18, 2015, http://ftw.usatoday .com/2015/09/researchers-find-evidence-of-cte-in-96-of-deceased-nfl-players-they -tested; Kevin Punsky, "Evidence Suggests Amateur Contact Sports Increase Risk of Degenerative Disorder," Mayo Clinic News Network, December 2, 2015, http://newsnetwork .mayoclinic.org/discussion/mayo-clinic-cte-fl-release/.

10. D. R. Weir, J. S. Jackson, and A. Sonnega, "National Football League Player Care Foundation: Study of Retired NFL Players," Institute for Social Research, University

of Michigan, September 10, 2009, http://www.ns.umich.edu/Releases/2009/Sep09/FinalReport.pdf.

11. Eric Sondheiemer, "High School Football Coaches See Fear of Injuries Draining Talent Pool," *Los Angeles Times,* September 24, 2015, http://www.latimes.com/sports/highschool/la-sp-freshman-football-sondheimer-20150925-column.html.

12. John Breech, "Players Make September First Arrest-Free Month in Six Years," CBS Sports, October 2, 2015, http://www.cbssports.com/nfl/eye-on-football/25325024/nfl-rarity-players-make-september-first-arrest-free-month-in-six-years.

13. D. G. Amen et al., "Reversing Brain Damage in Former NFL Players: Implications for Traumatic Brain Injury and Substance Abuse Rehabilitation," *Journal of Psychoactive Drugs* 43, no. 1 (January–March 2011): 1–5, doi: 10.1080/02791072.2011.566489.

14. Steven Reinberg, "Failing Sense of Smell Might Be Alzheimer's Warning," WebMD Archives, November 16, 2015, http://www.webmd.com/alzheimers/news/20151116/failing-sense-of-smell-might-be-alzheimers-warning; M. Quarmley et al., "Odor Identification Screening Improves Diagnostic Classification in Incipient Alzheimer's Disease," *Journal of Alzheimer's Disease* 55, no. 4 (November 18, 2016): 1497–507, doi: 10.3233/JAD-160842; M. H. Tabert et al., "A 10-Item Smell Identification Scale Related to Risk for Alzheimer's Disease," *Annals of Neurology* 58, no. 1 (July 2005): 155–60, doi: 10.1002/ana.20533.

15. A. Wu, Z. Ying, and F. Gomez-Pinilla, "Exercise Facilitates the Action of Dietary DHA on Functional Recovery after Brain Trauma," *Neuroscience* 248 (September 17, 2013): 655–63, doi: 10.1016/j.neuroscience.2013.06.041; A. Wu, Z. Ying, and F. Gomez-Pinilla, "Omega-3 Fatty Acids Supplementation Restores Mechanisms That Maintain Brain Homeostasis in Traumatic Brain Injury," *Journal of Neurotrauma* 24, no. 10 (October 2007): 1587–95, doi: 10.1089/neu.2007.0313.

16. R. Agrawal et al., "Dietary Fructose Aggravates the Pathobiology of Traumatic Brain Injury by Influencing Energy Homeostasis and Plasticity," *Journal of Cerebral Blood Flow and Metabolism* 36, no. 5 (May 2016): 941–53.

17. H. L. Ling et al., "Mixed Pathologies Including Chronic Traumatic Encephalopathy Account for Dementia in Retired Association Football (Soccer) Players," *Acta Neuropathologica* 133, no. 3 (March 2017): 337–52, doi:10.1007/s00401-017-1680-3.

18. I. Konstantinidis, E. Tsakiropoulous, and J. Constantinidis, "Long Term Effects of Olfactory Training in Patients with Post-Infectious Olfactory Loss," *Rhinology* 54, no. 2 (June 2016): 170–75, doi: 10.4193/Rhin15.264.

19. Sharon Amos, "Smell Training for Anosmia," *Saga,* October 22, 2013, http://www.saga.co.uk/magazine/health-wellbeing/treatments/smell-training-for-anosmia.

20. F. Samini et al., "Curcumin Pretreatment Attenuates Brain Lesion Size and Improves Neurological Function Following Traumatic Brain Injury in the Rat," *Pharmacology, Biochemistry, and Behavior* 110 (September 2013): 238–44, doi: 10.1016/j.pbb.2013.07.019; T. E. Sullivan et al., "Effects of Olfactory Stimulation on the Vigilance Performance of Individuals with Brain Injury," *Journal of Clinical and Experiential Neuropsychology* 20, no. 2 (April 1998): 227–36, doi: 10.1076/jcen.20.2.227.1175.

CHAPTER 10: T IS FOR TOXINS

1. T. Parrón et al., "Association between Environmental Exposure to Pesticides and Neurodegenerative Diseases," *Toxicology and Applied Pharmacology* 256, no. 3 (November 1, 2011): 379–85, doi: 10.1016/j.taap.2011.05.006.

2. "Advice about Eating Fish: What Pregnant Women and Parents Should Know," Food and Drug Administration, https://www.fda.gov/downloads/Food/FoodborneIllness/Contaminants/Metals/UCM536321.pdf.

3. C. Gasnier et al., "Glyphosate-Based Herbicides Are Toxic and Endocrine Disruptors in Human Cell Lines," *Toxicology* 262, no. 3 (August 21, 2009): 184–91, doi: 10.1016/j.tox.2009.06.006.

4. Ki-Su Kim et al., "Associations between Organochlorine Pesticides and Cognition in U.S.

Elders: National Health and Nutrition Examination Survey 1999–2002," *Environment International* 75 (February 2015): 87–92, doi: 10.1016/j.envint.2014.11.003.

5. C. T. DellaValle et al., "Dietary Nitrate and Nitrite Intake and Risk of Colorectal Cancer in the Shanghai Women's Health Study," *International Journal of Cancer* 134, no. 12 (June 15, 2014): 2917–26, 10.1002/ijc.28612; Suzanne M. de la Monte et al., "Epidemiological Trends Strongly Suggest Exposures as Etiologic Agents in the Pathogenesis of Sporadic Alzheimer's Disease, Diabetes Mellitus, and Non-Alcoholic Steatohepatitis," *Journal of Alzheimer's Disease* 17, no. 3 (July 1, 2009): 519–29, doi: 10.3233/JAD-2009-1070.

6. "The Health Costs of Beauty: EDCs in Personal Care Products and the HERMOSA Study," Collaborative on Health and the Environment website, March 22, 2016, accessed May 5, 2017, http://www.healthandenvironment.org/partnership_calls/18271.

7. H. Chen et al., "Living Near Major Roads and the Incidence of Dementia, Parkinson's Disease, and Multiple Sclerosis: A Population-Based Cohort Study," *Lancet* 389, no. 10070 (February 18, 2017): 718–26, doi: 10.1016/S0140-6736(16)32399-6.

8. Washington University School of Medicine in St. Louis, "Low Levels of Manganese in Welding Fumes Cause Neurological Problems," *ScienceDaily*, December 28, 2016, www.sciencedaily.com/releases/2016/12/161228171126.htm.

9. Charlotte Bergkvist et al., "Dietary Exposure to Polychlorinated Biphenyls and Risk of Myocardial Infarction: A Population-Based Prospective Cohort Study," *International Journal of Cardiology* 183 (March 15, 2015): 242–48.

10. José R. Suárez-Lopez et al., "Persistent Organic Pollutants in Young Adults and Changes in Glucose Related Metabolism over a 23-Year Follow-Up," *Environmental Research* 137 (February 2015): 485–94.

11. Joseph Pizzorno enumerates a number of these negative effects in his book *The Toxin Solution* (New York: Harper Collins, 2017), 23–25.

12. "The Health Costs of Beauty," http://www.healthandenvironment.org/partnership _calls/18271.

13. Stacy Malkan, "Johnson & Johnson Is Just the Tip of the Toxic Iceberg," *Time*, March 2, 2016, http://time.com/4239561/johnson-and-johnson-toxic-ingredients/.

14. G. L. LoSasso, L. J. Rapport, and B. N. Axelrod, "Neuropsychological Symptoms Associated with Low-Level Exposure to Solvents and (Meth)Acrylates among Nail Technicians," *Neuropsychiatry, Neuropsychology, and Behavioral Neurology* 14, no. 3 (July–September 2001): 183–89.

15. M. Kawahara and M. Kato-Negishi, "Link between Aluminum and the Pathogenesis of Alzheimer's Disease: The Integration of the Aluminum and Amyloid Cascade Hypotheses," *International Journal of Alzheimer's Disease* 2011 (March 8, 2011): 276393, doi: 10.4061/2011/276393; S. Davenward et al., "Silicon-Rich Mineral Water as a Non-Invasive Test of the 'Aluminum Hypothesis' in Alzheimer's Disease," *Journal of Alzheimer's Disease* 33, no. 2 (2013): 423–30; S. Maya et al., "Multifaceted Effects of Aluminium in Neurodegenerative Diseases: A Review," *Biomedicine and Pharmacotherapy* 83 (October 2016): 746–54, doi: 10.1016/j.biopha.2016.07.035; T. P. Flaten, "Aluminium as a Risk Factor in Alzheimer's Disease, with Emphasis on Drinking Water," *Brain Research Bulletin* 55, no. 2 (May 15, 2001): 187–96.

16. M. Fenech, A. Nersesyan, and S. Knasmueller, "A Systematic Review of the Association Between Occupational Exposure to Formaldehyde and Effects on Chromosomal DNA Damage Measured Using the Cytokinesis-Block Micronucleus Assay in Lymphocytes," *Mutation Research* 770, part A (October–December 2016): 46–57, doi: 10.1016/j.mrrev .2016.04.005.

17. A. Pontén and M. Bruze, "Formaldehyde," *Dermatitis* 26, no. 1 (January–February 2015): 3–6, doi: 10.1097/DER.0000000000000075.

18. P. D. Darbre and P. W. Harvey, "Parabens Can Enable Hallmarks and Characteristics of Cancer in Human Breast Epithelial Cells: A Review of the Literature with Reference to New Exposure Data and Regulatory Status," *Journal of Applied Toxicology* 34, no. 9 (September 2014): 925–38, doi: 10.1002/jat.3027.

19. P. Erkekoglu and B. Kocer-Gumusel, "Genotoxicity of Phthalates," *Toxicology Mechanisms and Methods* 24, no. 9 (December 2014): 616–26, doi: 10.3109/15376516.2014.960987.

20. P. Factor-Litvak et al., "Persistent Associations between Maternal Prenatal Exposure to Phthalates on Child IQ at Age 7 Years," *PLOS One* 9, no. 12 (December 10, 2014): e114003, doi: 10.1371/journal.pone.0114003.

21. C. A. Smith and M. R. Holahan, "Reduced Hippocampal Dendritic Spine Density and BDNF Expression Following Acute Postnatal Exposure to Di(2-Ethylhexyl) Phthalate in Male Long Evans Rats," *PLOS One* 9, no. 10 (October 8, 2014): e109522, doi: 10.1371/journal.pone.0109522.

22. "Ethylene Glycol," The Carcinogenic Potency Project, last updated October 3, 2007, accessed May 26, 2017, https://toxnet.nlm.nih.gov/cpdb/chempages/ETHYLENE%20GLYCOL.html.

23. Agency for Toxic Substances and Disease Registry, "Propylene Glycol," Organic Natural Health website, September 1997, accessed May 5, 2017, http://www.health-report.co.uk/ethylene_glycol_propylene_glycol.html.

24. US Food and Drug Administration, "5 Things to Know about Triclosan," US Food and Drug Administration website, last updated September 2, 2016, http://www.fda.gov/ForConsumers/ConsumerUpdates/ucm205999.htm; M. Axelstad et al., "Triclosan Exposure Reduces Thyroxine Levels in Pregnant and Lactating Rat Dams and in Directly Exposed Offspring," *Food and Chemical Toxicology* 59 (September 2013): 534–40, doi: 10.1016/j.fct.2013.06.050.

25. A. L. Yee and J. A. Gilbert, "Is Triclosan Harming Your Microbiome?" *Science* 353, no. 6297 (July 22, 2016), 348–49, doi: 10.1126/science.aag2698.

26. Kang-sheng Liu et al., "Neurotoxicity and Biomarkers of Lead Exposure: A Review," *Chinese Medical Sciences Journal* 28, no. 3 (September 2013): 178–88, doi: 10.1016/S1001-9294(13)60045-0.

27. "Don't Pucker Up: Lead in Lipstick," Campaign for Safe Cosmetics website, accessed May 5, 2017, http://www.safecosmetics.org/about-us/media/news-coverage/dont-pucker-up-lead-in-lipstick/.

28. Sa Liu, S. Katharine Hammond, and Ann Rojas-Cheatham, "Concentrations and Potential Health Risks of Metals in Lip Products," *Environmental Health Perspectives* 121, no. 6 (June 2013): 701–10, doi: 10.1289/ehp.1205518.

29. A. Ott et al., "Smoking and Risk of Dementia and Alzheimer's Disease in a Population-Based Cohort Study: The Rotterdam Study," *Lancet* 351, no. 9119 (June 20, 1998): 1840–43, doi: 10.1016/S0140-6736(97)07541-7.

30. "Tobacco and Dementia," World Health Organization, June 2014, http://apps.who.int/iris/bitstream/10665/128041/1/WHO_NMH_PND_CIC_TKS_14.1_eng.pdf.

31. K. J. Anstey, H. A. Mack, and N. Cherbuin, "Alcohol Consumption as a Risk Factor for Dementia and Cognitive Decline: Meta-Analysis of Prospective Studies," *American Journal of Geriatric Psychiatry* 17, no. 7 (July 2009): 542–55, doi: 10.1097/JGP.0b013e3181a2fd07; R. Peters et al., "Alcohol, Dementia and Cognitive Decline in the Elderly: A Systematic Review," *Age and Ageing* 37, no. 5 (September 2008): 505–12, doi: 10.1093/ageing/afn095; E. J. Neafsey and M. A. Collins, "Moderate Alcohol Consumption and Cognitive Risk," *Neuropsychiatric Disease and Treatment* 7 (2011): 465–84, doi: https://doi.org/10.2147/NDT.S23159.

32. Anya Topiwala et al., "Moderate Alcohol Consumption as Risk Factor for Adverse Brain Outcomes and Cognitive Decline: Longitudinal Cohort Study," *BMJ* 357 (June 6, 2017), doi: https://doi.org/10.1136/bmj.j2353.

33. E. P. Handing et al., "Midlife Alcohol Consumption and Risk of Dementia over 43 Years of Follow-Up: A Population-Based Study from the Swedish Twin Registry," *Journals of Gerontology, Series A: Biological Sciences and Medical Sciences* 70, no. 10 (October 2015): 1248–54, doi: 10.1093/gerona/glv038.

34. J. Ding et al., "Alcohol Intake and Cerebral Abnormalities on Magnetic Resonance Imaging in a Community-Based Population of Middle-Aged Adults: The Atherosclerosis

Risk in Communities (ARIC) Study," *Stroke* 35, no. 1 (January 2004): 16–21, doi: 10.1161/01.STR.0000105929.88691.8E.

35. J. Connor, "Alcohol Consumption as a Cause of Cancer," *Addiction* 112, no. 2 (February 2017): 222–28, doi: 10.1111/add.13477.

36. Daniel G. Amen et al., "Discriminative Properties of Hippocampal Hypoperfusion in Marijuana Users Compared to Healthy Controls: Implications for Marijuana Administration in Alzheimer's Dementia," *Journal of Alzheimer's Disease* 56, no. 1 (2017): 261–73, doi: 10.3233/JAD-160833.

37. Edward A. Bittner, Yun Yue, and Zhongcong Xie, "Brief Review: Anesthetic Neurotoxicity in the Elderly, Cognitive Dysfunction and Alzheimer's Disease," *Canadian Journal of Anesthesia* 58, no. 2 (February 2011): 216–23, doi: 10.1007/s12630-010-9418-x; C. W. Chen et al., "Increased Risk of Dementia in People with Previous Exposure to General Anesthesia: A Nationwide Population-Based Case-Control Study," *Alzheimer's and Dementia* 10, no. 2 (March 2014): 196–204, doi: http://dx.doi.org/10.1016/j.jalz .2013.05.1766.

38. Barynia Backeljauw et al., "Cognition and Brain Structure Following Early Childhood Surgery with Anesthesia," *Pediatrics* 136, no. 1 (July 2015), doi: 10.1542/peds.2014-3526.

39. N. Efimova et al., "Changes in Cerebral Blood Flow and Cognitive Function in Patients Undergoing Coronary Bypass Surgery with Cardiopulmonary Bypass," *Kardiologiia* 55, no. 6 (2015): 40–46.

40. I. H. Stanley, M. A. Hom, and T. E. Joiner, "A Systematic Review of Suicidal Thoughts and Behaviors among Police Officers, Firefighters, EMTs, and Paramedics," *Clinical Psychology Review* 44 (March 2016): 25–44, doi: 10.1016/j.cpr.2015.12.002.

41. University of Rochester Medical Center, "Chemotherapy's Damage to the Brain Detailed," *ScienceDaily*, April 22, 2008, www.sciencedaily.com/releases/2008/04/080422103947.htm.

42. Philip J. Landrigan and Charles Benbrook, "GMOs, Herbicides, and Public Health," *New England Journal of Medicine* 373, no. 8 (August 20, 2015): 693–95, doi: 10.1056 /NEJMp1505660.

43. Dana Loomis et al., "Carcinogenicity of Lindane, DDT, and 2,4-Dichlorophenoxyacetic Acid," *Lancet Oncology* 16, no. 8 (June 23, 2015): 891–92, doi: 10.1016/S1470-2045(15)00081-9.

44. L. A. Frassetto, R. C. Morris Jr., and A. Sebastian, "Effect of Age on Blood Acid-Base Composition in Adult Humans: Role of Age-Related Renal Functional Decline," *American Journal of Physiology* 271, no. 6, part 2 (December 1996): F1114–22.

45. Alena Hall, "What Happened after One Family Went Organic for Just Two Weeks," *Huffington Post*, May 14, 2015, http://www.huffingtonpost.com/2015/05/14/the-organic -effect_n_7244000.html; Jörgen Magnér et al., "Human Exposure to Pesticides from Food: A Pilot Study," Coop Sverige AB (January 2015), https://www.coop.se/contentassets /dc9bd9f95773402997e4aca0c11b8274/coop-ekoeffekten_rapport_eng.pdf.

46. Cynthia L. Curl, Richard A. Fenske, and Kai Elgethun, "Organophosphorus Pesticide Exposure of Urban and Suburban Preschool Children with Organic and Conventional Diets," *Environmental Health Perspectives* 111, no. 3 (March 2003): 377–82.

47. W. Wulaningsih et al., "Investigating Nutrition and Lifestyle Factors as Determinants of Abdominal Obesity: An Environment-Wide Study," *International Journal of Obesity* 41, no. 2 (February 2017): 340–47, doi: 10.1038/ijo.2016.203; S. P. Fowler, "Low-Calorie Sweetener Use and Energy Balance: Results from Experimental Studies in Animals, and Large-Scale Prospective Studies in Humans," *Physiology and Behavior* 164, part B (October 1, 2016): 517–23, doi: 10.1016/j.physbeh.2016.04.047; M. Paolini et al., "Aspartame, a Bittersweet Pill," *Carcinogenesis* (February 24, 2016), doi: 10.1093/carcin/bgw025; M. Soffritti et al., "The Carcinogenic Effects of Aspartame: The Urgent Need for Regulatory Re-evaluation," *American Journal of Industrial Medicine* 57, no. 4 (April 2014): 383–97, doi: 10.1002 /ajim.22296.

48. Jodi E. Nettleton, Raylene A. Reimer, and Jane Shearer, "Reshaping the Gut Microbiota: Impact of Low Calorie Sweeteners and the Link to Insulin Resistance?" *Physiology and Behavior* 164, part B (October 1, 2016): 488–93, doi: 10.1002/ajim.22296; J. Suez et al.,

"Artificial Sweeteners Induce Glucose Intolerance by Altering the Gut Microbiota," *Nature* 514, no. 7521 (October 9, 2014): 181–86, doi: 10.1038/nature13793.

49. D. E. King, A. G. Mainous III, and C. A. Lambourne, "Trends in Dietary Fiber Intake in the United States, 1999–2008," *Journal of the Academy of Nutrition and Dietetics* 112, no. 5 (May 2012): 642–48, doi: 10.1016/j.jand.2012.01.019.

50. Sarah Yang, "Teen Girls See Big Drop in Chemical Exposure with Switch in Cosmetics," *Berkeley News*, March 7, 2016, http://news.berkeley.edu/2016/03/07/cosmetics -chemicals/.

51. S. S. Zhou et al., "The Skin Function: A Factor of Anti-Metabolic Syndrome," *Diabetology and Metabolic Syndrome* 4, no. 1 (April 26, 2012): 15, doi: 10.1186/1758-5996-4-15.

52. Margaret E. Sears, Kathleen J. Kerr, and Riina I. Bray, "Arsenic, Cadmium, Lead, and Mercury in Sweat: A Systematic Review," *Journal of Environmental and Public Health* 2012 (2012): article ID 184745, doi: 10.1155/2012/184745; S. J. Genuis et al., "Blood, Urine, and Sweat (BUS) Study: Monitoring and Elimination of Bioaccumulated Toxic Elements," *Archives of Environmental Contamination and Toxicology* 61, no. 2 (August 2011): 344–57, doi: 10.1007/s00244-010-9611-5.

53. Margaret E. Sears and Stephen J. Genuis, "Environmental Determinants of Chronic Disease and Medical Approaches: Recognition, Avoidance, Supportive Therapy, and Detoxification," *Journal of Environmental and Public Health* 2012 (2012): article ID 356798, doi: 10.1155/2012/356798; H. Lew and A. Quintanilha, "Effects of Endurance Training and Exercise on Tissue Antioxidative Capacity and Acetaminophen Detoxification," *European Journal of Drug Metabolism and Pharmacokinetics* 16, no. 1 (January–March 1991): 59–68, doi: 10.1007/BF03189876; C. K. Sen, "Glutathione Homeostasis in Response to Exercise Training and Nutritional Supplements," *Molecular and Cellular Biochemistry* 196, nos. 1–2 (June 1999): 31–42; M. O. Murphy et al., "Exercise Protects against PCB-Induced Inflammation and Associated Cardiovascular Risk Factors," *Environmental Science and Pollution Research International* 23, no. 3 (February 2016): 2201–11; S. J. Genuis et al., "Human Elimination of Phthalate Compounds: Blood, Urine, and Sweat (BUS) Study," *Scientific World Journal* 2012 (2012): article ID 615068, doi: 10.1100/2012/615068; S. J. Genuis et al., "Human Excretion of Bisphenol A: Blood, Urine, and Sweat (BUS) Study," *Journal of Environmental and Public Health* 2012 (2012): article ID 185731, doi: 10.1155/2012/185731.

54. K. H. Kilburn, R. H. Warshaw, and M. G. Shields, "Neurobehavioral Dysfunction in Firemen Exposed to Polychlorinated Biphenyls (PCBs): Possible Improvement after Detoxification," *Archives of Environmental Health* 44, no. 6 (November–December 1989): 345–50, doi: 10.1080/00039896.1989.9935904.

55. T. Laukkanen et al., "Sauna Bathing Is Inversely Associated with Dementia and Alzheimer's Disease in Middle-Aged Finnish Men," *Age and Ageing* 46, no. 2 (March 1, 2017): 245–49, doi: 10.1093/ageing/afw212.

56. T. Laukkanen et al., "Association between Sauna Bathing and Fatal Cardiovascular and All-Cause Mortality Events," *JAMA Internal Medicine* 175, no. 4 (April 2015): 542–48, doi: 10.1001/jamainternmed.2014.8187.

57. K. F. Koltyn et al., "Changes in Mood State Following Whole-Body Hyperthermia," *International Journal of Hyperthermia* 8, no. 3 (May 1992): 305–7, doi: 10.3109 /02656739209021785; K. Kukkonen-Harjula and K. Kauppinen, "How the Sauna Affects the Endocrine System," *Annals of Clinical Research* 20, no. 4 (1988): 262–66; D. Jezová et al., "Rise in Plasma Beta-Endorphin and ACTH in Response to Hyperthermia in Sauna," *Hormone and Metabolic Research* 17, no. 12 (December 1985): 693–94; K. Kukkonen-Harjula et al., "Haemodynamic and Hormonal Responses to Heat Exposure in a Finnish Sauna Bath," *European Journal of Applied Physiology and Occupational Physiology* 58, no. 5 (1989): 543–50, doi: 10.1007/BF02330710; S. Kokura et al., "Whole Body Hyperthermia Improves Obesity-Induced Insulin Resistance in Diabetic Mice," *International Journal of Hyperthermia* 23, no. 3 (May 2007): 259–65, doi: 10.1080/02656730601176824.

58. T. Laukkanen et al., "Association between Sauna Bathing and Fatal Cardiovascular and All-Cause Mortality Events," 542–48.

59. R. J. Flanagan and T. J. Meredith, "Use of N-Acetylcysteine in Clinical Toxicology," *American Journal of Medicine* 91, no. 3C (September 1991): 131S–139S.

60. R. Kirchhoff et al., "Increase in Choleresis by Means of Artichoke Extract," *Phytomedicine* 1, no. 2 (September 1994): 107–15, doi: 10.1016/S0944-7113(11)80027-9.

61. S. M. Mansour et al., "*Ginkgo biloba* Extract (EGb 761) Normalizes Hypertension in 2K, 1C Hypertensive Rats: Role of Antioxidant Mechanisms, ACE Inhibiting Activity and Improvement of Endothelial Dysfunction," *Phytomedicine* 18, nos. 8–9 (June 15, 2011): 641–47, doi: 10.1016/j.phymed.2011.01.014.

62. K. Cavuşoğlu et al., "Protective Effect of Ginkgo biloba L. Leaf Extract against Glyphosate Toxicity in Swiss Albino Mice," *Journal of Medicinal Food* 14, no. 10 (October 2011): 1263–72, doi: 10.1089/jmf.2010.0202.

63. X. Liu and K. Lv, "Cruciferous Vegetables Intake Is Inversely Associated with Risk of Breast Cancer: A Meta-analysis," *Breast* 22, no. 3 (June 2013): 309–13, doi: 10.1016/j.breast.2012.07.013.

64. P. L. Crowell and M. N. Gould, "Chemoprevention and Therapy of Cancer by *d*-Limonene," *Critical Reviews in Oncogenesis* 5, no. 1 (1994): 1–22, doi: 10.1615/CritRevOncog.v5.i1.10.

65. J. NM et al., "Beyond the Flavour: A De-Flavoured Polyphenol Rich Extract of Clove Buds (Syzygium Aromaticum L) as a Novel Dietary Antioxidant Ingredient," *Food & Function* 6, no. 10 (October 2015): 3373–82, doi: 10.1039/c5fo00682a; E. A. Offord et al., "Mechanisms Involved in the Chemoprotective Effects of Rosemary Extract Studied in Human Liver and Bronchial Cells," *Cancer Letters* 114, nos. 1–2 (March 19, 1997): 275–81; A. Ganjre et al., "Anti-Carcinogenic and Anti-Bacterial Properties of Selected Spices: Implications in Oral Health," *Clinical Nutrition Research* 4, no. 4 (October 2015): 209–15, doi: 10.7762/cnr.2015.4.4.209.

CHAPTER 11: M IS FOR MENTAL HEALTH

1. W. Katon et al., "Effect of Depression and Diabetes Mellitus on the Risk for Dementia: A National Population-Based Cohort Study," *JAMA Psychiatry* 72, no. 6 (June 2015): 612–19, doi: 10.1001/jamapsychiatry.2015.0082; J. da Silva et al., "Affective Disorders and Risk of Developing Dementia: Systematic Review," *British Journal of Psychiatry* 202, no. 3 (March 2013): 177–86, doi: 10.1192/bjp.bp.111.101931; Osvaldo P. Almeida et al., "Risk of Dementia and Death in Community-Dwelling Older Men with Bipolar Disorder," *British Journal of Psychiatry* 209, no. 2 (August 2016): 121–26, doi: 10.1192/bjp.bp.115.180059; M. H. Chen et al., "Risk of Subsequent Dementia among Patients with Bipolar Disorder or Major Depression: A Nationwide Longitudinal Study in Taiwan," *Journal of the American Medical Directors Association* 16, no. 6 (June 1, 2015): 504–8, doi: 10.1016/j.jamda.2015.01.084; A. R. Ribe et al., "Long-Term Risk of Dementia in Persons with Schizophrenia: A Danish Population-Based Cohort Study," *JAMA Psychiatry* 72, no. 11 (November 2015): 1095–101, doi: 10.1001/jamapsychiatry.2015.1546; K. Yaffe et al., "Posttraumatic Stress Disorder and Risk of Dementia among US Veterans," *Archives of General Psychiatry* 67, no. 6 (June 2010): 608–13, doi: 10.1001/archgenpsychiatry.2010.61; T. Y. Wang et al., "Risk for Developing Dementia among Patients with Posttraumatic Stress Disorder: A Nationwide Longitudinal Study," *Journal of Affective Disorders* 205 (November 15, 2016): 306–10, doi: 10.1016/j.jad.2016.08.013; A. Golimstok et al., "Previous Adult Attention-Deficit and Hyperactivity Disorder Symptoms and Risk of Dementia with Lewy Bodies: A Case-Control Study," *European Journal of Neurology* 18, no. 1 (January 2011): 78–84, doi: 10.1111/j.1468-1331.2010.03064.x; L. Johansson et al., "Common Psychosocial Stressors in Middle-Aged Women Related to Longstanding Distress and Increased Risk of Alzheimer's Disease: A 38-Year Longitudinal Population Study," *BMJ Open* 3, no. 9 (September 2013): e003142, doi: 10.1136/bmjopen-2013-003142; L. Johansson et al., "Midlife Personality and Risk of Alzheimer Disease and Distress: A 38-Year Follow-Up," *Neurology* 83, no. 17 (October 21, 2014): 1538–44, doi: 10.1212/WNL.0000000000000907; Kate Kelland, "Study Finds How Stress Raises Heart Disease and Stroke Risk," *Reuters*, January 11, 2017, http://www.reuters.com/article/us-health-heart-stress-idUSKBN14V2T3.

2. Lizzie Parry, "Head Rules Your Heart: Depression Is 'AS Dangerous as Being FAT— Causing Almost One in Five Heart Deaths,'" *Sun*, January 16, 2017, https://www.thesun .co.uk/living/2627090/depression-is-as-dangerous-as-being-fat-causing-almost-one -in-five-heart-deaths/; E. R. Walker, R. E. McGee, and B. G. Druss, "Mortality in Mental Disorders and Global Disease Burden Implications: A Systematic Review and Meta-Analysis," *JAMA Psychiatry* 72, no. 4 (April 2015): 334–41, doi: 10.1001/jamapsychiatry .2014.2502.

3. M. L. Alosco, A. Fedor, and J. Gunstad, "Attention Deficit Hyperactivity Disorder as a Risk Factor for Concussions in NCAA Division-1 Athletes," *Brain Injury* 28, no. 4 (February 2014): 472–74, doi: 10.3109/02699052.2014.887145; A. Raziel, N. Sakran, and D. Goitein, "The Relationship between Attention Deficit Hyperactivity Disorders (ADHD) and Obesity," *Harefuah* 153, no. 9 (September 2014): 541–45, 557; Søren Dalsgaard et al., "Mortality in Children, Adolescents, and Adults with Attention Deficit Hyperactivity Disorder: A Nationwide Cohort Study," *Lancet* 385, no. 9983 (May 30, 2015): 2190–96, doi: 10.1016 /S0140-6736(14)61684-6; Duke Medicine, "ADHD Treatment Associated with Lower Smoking Rates," *ScienceDaily*, May 12, 2014, www.sciencedaily.com/releases/2014/05 /140512101304.htm.

4. A. Golimstok et al., "Previous Adult Attention-Deficit and Hyperactivity Disorder Symptoms and Risk of Dementia with Lewy Bodies: A Case-Control Study," *European Journal of Neurology* 18, no. 1 (January 2011): 78–84, doi: 10.1111/j.1468-1331.2010.03064.x.

5. K. Yaffe et al., "Depressive Symptoms and Cognitive Decline in Nondemented Elderly Women," *Archives of General Psychiatry* 56, no. 5: 425–30, doi:10.1001/archpsyc.56.5.425.

6. F. F. de Oliveira et al., "Risk Factors for Age at Onset of Dementia Due to Alzheimer's Disease in a Sample of Patients with Low Mean Schooling from São Paulo, Brazil," *International Journal of Geriatric Psychiatry* 29, no. 10 (October 2014): 1033–39, doi: 10.1002/gps.4094; Ismail Zahinoor et al., "Prevalence of Depression in Patients with Mild Cognitive Impairment: A Systematic Review and Meta-Analysis," *JAMA Psychiatry* 74, no. 1 (2017), 58–67, doi: 10.1001/jamapsychiatry.2016.3162.

7. D. G. Amen et al., "Classification of Depression, Cognitive Disorders, and Co-Morbid Depression and Cognitive Disorders with Perfusion SPECT Neuroimaging," *Journal of Alzheimer's Disease* 57, no. 1 (February 10, 2017): 253–66.

8. A. P. Silva et al., "Measurement of the Effect of Physical Exercise on the Concentration of Individuals with ADHD," *PLOS One* 10, no. 3 (March 24, 2015): e0122119, doi: 10.1371/journal.pone.0122119; Beron W. Z. Tan et al., "Meta-Analytic Review of the Efficacy of Physical Exercise Interventions on Cognition in Individuals with Autism Spectrum Disorder and ADHD," *Journal of Autism and Developmental Disorders* 46, no. 9 (September 2016): 3126–43, doi: 0.1007/s10803-016-2854-x; B. Hoza et al., "A Randomized Trial Examining the Effects of Aerobic Physical Activity on Attention-Deficit/Hyperactivity Disorder Symptoms in Young Children," *Journal of Abnormal Child Psychology* 43, no. 4 (May 2015): 655–67, doi: 10.1007/s10802-014-9929-y.

9. S. B. Cooper et al., "Breakfast Glycaemic Index and Exercise: Combined Effects on Adolescents' Cognition," *Physiology & Behavior* 139 (February 2015): 104–11, doi: 10.1016/j.physbeh.2014.11.024; J. Ingwersen et al., "A Low Glycaemic Index Breakfast Cereal Preferentially Prevents Children's Cognitive Performance from Declining throughout the Morning," *Appetite* 49, no. 1 (July 2007): 240–44, doi: 10.1016/j.appet .2006.06.009.

10. J. Knapen et al., "Exercise Therapy Improves Both Mental and Physical Health in Patients with Major Depression," *Disability and Rehabilitation* 37, no. 16 (2015): 1490–95, doi: 10.3109/09638288.2014.972579; C. Battaglia et al., "Participation in a 9-Month Selected Physical Exercise Programme Enhances Psychological Well-Being in a Prison Population," *Criminal Behaviour and Mental Health* 25, no. 5 (December 2015): 343–54, doi: 10.1002/cbm.1922.

11. M. Hosseinzadeh et al., "Empirically Derived Dietary Patterns in Relation to Psychological Disorders," *Public Health Nutrition* 19, no. 2 (February 2016): 204–17, doi: 10.1017 /S136898001500172X.

12. K. Niu et al., "A Tomato-Rich Diet Is Related to Depressive Symptoms among an Elderly Population Aged 70 Years and Over: A Population-Based, Cross-Sectional Analysis," *Journal of Affective Disorders* 144, nos. 1–2 (January 10, 2013): 165–70, doi: 10.1016/j .jad.2012.04.040.

13. R. T. Ackermann and J. W. Williams Jr., "Rational Treatment Choices for Non-Major Depressions in Primary Care: An Evidence-Based Review," *Journal of General Internal Medicine* 17, no. 4 (April 2002): 293–301.

14. A. S. Yeung et al., "A Pilot Study of Acupuncture Augmentation Therapy in Antidepressant Partial and Non-Responders with Major Depressive Disorder," *Journal of Affective Disorders* 130, nos. 1–2 (April 2011): 285–89, doi: 10.1016/j.jad.2010.07.025; J. Wu et al., "Acupuncture for Depression: A Review of Clinical Applications," *Canadian Journal of Psychiatry* 57, no. 7 (July 2012): 397–405, doi: 10.1177/070674371205700702.

15. G. I. Papakostas et al., "L-Methylfolate as Adjunctive Therapy for SSRI-Resistant Major Depression: Results of Two Randomized, Double-Blind, Parallel-Sequential Trials," *American Journal of Psychiatry* 169, no. 12 (December 2012): 1267–74, doi: 10.1176/appi .ajp.2012.11071114.

16. A. S. de Sá Filho et al., "Potential Therapeutic Effects of Physical Exercise for Bipolar Disorder," *CNS and Neurological Disorders Drug Targets* 14, no. 10 (2015): 1255–59.

17. L. Chen et al., "Eye Movement Desensitization and Reprocessing versus Cognitive-Behavioral Therapy for Adult Posttraumatic Stress Disorder: Systematic Review and Meta-Analysis," *Journal of Nervous and Mental Disease* 203, no. 6 (June 2015): 443–51, doi: 10.1097/NMD.0000000000000306.

18. D. J. Kearney et al., "Loving-Kindness Meditation for Posttraumatic Stress Disorder: A Pilot Study," *Journal of Traumatic Stress* 26, no. 4 (August 2013): 426–34, doi: 10.1002 /jts.21832; D. J. Kearney et al., "Loving-Kindness Meditation and the Broaden-and-Build Theory of Positive Emotions among Veterans with Posttraumatic Stress Disorder," *Medical Care* 52, no. 12, suppl. 5 (December 2014): S32–38, doi: 10.1097/MLR .0000000000000221.

19. Mayo Clinic Staff, "Exercise and Stress: Get Moving to Manage Stress," Mayo Clinic website, April 16, 2015, http://www.mayoclinic.org/healthy-lifestyle/stress-management /in-depth/exercise-and-stress/art-20044469.

20. J. N. Belding et al., "Social Buffering by God: Prayer and Measures of Stress," *Journal of Religion and Health* 49, no. 2 (June 2010): 179–87, doi: 10.1007/s10943-009-9256-8; K. Bluth, P. N. Roberson, and S. A. Gaylord, "A Pilot Study of a Mindfulness Intervention for Adolescents and the Potential Role of Self-Compassion in Reducing Stress," *Explore* 11, no. 4 (July–August 2015): 292–95, doi: 10.1016/j.explore.2015.04.005; W. Turakitwanakan et al., "Effects of Mindfulness Meditation on Serum Cortisol of Medical Students," *Journal of the Medical Association of Thailand* 96, suppl. 1 (January 2013): S90–95.

21. R. A. Emmons and M. E. McCullough, "Counting Blessings versus Burdens: An Experimental Investigation of Gratitude and Subjective Well-Being in Daily Life," *Journal of Personality and Social Psychology* 84, no. 2 (February 2003): 377–89.

22. Marjorie Ingall, "Chocolate Can Do Good Things for Your Heart, Skin and Brain," *Health Magazine*, December 22, 2006, http://www.cnn.com/2006/HEALTH/12/20/health .chocolate/.

23. H. J. Trappe and G. Voit, "The Cardiovascular Effect of Musical Genres," *Deutsches Arzteblatt International* 113, no. 20 (May 20, 2016): 347–52, doi: 10.3238/arztebl.2016.0347.

24. Erin Brodwin, "Psychologists Discover the Simplest Way to Boost Your Mood," *Business Insider,* April 3, 2015, http://www.businessinsider.com/how-to-boost-your-mood-2015-4.

25. K. Kimura et al., "L-Theanine Reduces Psychological and Physiological Stress Responses," *Biological Psychology* 74, no. 1 (January 2007): 39–45, doi: 10.1016/j.biopsycho.2006.06.006.

26. M. Rudd, K. D. Vohs, and J. Aaker, "Awe Expands People's Perception of Time, Alters Decision Making, and Enhances Well-Being," *Psychological Science* 23, no. 10 (October 1, 2012): 1130–36, doi: 10.1177/0956797612438731.

27. Y. Miyazaki et al., "Preventive Medical Effects of Nature Therapy," *Nihon Eiseigaku Zasshi* 66, no. 4 (September 2011): 651–56; G. N. Bratman et al., "Nature Experience Reduces Rumination and Subgenual Prefrontal Cortex Activation," *Proceedings of the National Academy of Sciences in the United States of America* 112, no. 28 (July 14, 2015): 8567–72, doi: 10.1073/pnas.1510459112.

28. Stephanie Slon, "7 Health Benefits of Going Barefoot Outside," mindbodygreen website, March 29, 2012, http://www.mindbodygreen.com/0-4369/7-Health-Benefits-of-Going-Barefoot-Outside.html.

29. L. Taruffi and S. Koelsch, "The Paradox of Music-Evoked Sadness: An Online Survey," *PLOS One* 9, no. 10 (October 20, 2014): e110490, doi: 10.1371/journal.pone.0110490.

30. Y. H. Liu et al., "Effects of Music Listening on Stress, Anxiety, and Sleep Quality for Sleep-Disturbed Pregnant Women," *Women & Health* 56, no. 3 (2016): 296–311, doi: 10.1080/03630242.2015.1088116.

31. Travis Bradberry, "How Complaining Rewires Your Brain for Negativity," *Huffington Post* blog, December 26, 2016, http://www.huffingtonpost.com/dr-travis-bradberry/how-complaining-rewires-y_b_13634470.html.

32. "Can You Catch Depression? Being Surrounded by Gloomy People Can Make You Prone to Illness," *Daily Mail,* April 19, 2013, http://www.dailymail.co.uk/health/article-2311523/Can-CATCH-depression-Being-surrounded-gloomy-people-make-prone-illness-say-scientists.html.

33. Ryan T. Howell et al., "Momentary Happiness: The Role of Psychological Need Satisfaction," *Journal of Happiness Studies* 12, no. 1 (March 2011): 1–15, doi: 10.1007/s10902-009-9166-1.

34. Carolyn Gregoire, "Older People Are Happier Than You. Why?" *Huffington Post,* April 24, 2015, http://www.cnn.com/2015/04/24/health/old-people-happy/.

35. M. Mela et al., "The Influence of a Learning to Forgive Programme on Negative Affect among Mentally Disordered Offenders," *Criminal Behaviour and Mental Health* 27, no. 2 (April 2017): 162–75, doi: 10.1002/cbm.1991.

36. L. Bolier et al., "Positive Psychology Interventions: A Meta-Analysis of Randomized Controlled Studies," *BMC Public Health* 13 (February 8, 2013): 119, doi: 10.1186/1471-2458-13-119.

37. Paul Bentley, "What Really Makes Us Happy? How Spending Time with Your Friends Is Better for You Than Being with Family," *Daily Mail,* June 30, 2013, http://www.dailymail.co.uk/news/article-2351870/What-really-makes-happy-How-spending-time-friends-better-family.html.

38. David G. Blanchflower and Andrew J. Oswald, "Money, Sex, and Happiness: An Empirical Study," *Scandinavian Journal of Economics* 106, no. 3 (2004): 393–415, doi: 10.3386/w10499.

39. Maud Purcell, "The Health Benefits of Journaling," Psych Central website, May 17, 2016, https://psychcentral.com/lib/the-health-benefits-of-journaling/.

40. Xianglong Zeng et al., "The Effect of Loving-Kindness Meditation on Positive Emotions: A Meta-Analytic Review," *Frontiers in Psychology* 6 (November 3, 2015): 1693, doi: 10.3389/fpsyg.2015.01693; Barbara L. Fredrickson et al., "Open Hearts Build Lives: Positive Emotions, Induced through Loving-Kindness Meditation, Build Consequential Personal Resources," *Journal of Personality and Social Psychology* 95, no. 5 (November 2008): 1045–62.

41. J. W. Carson et al., "Loving-Kindness Meditation for Chronic Low Back Pain: Results from a Pilot Trial," *Journal of Holistic Nursing* 23, no. 3 (September 2005): 287–304; M. E. Tonelli and A. B. Wachholtz, "Meditation-Based Treatment Yielding Immediate Relief for Meditation-Naïve Migraineurs," *Pain Management Nursing* 15, no. 1 (March 2014): 36–40; Kearney et al., "Loving-Kindness Meditation for Posttraumatic Stress Disorder," 426–34; A. J. Stell and T. Farsides, "Brief Loving-Kindness Meditation Reduces Racial Bias, Mediated by Positive Other-Regarding Emotions," *Motivation and Emotion* 40, no. 1 (2016): 140–47, doi: 10.1007/s11031-015-9514-x.

42. M. K. Leung et al., "Increased Gray Matter Volume in the Right Angular and Posterior

Parahippocampal Gyri in Loving-Kindness Meditators," *Social Cognitive and Affective Neuroscience* 8, no. 1 (January 2013): 34–39; B. E. Kok et al., "How Positive Emotions Build Physical Health: Perceived Positive Social Connections Account for the Upward Spiral between Positive Emotions and Vagal Tone," *Psychological Science* 24, no. 7 (July 1, 2013): 1123–32.

43. E. Hawkey and J. T. Nigg, "Omega3 Fatty Acid and ADHD: Blood Level Analysis and Meta-Analytic Extension of Supplementation Trials," *Clinical Psychology Review* 34, no. 6 (August 2014): 496–505, doi: 10.1016/j.cpr.2014.05.005; C. M. Milte et al., "Increased Erythrocyte Eicosapentaenoic Acid and Docosahexaenoic Acid Are Associated with Improved Attention and Behavior in Children with ADHD in a Randomized Controlled Three-Way Crossover Trial," *Journal of Attention Disorders* 19, no. 11 (November 2015): 954–64, doi: 10.1177/1087054713510562; K. Widenhorn-Müller et al., "Effect of Supplementation with Long-Chain ω-3 Polyunsaturated Fatty Acids on Behavior and Cognition in Children with Attention Deficit/Hyperactivity Disorder (ADHD): A Randomized Placebo-Controlled Intervention Trial," *Prostaglandins, Leukotrienes, and Essential Fatty Acids* 91, nos. 1–2 (July–August 2014): 49–60, doi: 10.1016/j.plefa.2014.04.004; H. Perera et al., "Combined ω3 and ω6 Supplementation in Children with Attention-Deficit Hyperactivity Disorder (ADHD) Refractory to Methylphenidate Treatment: A Double-Blind, Placebo-Controlled Study," *Journal of Child Neurology* 27, no. 6 (June 2012): 747–53, doi: 10.1177/0883073811435243; D. J. Bos et al., "Reduced Symptoms of Inattention after Dietary Omega-3 Fatty Acid Supplementation in Boys with and without Attention Deficit/Hyperactivity Disorder," *Neuropsychopharmacology* 40, no. 10 (September 2015): 2298–306, doi: 10.1038/npp.2015.73.

44. P. Toren et al., "Zinc Deficiency in Attention-Deficit Hyperactivity Disorder," *Biological Psychiatry* 40, no. 12 (December 15, 1996): 1308–10, doi: 10.1016/S0006-3223(96)00310-1; O. Oner et al., "Effects of Zinc and Ferritin Levels on Parent and Teacher Reported Symptom Scores in Attention Deficit Hyperactivity Disorder," *Child Psychiatry and Human Development* 41, no. 4 (August 2010): 441–47, doi: 10.1007/s10578-010-0178-1; O. Yorbik et al., "Potential Effects of Zinc on Information Processing in Boys with Attention Deficit Hyperactivity Disorder," *Progress in Neuropsychopharmacology & Biological Psychiatry* 32, no. 3 (April 1, 2008): 662–67, doi: 10.1016/j.pnpbp.2007.11.009; S. Akhondzadeh, M. R. Mohammadi, and M. Khademi, "Zinc Sulfate as an Adjunct to Methylphenidate for the Treatment of Attention Deficit Hyperactivity Disorder in Children: A Double Blind and Randomized Trial," *BMC Psychiatry* 4 (April 8, 2004): 9, doi: 10.1186/1471-244X-4-9.

45. M. Mousain-Bosc et al., "Improvement of Neurobehavioral Disorders in Children Supplemented with Magnesium-Vitamin B6. I. Attention Deficit Hyperactivity Disorders," *Magnesium Research* 19, no. 1 (March 2006): 46–52; A. Ghanizadeh, "A Systematic Review of Magnesium Therapy for Treating Attention Deficit Hyperactivity Disorder," *Archives of Iranian Medicine* 16, no. 7 (July 2013): 412–17, doi: 013167/AIM.0010; M. Huss, A. Völp, and M. Stauss-Grabo, "Supplementation of Polyunsaturated Fatty Acids, Magnesium and Zinc in Children Seeking Medical Advice for Attention-Deficit/Hyperactivity Problems—An Observational Cohort Study," *Lipids in Health & Disease* 9 (September 24, 2010): 105, doi: 10.1186/1476-511X-9-105.

46. J. S. Halterman et al., "Iron Deficiency and Cognitive Achievement among School-Aged Children and Adolescents in the United States," *Pediatrics* 107, no. 6 (June 2001): 1381–86.

47. S. Hirayama et al., "The Effect of Phosphatidylserine Administration on Memory and Symptoms of Attention-Deficit Hyperactivity Disorder: A Randomised, Double-Blind, Placebo-Controlled Clinical Trial," *Journal of Human Nutrition and Dietetics* 27, suppl. 2 (April 2014): 284–91, doi: 10.1111/jhn.12090; I. Manor et al., "The Effect of Phosphatidylserine Containing Omega3 Fatty-Acids on Attention-Deficit Hyperactivity Disorder Symptoms in Children: A Double-Blind Placebo-Controlled Trial, Followed by an Open-Label Extension," *European Psychiatry* 27, no. 5 (July 2012): 335–42, doi: 10.1016/j.eurpsy.2011.05.004.

48. Giuseppe Grosso et al., "Role of Omega-3 Fatty Acids in the Treatment of Depressive Disorders: A Comprehensive Meta-Analysis of Randomized Clinical Trials," *PLOS One* 9,

no. 5 (May 7, 2014): e96905, doi: 10.1371/journal.pone.0096905; B. Hallahan et al., "Efficacy of Omega-3 Highly Unsaturated Fatty Acids in the Treatment of Depression," *British Journal of Psychiatry* 209, no. 3 (September 2016): 192–201, doi: 10.1192/bjp .bp.114.160242; J. G. Martins, "EPA but Not DHA Appears to Be Responsible for the Efficacy of Omega-3 Long Chain Polyunsaturated Fatty Acid Supplementation in Depression: Evidence from a Meta-Analysis of Randomized Controlled Trials," *Journal of the American College of Nutrition* 28, no. 5 (October 2009): 525–42.

49. M. H. Rapaport et al., "Inflammation as a Predictive Biomarker for Response to Omega-3 Fatty Acids in Major Depressive Disorder: A Proof of Concept Study," *Molecular Psychiatry* 21, no. 1 (January 2016): 71–79, doi: 10.1038/mp.2015.22.

50. D. J. Carpenter, "St. John's Wort and S-Adenosyl Methionine as 'Natural' Alternatives to Conventional Antidepressants in the Era of the Suicidality Boxed Warning: What Is the Evidence for Clinically Relevant Benefit?" *Alternative Medicine Review* 16, no. 1 (March 2011): 17–39; G. I. Papakostas et al., "S-Adenosyl Methionine (SAMe) Augmentation of Serotonin Reuptake Inhibitors for Antidepressant Nonresponders with Major Depressive Disorder: A Double-Blind, Randomized Clinical Trial," *American Journal of Psychiatry* 167, no. 8 (August 2010): 942–48, doi: 10.1176/appi.ajp.2009.09081198; J. Sarris et al., "S-Adenosyl Methionine (SAMe) versus Escitalopram and Placebo in Major Depression RCT: Efficacy and Effects of Histamine and Carnitine as Moderators of Response," *Journal of Affective Disorders* 164 (August 2014): 76–81, doi: 10.1016/j.jad.2014.03.041; J. Sarris et al., "Is S-Adenosyl Methionine (SAMe) for Depression Only Effective in Males? A Re-Analysis of Data from a Randomized Clinical Trial," *Pharmacopsychiatry* 48, nos. 4–5 (July 2015): 141–44, doi: 10.1055/s-0035-1549928.

51. A. L. Lopresti and P. D. Drummond, "Efficacy of Curcumin, and a Saffron/Curcumin Combination for the Treatment of Major Depression: A Randomised, Double-Blind, Placebo-Controlled Study," *Journal of Affective Disorders* 207 (January 1, 2017): 188–96, doi: 10.1016/j.jad.2016.09.047.

52. Z. Sepehrmanesh et al., "Vitamin D Supplementation Affects the Beck Depression Inventory, Insulin Resistance, and Biomarkers of Oxidative Stress in Patients with Major Depressive Disorder: A Randomized, Controlled Clinical Trial," *Journal of Nutrition* 146, no. 2 (February 2016): 243–48, doi: 10.3945/jn.115.218883; H. Mozaffari-Khosravi et al., "The Effect of 2 Different Single Injections of High Dose of Vitamin D on Improving the Depression in Depressed Patients with Vitamin D Deficiency: A Randomized Clinical Trial," *Journal of Clinical Psychopharmacology* 33, no. 3 (June 2013): 378–85, doi: 10.1097 /JCP.0b013e31828f619a.

53. Christa Sgobba, "This Over-the-Counter Tablet Can Blast through Your Blues in Just 2 Weeks," *Men's Health*, June 28, 2017, http://www.menshealth.com/health/magnesium -for-depression.

54. R. K. McNamara et al., "Adolescents with or at Ultra-High Risk for Bipolar Disorder Exhibit Erythrocyte Docosahexaenoic Acid and Eicosapentaenoic Acid Deficits: A Candidate Prodromal Risk Biomarker," *Early Intervention in Psychiatry* 10, no. 3 (June 2016): 203–11, doi: 10.1111/eip.12282; J. Sarris, D. Mischoulon, and I. Schweitzer, "Omega-3 for Bipolar Disorder: Meta-Analyses of Use in Mania and Bipolar Depression," *Journal of Clinical Psychiatry* 73, no. 1 (January 2012): 81–86, doi: 10.4088/JCP.10r06710.

55. R. K. Sripada et al., "DHEA Enhances Emotion Regulation Neurocircuits and Modulates Memory for Emotional Stimuli," *Neuropsychopharmacology* 38, no. 9 (August 2013): 1798–807, doi: 10.1038/npp.2013.79.

56. R. S. Khan et al., "Effect of a Serotonin Precursor and Uptake Inhibitor in Anxiety Disorders: A Double-Blind Comparison of 5-Hydroxytryptophan, Clomipramine and Placebo," *International Clinical Pharmacology* 2, no. 1 (January 1987): 33–45; A. Ghajar et al., "Crocus Sativus L. versus Citalopram in the Treatment of Major Depressive Disorder with Anxious Distress: A Double-Blind, Controlled Clinical Trial," *Pharmacopsychiatry* (October 4, 2016), doi: 10.1055/s-0042-116159; H. Fukui, K. Toyoshima, and R. Komaki, "Psychological and Neuroendocrinological Effects of Odor of Saffron (Crocus Sativus)," *Phytomedicine* 18, nos. 8–9 (June 15, 2011): 726–30, doi: 10.1016/j.phymed.2010.11.013.

57. A. M. Abdou et al., "Relaxation and Immunity Enhancement Effects of Gamma-Aminobutyric Acid (GABA) Administration in Humans," *Biofactors* 26, no. 3 (2006): 201–8; A. Yoto et al., "Oral Intake of Y-aminobutyric Acid Affects Mood and Activities of Central Nervous System during Stressed Condition Induced by Mental Tasks," *Amino Acids* 43, no. 3 (September 2012): 1331–37, doi: 10.1007/s00726-011-1206-6; B. S. Weeks et al., "Formulations of Dietary Supplements and Herbal Extracts for Relaxation and Anxiolytic Action: Relarian," *Medical Science Monitor* 15, no. 11 (November 2009): RA256–62; K. Kimura et al., "L-Theanine Reduces Psychological and Physiological Stress Responses," 39–45.

58. D. M. Lovinger, "Serotonin's Role in Alcohol's Effects on the Brain," *Alcohol Health and Research World* 21, no. 2 (1997): 114–20.

59. R. P. Sharma and R. A. Coulombe Jr., "Effects of Repeated Doses of Aspartame on Serotonin and Its Metabolite in Various Regions of the Mouse Brain," *Food and Chemical Toxicology* 25, no. 8 (August 1987): 565–68.

60. "Foods That Fight Winter Depression," WebMD, accessed May 30, 2017, http://www.webmd.com/depression/features/foods-that-fight-winter-depression#1.

61. A. Ghajar et al., "Crocus Sativus L. versus Citalopram"; H. A. Hausenblas et al., "A Systematic Review of Randomized Controlled Trials Examining the Effectiveness of Saffron (Crocus Sativus L.) on Psychological and Behavioral Outcomes," *Journal of Integrative Medicine* 13, no. 4 (July 2015): 231–40, doi: 10.1016/S2095-4964(15)60176-5; S. K. Kulkarni, M. K. Bhutani, and M. Bishnoi, "Antidepressant Activity of Curcumin: Involvement of Serotonin and Dopamine System," *Psychopharmacology* 201, no. 3 (December 2008): 435–42, doi: 10.1007/s00213-008-1300-y; A. L. Lopresti et al., "Curcumin for the Treatment of Major Depression: A Randomised, Double-Blind, Placebo Controlled Study," *Journal of Affective Disorders* 167 (2014): 368–75, doi: 10.1016/j.jad.2014.06.001; A. L. Lopresti and P. D. Drummond, "Efficacy of Curcumin, and a Saffron/Curcumin Combination for the Treatment of Major Depression," 188–96; S. Barker et al., "Improved Performance on Clerical Tasks Associated with Administration of Peppermint Odor," *Perceptual and Motor Skills* 97, no. 3, part 1 (December 2003): 1007–10, doi: 10.2466/pms.2003.97.3.1007; P. R. Zoladz and B. Raudenbush, "Cognitive Enhancement through Stimulation of the Chemical Senses," *North American Journal of Psychology* 7, no. 1 (April 2005): 125–40; H. M. Chen and H. W. Chen, "The Effect of Applying Cinnamon Aromatherapy for Children with Attention Deficit Hyperactivity Disorder," *Journal of Chinese Medicine* 19, no. 112 (2008): 27–34; "Study Finds That Peppermint and Cinnamon Lower Drivers' Frustration and Increase Alertness," Wheeling Jesuit University website, accessed May 30, 2017, http://www.wju.edu/about/adm_news_story.asp?iNewsID=1882&strBack=/about/adm_news_archive.asp.

62. S. K. Kulkarni, M. K. Bhutani, and M. Bishnoi, "Antidepressant Activity of Curcumin": 435–42; T. Yamada et al., "Effects of Theanine, r-glutamylethylamide, on Neurotransmitter Release and Its Relationship with Glutamic Acid Neurotransmission," *Nutritional Neuroscience* 8, no. 4 (August 2005): 219–26, doi: 10.1080/10284150500170799.

63. Diana L. Walcutt, "Chocolate and Mood Disorders," Psych Central website, accessed May 30, 2017, https://psychcentral.com/blog/archives/2009/04/27/chocolate-and-mood-disorders/; A. A. Sunni and R. Latif, "Effects of Chocolate Intake on Perceived Stress; a Controlled Clinical Study," *International Journal of Health Sciences (Qassim)* 8, no. 4 (October 2014): 393–401.

64. University of Warwick, "Fruit and Veggies Give You the Feel-Good Factor," *ScienceDaily*, July 10, 2016, www.sciencedaily.com/releases/2016/07/160710094239.htm.

65. L. Stojanovska et al., "Maca Reduces Blood Pressure and Depression, in a Pilot Study in Postmenopausal Women," *Climacteric* 18, no. 1 (February 2015): 69–78, doi: 10.3109/13697137.2014.929649.

66. Cornell University, "Omega-3 Fatty Acids: Good for the Heart, and (Maybe) Good for the Brain," *ScienceDaily*, November 8, 2004, www.sciencedaily.com/releases/2004/11/041108024221.htm.

CHAPTER 12: I IS FOR IMMUNITY/INFECTION ISSUES

1. Y. H. Peng et al., "Adult Asthma Increases Dementia Risk: A Nationwide Cohort Study," *Journal of Epidemiology and Community Health* 69, no. 2 (February 2015): 123–28, doi: 10.1136/jech-2014-204445; M. Rusanen et al., "Chronic Obstructive Pulmonary Disease and Asthma and the Risk of Mild Cognitive Impairment and Dementia: A Population Based CAIDE Study," *Current Alzheimer Research* 10, no. 5 (June 2013): 549–55.

2. R. C. Chou et al., "Treatment for Rheumatoid Arthritis and Risk of Alzheimer's Disease: A Nested Case-Control Analysis," *CNS Drugs* 30, no. 11 (November 2016): 1111–20, doi: 10.1007/s40263-016-0374-z.

3. Y. R. Lin et al., "Increased Risk of Dementia in Patients with Systemic Lupus Erythematosus: A Nationwide Population-Based Cohort Study," *Arthritis Care and Research* 68, no. 12 (December 2016): 1774–79, doi: 10.1002/acr.22914.

4. Dennis Thompson, "Immune Disorders Such as MS, Psoriasis May Be Tied to Dementia Risk," *HealthDay*, March 1, 2017, https://consumer.healthday.com/diseases-and-conditions -information-37/immune-disorder-news-404/immune-disorders-such-as-ms-psoriasis -may-be-tied-to-dementia-risk-720235.html.

5. K. Abuabara et al., "Cause-Specific Mortality in Patients with Severe Psoriasis: A Population-Based Cohort Study in the U.K.," *British Journal of Dermatology* 163, no. 3 (September 2010): 586–92, doi: 10.1111/j.1365-2133.2010.09941.x.

6. R. F. Itzhaki et al., "Microbes and Alzheimer's Disease," *Journal of Alzheimer's Disease* 51, no. 4 (2016): 979–84, doi: 10.3233/JAD-160152.

7. A. J. Steel and G. D. Eslick, "Herpes Viruses Increase the Risk of Alzheimer's Disease: A Meta-Analysis," *Journal of Alzheimer's Disease* 47, no. 2 (2015): 351–64, doi: 10.3233 /JAD-140822; T. E. Strandberg et al., "Cognitive Impairment and Infectious Burden in the Elderly," *Archives of Gerontology and Geriatrics*, suppl. 9 (2004): 419–23, doi: 10.1016/j .archger.2004.04.053.

8. Dana Parish, "'A Slow Slipping Away'—Kris Kristofferson's Long-Undiagnosed Battle with Lyme Disease," *Huffington Post*, July 6, 2016, http://www.huffingtonpost.com /entry/a-slow-slipping-away-kris-kristoffersons-long_us_577c047be4b00a3ae4ce6609.

9. C. J. Carter, "Toxoplasmosis and Polygenic Disease Susceptibility Genes: Extensive *Toxoplasma Gondii* Host/Pathogen Interactome Enrichment in Nine Psychiatric or Neurological Disorders," *Journal of Pathogens* 2013 (2013): article 965046, doi: http://dx.doi.org/10.1155/2013/965046.

10. Ed Yong, "Zombie Roaches and Other Parasite Tales," TED Talk, March 2014, https://www .ted.com/talks/ed_yong_suicidal_wasps_zombie_roaches_and_other_tales_of_parasites.

11. F. Blanc et al., "Lyme Neuroborreliosis and Dementia," *Journal of Alzheimer's Disease* 41, no. 4 (2014): 1087–93, doi: 10.3233/JAD-130446.

12. J. C. McArthur, "HIV Dementia: An Evolving Disease," *Journal of Neuroimmunology* 157, nos. 1–2 (December 2004): 3–10, doi: 10.1016/j.jneuroim.2004.08.042.

13. J. Miklossy, "Historic Evidence to Support a Causal Relationship between Spirochetal Infections and Alzheimer's Disease," *Frontiers in Aging Neuroscience* 7 (April 16, 2015): 46, doi: 10.3389/fnagi.2015.00046.

14. S. A. Harris and E. A. Harris, "Herpes Simplex Virus Type 1 and Other Pathogens Are Key Causative Factors in Sporadic Alzheimer's Disease," *Journal of Alzheimer's Disease* 48, no. 2 (2015): 319–53, doi: 10.3233/JAD-142853; A. J. Steel and G. D. Eslick, "Herpes Viruses Increase the Risk of Alzheimer's Disease," 351–64.

15. L. L. Barnes et al., "Cytomegalovirus Infection and Risk of Alzheimer Disease in Older Black and White Individuals," *Journal of Infectious Diseases* 211, no. 2 (January 15, 2015): 230–37, doi: 10.1093/infdis/jiu437.

16. S. M. Shim et al., "Elevated Epstein-Barr Virus Antibody Level Is Associated with Cognitive Decline in the Korean Elderly," *Journal of Alzheimer's Disease* 55, no. 1 (2017): 293–301, doi: 10.3233/JAD-160563.

17. M. Mahami-Oskouei et al., "Toxoplasmosis and Alzheimer: Can Toxoplasma Gondii Really

Be Introduced as a Risk Factor in Etiology of Alzheimer?" *Parasitology Research* 115, no. 8 (August 2016): 3169–74, doi: 10.1007/s00436-016-5075-5.

18. T. Shindler-Itskovitch et al., "A Systematic Review and Meta-Analysis of the Association between Helicobacterpylori Infection and Dementia," *Journal of Alzheimer's Disease* 52, no. 4 (April 15, 2016): 1431–42, doi: 10.3233/JAD-160132.

19. Priya Maheshwari and Guy D. Eslick, "Bacterial Infection and Alzheimer's Disease: A Meta-Analysis," *Journal of Alzheimer's Disease* 43, no. 3 (2015): 957–66, doi: 10.3233 /JAD-140621.

20. B. Porcelli et al., "Association between Stressful Life Events and Autoimmune Diseases: A Systematic Review and Meta-Analysis of Retrospective Case-Control Studies," *Autoimmunity Reviews* 15, no. 4 (April 2016): 325–34, doi: 10.1016/j.autrev.2015.12.005; A. Matos-Santos et al., "Relationship between the Number and Impact of Stressful Life Events and the Onset of Graves' Disease and Toxic Nodular Goitre," *Clinical Endocrinology* 55, no. 1 (July 2001): 15–19; D. C. Mohr et al., "Association between Stressful Life Events and Exacerbation in Multiple Sclerosis: A Meta-Analysis," *BMJ* 328 (March 25, 2004): 731, doi: https://doi.org/10.1136/bmj.38041.724421.55.

21. L. S. Berk et al., "Modulation of Neuroimmune Parameters during the Eustress of Humor-Associated Mirthful Laughter," *Alternative Therapies in Health and Medicine* 7, no. 2 (March 2001): 62–72, 74–6; K. H. Ryu, H. S. Shin, and E. Y. Yang, "Effects of Laughter Therapy on Immune Responses in Postpartum Women," *Journal of Alternative and Complementary Medicine* 21, no. 12 (December 2015): 781–88, doi: 10.1089/acm .2015.0053; N. Cousins, "Anatomy of an Illness (as Perceived by the Patient)," *New England Journal of Medicine* 295 (December 23, 1976): 1458–63, doi: 10.1056 /NEJM197612232952605.

22. S. P. Wasser, "Medicinal Mushrooms as a Source of Antitumor and Immunomodulating Polysaccharides," *Applied Microbiology and Biotechnology* 60, no. 3 (November 2002): 258–74.

23. Peter Roupas et al., "The Role of Edible Mushrooms in Health: Evaluation of the Evidence," *Journal of Functional Foods* 4, no. 4 (October 2012): 687–709; S. Patel and A. Goyal, "Recent Developments in Mushrooms as Anti-Cancer Therapeutics: A Review," *3 Biotech* 2, no. 1 (March 2012): 1–15; L. Ren, C. Perera, and Y. Hemar, "Antitumor Activity of Mushroom Polysaccharides: A Review," *Food & Function* 3, no. 11 (November 2012): 1118–30; D. Gunawardena et al., "Anti-Inflammatory Effects of Five Commercially Available Mushroom Species Determined in Lipopolysaccharide and Interferon-γ Activated Murine Macrophages," *Food Chemistry* 148 (April 2014): 92–96.

24. M. Nagano et al., "Reduction of Depression and Anxiety by 4 Weeks Hericium Erinaceus Intake," *Biomedical Research* 31, no. 4 (August 2010): 231–37; K. Mori et al., "Improving Effects of the Mushroom Yamabushitake (Hericium erinaceus) on Mild Cognitive Impairment: A Double-Blind Placebo-Controlled Clinical Trial," *Phytotherapy Research* 23, no. 3 (March 2009): 367–72, doi: 10.1002/ptr.2634.

25. X. Dai et al., "Consuming Lentinula Edodes (Shiitake) Mushrooms Daily Improves Human Immunity: A Randomized Dietary Intervention in Healthy Young Adults," *Journal of the American College of Nutrition* 34, no. 6 (2015): 478–87, doi: 10.1080/07315724.2014.950391; M. J. Feeney et al., "Mushrooms and Health Summit Proceedings," *Journal of Nutrition* 144, no. 7 (July 2014): 1128S–36S, doi: 10.3945/jn.114.190728; J. M. Gaullier et al., "Supplementation with a Soluble β-glucan Exported from Shiitake Medicinal Mushroom, Lentinus Edodes (Berk.) Singer Mycelium: A Crossover, Placebo-Controlled Study in Healthy Elderly," *International Journal of Medicinal Mushrooms* 13, no. 4 (2011): 319–26.

26. B. S. Sanodiya et al., "Ganoderma Lucidum: A Potent Pharmacological Macrofungus," *Current Pharmaceutical Biotechnology* 10, no. 8 (December 2009): 717–42; H. Zhao et al., "Spore Powder of Ganoderma lucidum Improves Cancer-Related Fatigue in Breast Cancer Patients Undergoing Endocrine Therapy: A Pilot Clinical Trial," *Evidence-Based Complementary and Alternative Medicine* 2012 (2012): 809614, doi: 10.1155/2012/809614.

27. X. T. Li et al., "Protective Effects on Mitochondria and Anti-Aging Activity of

Polysaccharides from Cultivated Fruiting Bodies of Cordyceps Militaris," *American Journal of Chinese Medicine* 38, no. 6 (2010): 1093–106, doi: 10.1142/S0192415X10008494.

28. S. S. Percival, "Aged Garlic Extract Modifies Human Immunity," *Journal of Nutrition* 146, no. 2 (February 2016): 433S–36S, doi: 10.3945/jn.115.210427; C. S. Charron et al., "A Single Meal Containing Raw, Crushed Garlic Influences Expression of Immunity- and Cancer-Related Genes in Whole Blood of Humans," *Journal of Nutrition* 145, no. 11 (November 2015): 2448–55, doi: 10.3945/jn.115.215392.

29. C. A. Rowe et al., "Regular Consumption of Concord Grape Juice Benefits Human Immunity," *Journal of Medicinal Food* 14, nos. 1–2 (January–February 2011): 69–78, doi: 10.1089/jmf.2010.0055; S. Zunino, "Type 2 Diabetes and Glycemic Response to Grapes or Grape Products," *Journal of Nutrition* 139, no. 9 (September 2009): 1794S–800S, doi: 10.3945/jn.109.107631; M. P. Nantz et al., "Immunity and Antioxidant Capacity in Humans Is Enhanced by Consumption of a Dried, Encapsulated Fruit and Vegetable Juice Concentrate," *Journal of Nutrition* 136, no. 10 (October 2006): 2606–10.

30. M. Karsch-Völk, B. Barrett, and K. Linde, "*Echinacea* for Preventing and Treating the Common Cold," *JAMA* 313, no. 6 (February 10, 2015): 618–19, doi: 10.1001/jama.2014.17145; K. I. Block and M. N. Mead, "Immune System Effects of Echinacea, Ginseng, and Astragalus: A Review," *Integrative Cancer Therapies* 2, no. 3 (September 2003): 247–67, doi: 10.1177/1534735403256419.

31. A. Dhur, P. Galan, and S. Hercberg, "Folate Status and the Immune System," *Progress in Food and Nutrition Science* 15, nos. 1–2 (1991): 43–60.

32. D. P. Cardinali et al., "Melatonin and the Immune System in Aging," *Neuroimmunomodulation* 15, nos. 4–6 (2008): 272–78, doi: 10.1159/000156470; A. Carrillo-Vico et al., "Melatonin: Buffering the Immune System," *International Journal of Molecular Sciences* 14, no. 4 (April 22, 2013): 8638–83, doi: 10.3390/ijms14048638.

33. A. T. Vieira, M. M. Teixeira, and F. S. Martins, "The Role of Probiotics and Prebiotics in Inducing Gut Immunity," *Frontiers in Immunology* 4 (December 12, 2013): 445, doi: 10.3389/fimmu.2013.00445; R. Sharma et al., "Dietary Supplementation of Milk Fermented with Probiotic Lactobacillus Fermentum Enhances Systemic Immune Response and Antioxidant Capacity in Aging Mice," *Nutrition Research* 34, no. 11 (November 2014): 968–81, doi: 10.1016/j.nutres.2014.09.006.

34. C. R. de Farias et al., "A Randomized-Controlled, Double-Blind Study of the Impact of Selenium Supplementation on Thyroid Autoimmunity and Inflammation with Focus on the GPx1 Genotypes," *Journal of Endocrinological Investigation* 38, no. 10 (October 2015): 1065–74, doi: 10.1007/s40618-015-0285-8; H. Steinbrenner et al., "Dietary Selenium in Adjuvant Therapy of Viral and Bacterial Infections," *Advances in Nutrition* 6 (January 2015): 73–82, doi: 10.3945/an.114.007575.

35. J. R. Mora, M. Iwata, and U. H. von Andrian, "Vitamin Effects on the Immune System: Vitamins A and D Take Centre Stage," *Nature Reviews: Immunology* 8, no. 9 (September 2008): 685–98, doi: 10.1038/nri2378; O. P. Garcia, "Effect of Vitamin A Deficiency on the Immune Response in Obesity," *Proceedings of the Nutrition Society* 71, no. 2 (May 2012): 290–97, doi: 10.1017/S0029665112000079.

36. Chad Robertson, "The Link between Vitamin C and Optimal Immunity," *Life Extension*, November 2015, http://www.lifeextension.com/magazine/2015/11/the-link-between-vitamin-c-and-optimal-immunity/page-01; M. De la Fuente et al., "Immune Function in Aged Women Is Improved by Ingestion of Vitamins C and E," *Canadian Journal of Physiology and Pharmacology* 76, no. 4 (April 1998): 373–80.

37. J. R. Mora, M. Iwata, and U. H. von Andrian, "Vitamin Effects on the Immune System: Vitamins A and D Take Centre Stage"; C. Aranow, "Vitamin D and the Immune System," *Journal of Investigative Medicine* 59, no. 6 (August 2011): 881–86, doi: 10.231/JIM.0b013e31821b8755; "Key Feature of Immune System Survived in Humans, Other Primates for 60 Million Years," EurekAlert! website, August 18, 2009, https://www.eurekalert.org/pub_releases/2009-08/osu-kfo081809.php; M. Urashima et al., "Randomized Trial of Vitamin D Supplementation to Prevent Seasonal Influenza A in

Schoolchildren," *American Journal of Clinical Nutrition* 91, no. 5 (May 2010): 1255–60, doi: 10.3945/ajcn.2009.29094.

38. S. Moriguchi and M. Muraga, "Vitamin E and Immunity," *Vitamins and Hormones* 59 (2000): 305–36.

39. J. B. Barnett et al., "Effect of Zinc Supplementation on Serum Zinc Concentration and T Cell Proliferation in Nursing Home Elderly: A Randomized, Double-Blind, Placebo-Controlled Trial," *American Journal of Clinical Nutrition* 103, no. 3 (March 2016): 942–51, doi: 10.3945/ajcn.115.115188; L. Kahmann et al., "Effect of Improved Zinc Status on T Helper Cell Activation and TH1/TH2 Ratio in Healthy Elderly Individuals," *Biogerontology* 7, nos. 5–6 (October–December 2006): 429–35, doi: 10.1007/s10522-006-9058-2; A. S. Prasad et al., "Effect of Zinc Supplementation on Incidence of Infections and Hospital Admissions in Sickle Cell Disease (SCD)," *American Journal of Hematology* 61, no. 3 (July 1999): 194–202.

40. J. Correale, M. C. Ysrraelit, and M. I. Gaitlán, "Immunomodulatory Effects of Vitamin D in Multiple Sclerosis," *Brain* 132, part 5 (May 2009): 1146–60.

41. Various scholarly articles supporting the value of vitamin D may be found at the GreenMedinfo website: http://www.greenmedinfo.com/substance/vitamin-d.

42. P. Knekt et al, "Serum 25-Hydroxyvitamin D Concentration and Risk of Dementia," *Epidemiology* 26, no. 6 (November 2014): 799–804.

43. Rathish Nair and Arun Maseeh, "Vitamin D: The 'Sunshine' Vitamin," *Journal of Pharmacology and Pharmacotherapeutics* 3, no. 2 (April–June 2012): 118–26.

44. P. Autier and S. Gandini, "Vitamin D Supplementation and Total Mortality: A Meta-Analysis of Randomized Controlled Trials," *Archives of Internal Medicine* 167, no. 16 (September 10, 2007): 1730–37.

45. Adrian R. Martineau et al., "Vitamin D Supplementation to Prevent Acute Respiratory Tract Infections: Systematic Review and Meta-analysis of Individual Participant Data," *BMJ* 356 (February 15, 2017): i6583.

46. A. Masoumi et al., "1alpha,25-dihydroxyvitamin D3 Interacts with Curcuminoids to Stimulate Amyloid-Beta Clearance by Macrophages of Alzheimer's Disease Patients," *Journal of Alzheimer's Disease* 17, no. 3 (2009): 703–17; S. Shab-Bidar et al., "Improvement of Vitamin D Status Resulted in Amelioration of Biomarkers of Systemic Inflammation in the Subjects with Type 2 Diabetes," *Diabetes Metabolism Research and Reviews* 28, no. 5 (July 2012): 424–30.

47. Albina Nowak et al., "Effect of Vitamin D3 on Self-Perceived Fatigue: A Double-Blind Randomized Placebo-Controlled Trial," *Medicine (Baltimore)* 95, no. 52 (December 2016): e5353.

48. Rathish Nair and Arun Maseeh, "Vitamin D: The 'Sunshine' Vitamin," 118–26.

49. E. Sohl et al., "The Impact of Medication on Vitamin D Status in Older Individuals," *European Journal of Endocrinology* 166, no. 3 (March 2012): 477–85.

50. C. Annweiler et al., "Effectiveness of the Combination of Memantine Plus Vitamin D on Cognition in Patients with Alzheimer Disease: A Pre-Post Pilot Study," *Cognitive and Behavioral Neurology* 25, no. 3 (September 2012): 121–27.

51. I. A. Myles, "Fast Food Fever: Reviewing the Impacts of the Western Diet on Immunity," *Nutrition Journal* 13 (June 17, 2014): 61, doi: 10.1186/1475-2891-13-61.

52. J. Todd et al., "The Antimicrobial Effects of Cinnamon Leaf Oil against Multi-Drug Resistant Salmonella Newport on Organic Leafy Greens," *International Journal of Food Microbiology* 166, no. 1 (August 16, 2013): 193–99, doi: 10.1016/j.ijfoodmicro.2013.06.021.

53. H. Hosseinzadeh et al., "Effects of Different Levels of Coriander (*Coriandrum sativum*) Seed Powder and Extract on Serum Biochemical Parameters, Microbiota, and Immunity in Broiler Chicks," *Scientific World Journal* 2014 (December 28, 2014): 628979, doi: http://dx.doi.org/10.1155/2014/628979.

54. X. Dai et al., "Consuming Lentinula Edodes (Shiitake) Mushrooms Daily Improves Human Immunity: A Randomized Dietary Intervention in Healthy Young

Adults," *Journal of the American College of Nutrition* 34, no. 6 (2015): 478–87, doi: 10.1080/07315724.2014.950391; J. M. Gaullier et al., "Supplementation with a Soluble β-glucan Exported from Shiitake Medicinal Mushroom, Lentinus Edodes (Berk.) Singer Mycelium: A Crossover, Placebo-Controlled Study in Healthy Elderly," *International Journal of Medicinal Mushrooms* 13, no. 4 (2011): 319–26.

55. L. C. Chandra et al., "White Button, Portabella, and Shiitake Mushroom Supplementation Up-Regulates Interleukin-23 Secretion in Acute Dextran Sodium Sulfate Colitis C57BL/6 Mice and Murine Macrophage J.744.1 Cell Line," *Nutrition Research* 33, no. 5 (May 2013): 388–96, doi: 10.1016/j.nutres.2013.02.009.

56. D. B. Haytowitz, "Vitamin D in Mushrooms," Beltsville Human Nutrition Research Center website, accessed June 6, 2017, https://www.ars.usda.gov/ARSUserFiles/80400525 /Articles/AICR09_Mushroom_VitD.pdf; Nick McDermott, "Mushrooms Can Provide As Much Vitamin D As Supplements—But Only if You Put Them in the Sun before You Eat Them," *Daily Mail*, April 22, 2013, http://www.dailymail.co.uk/health/article-2313062 /Mushrooms-provide-vitamin-D-supplements--sun-eat-them.html; "All About Vitamin D," Fresh Mushrooms website, accessed June 6, 2017, http://www.mushroominfo.com /all-about-vitamin-d/.

57. P. A. Engen et al., "The Gastrointestinal Microbiome: Alcohol Effects on the Composition of Intestinal Microbiota," *Alcohol Research: Current Reviews* 37, no. 2 (2015): 223–36.

CHAPTER 13: N IS FOR NEUROHORMONE DEFICIENCIES

1. J. J. Haggerty Jr., D. L. Evans, and A. J. Prange Jr., "Organic Brain Syndrome Associated with Marginal Hypothyroidism," *American Journal of Psychiatry* 143, no. 6 (June 1986): 785–86, doi: 10.1176/ajp.143.6.785.

2. Ridha Arem, *The Thyroid Solution: A Revolutionary Mind-Body Program for Regaining Your Emotional and Physical Health* (New York: Ballantine Books, 2007), 86–87.

3. Richard Shames and Karilee Shames, *Thyroid Mind Power: The Proven Case for Hormone-Related Depression, Anxiety, and Memory Loss* (New York: Rodale, 2011), 11.

4. L. Adly et al., "Serum Concentrations of Estrogens, Sex Hormone-Binding Globulin, and Androgens and Risk of Breast Cancer in Postmenopausal Women," *International Journal of Cancer* 119, no. 10 (November 15, 2006): 2402–7, doi: 10.1002/ijc.22203.

5. S. Deandrea et al., "Alcohol and Breast Cancer Risk Defined by Estrogen and Progesterone Receptor Status: A Case-Control Study," *Cancer Epidemiology, Biomarkers and Prevention* 17, no. 8 (August 2008): 2025–28, doi: 10.1158/1055-9965.EPI-08-0157.

6. S. S. Solden et al., "Immune Modulation of Multiple Sclerosis Patients Treated with the Pregnancy Hormone Estriol," *Journal of Immunology* 171, no. 11 (December 1, 2003): 6267–74, doi: 10.4049/jimmunol.171.11.6267.

7. J. Jones, W. D. Mosher, and K. Daniels, "Current Contraceptive Use in the United States, 2006–2010, and Changes in Patterns of Use since 1995," *National Health Statistics Reports*, no. 60 (October 18, 2012).

8. Loyola University Health System, "Increased Stroke Risk from Birth Control Pills, Review Finds," *ScienceDaily*, October 27, 2009, https://www.sciencedaily.com/releases/2009/10 /091026152820.htm.

9. R. A. Greene, "Estrogen and Cerebral Blood Flow: A Mechanism to Explain the Impact of Estrogen on the Incidence and Treatment of Alzheimer's Disease," *International Journal of Fertility and Women's Medicine* 45, no. 4 (July–August 2000): 253–57.

10. J. Ryan et al., "Characteristics of Hormone Therapy, Cognitive Function, and Dementia: The Prospective 3C Study," *Neurology* 73, no. 21 (November 24, 2009): 1729–37, doi: 10.1212/WNL.0b013e3181c34b0c.

11. Bushra Imtiaz et al., "Risk of Alzheimer's Disease among Users of Postmenopausal Hormone Therapy: A Nationwide Case-Control Study," *Maturitas* (published online January 9, 2017), http://dx.doi.org/10.1016/j.maturitas.2017.01.002.

12. C. Pergola et al., "Testosterone Suppresses Phospholipase D, Causing Sex Differences in

Leukotriene Biosynthesis in Human Monocytes," *FASEB Journal* 25, no. 10 (October 2011): 3377–87, doi: 10.1096/fj.11-182758.

13. Kevin T. Nead et al., "Androgen Deprivation Therapy and Future Alzheimer's Disease Risk," *Journal of Clinical Oncology* 34, no. 6 (February 20, 2016): 566–71, doi: 10.1200/JCO.2015 .63.6266.

14. L. Sun et al., "Meta-Analysis Suggests That Smoking Is Associated with an Increased Risk of Early Natural Menopause," *Menopause* 19, no. 2 (February 2012): 126–32, doi: 10.1097 /gme.0b013e318224f9ac.

15. A. M. Fernández-Alonso et al., "Obesity Is Related to Increased Menopausal Symptoms among Spanish Women," *Menopause International* 16, no. 3 (September 2010): 105–10, doi: 10.1258/mi.2010.010029.

16. Reini W. Bretvld et al., "Pesticide Exposure: The Hormonal Function of the Female Reproductive System Disrupted?" *Reproductive Biology and Endocrinology* 4, no. 30 (May 31, 2006), doi: 10.1186/1477-7827-4-30.

17. T. T. Wang et al., "Estrogen Receptor Alpha as a Target for Indole-3-Carbinol," *Journal of Nutritional Biochemistry* 17, no. 10 (October 2006): 659–64, doi: 10.1016/j.jnutbio.2005 .10.012.

18. G. A. Reed et al., "A Phase I Study of Indole-3-Carbinol in Women: Tolerability and Effects," *Cancer Epidemiology, Biomarkers and Prevention* 14, no. 8 (August 2005): 1953–60, doi: 10.1158/1055-9965.EPI-05-0121.

19. R. A. Karmali, "N-3 Fatty Acids and Cancer," *Journal of Internal Medicine* 225, no. S731 (December 1989): 197–200, doi: 10.1111/j.1365-2796.1989.tb01456.x.

20. H. L. Bradlow et al., "Indole-3-Carbinol: A Novel Approach to Breast Cancer Prevention," *Annals of the New York Academies of Sciences* 768 (September 30, 1995): 180–200.

CHAPTER 14: D IS FOR DIABESITY

1. M. Lutski et al., "Insulin Resistance and Future Cognitive Performance and Cognitive Decline in Elderly Patients with Cardiovascular Disease," *Journal of Alzheimer's Disease* 57, no. 2 (2017): 633–43, doi: 10.3233/JAD-161016.

2. E. Steen et al., "Impaired Insulin and Insulin-like Growth Factor Expression and Signaling Mechanisms in Alzheimer's Disease—Is This Type 3 Diabetes?," *Journal of Alzheimer's Disease* 7, no. 1 (February 2005): 63–80.

3. F. Pasquier et al., "Diabetes Mellitus and Dementia," *Diabetes & Metabolism* 32, no. 5, part 1 (November 2006): 403–14; K. Gudala et al., "Diabetes Mellitus and Risk of Dementia: A Meta-Analysis of Prospective Observational Studies," *Journal of Diabetes Investigation* 4, no. 6 (November 27, 2013): 640–50, doi: 10.1111/jdi.12087.

4. H. Niwa et al., "Clinical Analysis of Cognitive Function in Diabetic Patients by MMSE and SPECT," *Diabetes Research and Clinical Practice* 72, no. 2 (May 2006): 142–47; J. F. Jimenez-Bonilla et al., "Assessment of Cerebral Blood Flow in Diabetic Patients with No Clinical History of Neurological Disease," *Nuclear Medicine Communications* 17, no. 9 (September 1996): 790–94.

5. M. T. Heneka, A. Fink, and G. Doblhammer, "Effect of Pioglitazone Medication on the Incidence of Dementia," *Annals of Neurology* 78, no. 2 (August 2015): 284–94, doi: 10.1002 /ana.24439.

6. K. Plucińska et al., "Neuronal Human BACE1 Knockin Induces Systemic Diabetes in Mice," *Diabetologia* 59, no. 7 (July 2016): 1513–23, doi: 10.1007/s00125-016-3960-1.

7. Paul K. Crane et al., "Glucose Levels and Risk of Dementia," *New England Journal of Medicine* 369, no. 6 (August 8, 2013): 540–48, doi: 10.1056/NEJMoa1215740.

8. M. E. Mortby et al., "High 'Normal' Blood Glucose Is Associated with Decreased Brain Volume and Cognitive Performance in the 60s: The PATH through Life Study," *PLOS One* 8, no. 9 (September 4, 2013): e73697, doi: 10.1371/journal.pone.0073697; N. Cherubin, P. Sachdev, and K. J. Anstey, "Higher Normal Fasting Plasma Glucose Is Associated

with Hippocampal Atrophy: The PATH Study," *Neurology* 79, no. 10 (September 4, 2012): 1019–26, doi: 10.1212/WNL.0b013e31826846de.

9. A. Menke et al., "Prevalence of and Trends in Diabetes among Adults in the United States, 1988–2012," *JAMA* 314, no. 10 (2015): 1021–29, doi: 10.1001/jama.2015.10029.

10. Mark Hyman, *Eat Fat, Get Thin* (New York: Little Brown and Company, 2016), 4.

11. C. A. Raji et al., "Brain Structure and Obesity," *Human Brain Mapping* 31, no. 3 (March 2010): 353–64, doi: 10.1002/hbm.20870.

12. K. Willeumier, D. V. Taylor, and D. G. Amen, "Elevated Body Mass in National Football League Players Linked to Cognitive Impairment and Decreased Prefrontal Cortex and Temporal Pole Activity," *Translational Psychiatry* 2 (January 17, 2012): e68, doi: 10.1038 /tp.2011.67; K. Willeumier, D. V. Taylor, and D. G. Amen, "Elevated BMI Is Associated with Decreased Blood Flow in the Prefrontal Cortex Using SPECT Imaging in Healthy Adults," *Obesity* 19, no. 5 (May 2011): 1095–97, doi: 10.1038/oby.2011.16.

13. M. Kyrgiou et al., "Adiposity and Cancer at Major Anatomical Sites: Umbrella Review of the Literature," *BMJ* 356 (February 28, 2017): j477, doi: 10.1136/bmj.j477.

14. Susan Scutti, "Diabetes, Weight Gain Can Combine to Alter Brain, Study Says," CNN, April 28, 2017, http://www.cnn.com/2017/04/27/health/diabetes-brain-study/index.html; S. Yoon et al., "Brain Changes in Overweight/Obese and Normal-Weight Adults with Type 2 Diabetes Mellitus," *Diabetologia* 60, no. 7 (July 2017): 1207–17, doi: 10.1007 /s00125-017-4266-7.

15. R. A. Whitmer, "The Epidemiology of Adiposity and Dementia," *Current Alzheimer Research* 4, no. 2 (April 2007): 117–22.

16. J. Gunstad et al., "Elevated Body Mass Index Is Associated with Executive Dysfunction in Otherwise Healthy Adults," *Comprehensive Psychiatry* 48, no. 1 (January–February 2007): 57–61, doi: 10.1016/j.comppsych.2006.05.001.

17. D. O. Clark et al., "Does Body Mass Index Modify Memory, Reasoning, and Speed of Processing Training Effects in Older Adults," *Obesity* 24, no. 11 (November 2016): 2319–26, doi: 10.1002/oby.21631.

18. K. Willeumier et al., "Elevated Body Mass in National Football League Players Linked to Cognitive Impairment and Decreased Prefrontal Cortex and Temporal Pole Activity," e68.

19. K. Yaffe, "Metabolic Syndrome and Cognitive Disorders: Is the Sum Greater Than Its Parts?" *Alzheimer Disease and Associated Disorders* 21, no. 1 (April–June 2007): 167–71, doi: 10.1097/WAD.0b013e318065bfd6.

20. G. Razay, V. Vreugdenil, and G. Wilcock, "The Metabolic Syndrome and Alzheimer Disease," *Archives of Neurology* 64, no. 1 (January 2007): 93–96, doi: 10.1001/archneur .64.1.93; M. Vanhanen et al., "Association of Metabolic Syndrome with Alzheimer Disease: A Population-Based Study," *Neurology* 67, no. 5 (September 12, 2006): 843–47, doi: 10.1212/01.wnl.0000234037.91185.99.

21. A. C. Birdsill et al., "Low Cerebral Blood Flow Is Associated with Lower Memory Function in Metabolic Syndrome," *Obesity* 21, no. 7 (July 2013): 1313–20, doi: 10.1002/oby.20170.

22. J. Tuomilehto et al., "Prevention of Type 2 Diabetes Mellitus by Changes in Lifestyle among Subjects with Impaired Glucose Tolerance," *New England Journal of Medicine* 344, no. 18 (May 3, 2001): 1343–50, doi: 10.1056/NEJM200105033441801.

23. Lara Howells et al., "Clinical Impact of Lifestyle Interventions for the Prevention of Diabetes: An Overview of Systemic Reviews," *BMJ Open* 6, no. 12 (December 21, 2016): e013806, doi: 10.1136/bmjopen-2016-013806.

24. Matthew P. Pase, "Sugary Beverage Intake and Preclinical Alzheimer's Disease in the Community," *Alzheimer's and Dementia* 17 (March 6, 2017): doi: 10.1016/j.jalz.2017.01.024.

25. A. G. Dulloo et al., "Twenty-Four-Hour Energy Expenditure and Urinary Catecholamines of Humans Consuming Low-to-Moderate Amounts of Medium-Chain Triglycerides: A Dose-Response Study in a Human Respiratory Chamber," *European Journal of Clinical Nutrition* 50, no. 3 (March 1996): 152–58.

26. C. J. Chiang et al., "Midlife Risk Factors for Subtypes of Dementia: A Nested Case-Control

Study in Taiwan," *American Journal of Geriatric Psychiatry* 15, no. 9 (September 2007): 762–71, doi: 10.1097/JGP.0b013e318050c98f; H. White et al., "Weight Change in Alzheimer's Disease," *Journal of the American Geriatrics Society* 44, no. 3 (March 1996): 265–72.

27. E. J. Shiroma et al., "Strength Training and the Risk of Type 2 Diabetes and Cardiovascular Disease," *Medicine and Science in Sports and Exercise* 49, no. 1 (January 2017): 40–46, doi: 10.1249/MSS.0000000000001063.

28. F. B. Hu et al., "Walking Compared with Vigorous Physical Activity and Risk of Type 2 Diabetes in Women: A Prospective Study," *JAMA* 282, no. 15 (October 20, 1999): 1433–39; C. J. Caspersen and J. E. Fulton, "Epidemiology of Walking and Type 2 Diabetes," *Medicine and Science in Sports and Exercise* 40, no. 7, suppl. (July 2008): S519–28, doi: 10.1249/MSS.0b013e31817c6737.

29. Artemis P. Simopoulos, "Dietary Omega-3 Fatty Acid Deficiency and High Fructose Intake in the Development of Metabolic Syndrome, Brain Metabolic Abnormalities, and Non-Alcoholic Fatty Liver Disease," *Nutrients* 5, no. 8 (July 26, 2013): 2901–23, doi: 10.3390/nu5082901.

30. L. Djoussé et al., "Plasma Omega-3 Fatty Acids and Incident Diabetes in Older Adults," *American Journal of Clinical Nutrition* 94, no. 2 (2011): 527–33, doi: 10.3945/ajcn.111.013334.

31. S. Sarbolouki et al., "Eicosapentaenoic Acid Improves Insulin Sensitivity in Overweight Type 2 Diabetes Mellitus Patients: A Double-Blind Randomised Clinical Trial," *Singapore Medical Journal* 54, no. 7 (2013): 387–90.

32. K. A. Brownley et al., "A Double-Blind, Randomized Pilot Trial of Chromium Picolinate for Binge Eating Disorder: Results of the Binge Eating and Chromium (BEACh) Study," *Journal of Psychosomatic Research* 75, no. 1 (July 2013): 36–42, doi: 10.1016/j.jpsychores.2013.03.092.

33. N. Suksomboon, N. Poolsup, and A. Yuwanakorn, "Systematic Review and Meta-Analysis of the Efficacy and Safety of Chromium Supplementation in Diabetes," *Journal of Clinical Pharmacy and Therapeutics* 39, no. 3 (June 2014): 292–306, doi: 10.1111/jcpt.12147; H. Rabinovitz et al., "Effect of Chromium Supplementation on Blood Glucose and Lipid Levels in Type 2 Diabetes Mellitus Elderly Patients," *International Journal for Vitamin and Nutrition Research* 74, no. 3 (May 2004): 178–82, doi: 10.1024/0300-9831.74.3.178; C. A. Albarracin et al., "Chromium Picolinate and Biotin Combination Improves Glucose Metabolism in Treated, Uncontrolled Overweight to Obese Patients with Type 2 Diabetes," *Diabetes/Metabolism Research and Reviews* 24, no. 1 (January–February 2008): 41–56; R. Krikorian et al., "Improved Cognitive-Cerebral Function in Older Adults with Chromium Supplementation," *Nutritional Neuroscience* 13, no. 3 (June 2010): 116–22, doi: 10.1179/147683010X12611460764084.

34. T. Lu et al., "Cinnamon Extract Improves Fasting Blood Glucose and Glycosylated Hemoglobin in Chinese Patients with Type 2 Diabetes," *Nutrition Research* 32, no. 6 (June 2012): 408–12, doi: 10.1016/j.nutres.2012.05.003; P. A. Davis and W. Yokoyama, "Cinnamon Intake Lowers Fasting Blood Glucose: Meta-Analysis," *Journal of Medicinal Food* 14, no. 9 (2011): 884–89, doi: 10.1089/jmf.2010.0180; A. Magistrelli and J. C. Chezem, "Effect of Ground Cinnamon on Postprandial Blood Glucose Concentration in Normal-Weight and Obese Adults," *Journal of the Academy of Nutrition and Dietetics* 112, no. 11 (November 2012): 1806–9, doi: 10.1016/j.jand.2012.07.037; Ashley N. Hoehn and Amy L. Stockert, "The Effects of *Cinnamomum Cassia* on Blood Glucose Values Are Greater Than Those of Dietary Changes Alone," *Nutrition and Metabolic Insights* 5 (2012): 77–83, doi: 10.4137/NMI.S10498.

35. M. L. Wahlqvist et al., "Cinnamon Users with Prediabetes Have a Better Fasting Working Memory: A Cross-Sectional Function Study," *Nutrition Research* 36, no. 4 (April 2016): 305–10, doi: 10.1016/j.nutres.2015.12.005.

36. A. Bast and G. R. Haenen, "Lipoic Acid: A Multifunctional Antioxidant," *BioFactors* 17, nos. 1–4 (2003): 207–13.

37. G. P. Biewenga, G. R. Haenen, and A. Bast, "The Pharmacology of the Antioxidant Lipoic Acid," *General Pharmacology* 29, no. 3 (September 1997): 315–31; L. Zhao and F. X. Hu,

"α-Lipoic Acid Treatment of Aged Type 2 Diabetes Mellitus Complicated with Acute Cerebral Infarction," *European Review for Medical and Pharmacological Sciences* 18, no. 23 (2014): 3715–19.

38. A. Maczurek et al., "Lipoic Acid as an Anti-Inflammatory and Neuroprotective Treatment for Alzheimer's Disease," *Advanced Drug Delivery Reviews* 60, nos. 13–14 (October–November 2008): 1463–70, doi: 10.1016/j.addr.2008.04.015.

39. M. D. Mitkov, I. Y. Aleksandrova, and M. M. Orbetzoya, "Effect of Transdermal Testosterone or Alpha-Lipoic Acid on Erectile Dysfunction and Quality of Life in Patients with Type 2 Diabetes Mellitus," *Folia Medica* 55, no. 1 (January–March 2013): 55–63.

40. V. Cappelli et al., "Evaluation of a New Association between Insulin-Sensitizers and α-Lipoic Acid in Obese Women Affected by PCOS," *Minerva Ginecologica* 65, no. 4 (August 2013): 425–33.

41. C. Y. Liu et al., "Effects of Green Tea Extract on Insulin Resistance and Glucagon-like Peptide 1 in Patients with Type 2 Diabetes and Lipid Abnormalities: A Randomized, Double-Blinded, and Placebo-Controlled Trial," *PLOS One* 9, no. 3 (March 10, 2014): e91163, doi: 10.1371/journal.pone.0091163.

42. A. H. Wu et al., "Effect of 2-Month Controlled Green Tea Intervention on Lipoprotein Cholesterol, Glucose, and Hormone Levels in Healthy Postmenopausal Women," *Cancer Prevention Research* 5, no. 3 (March 2012): 393–402, doi: 10.1158/1940-6207.CAPR-11-0407.

43. A. Hata et al., "Magnesium Intake Decreases Type 2 Diabetes Risk through the Improvement of Insulin Resistance and Inflammation: The Hisayama Study," *Diabetic Medicine: A Journal of the British Diabetic Association* 30, no. 12 (December 2013): 1487–94, doi: 10.1111/dme.12250; A. Hruby et al., "Higher Magnesium Intake Reduces Risk of Impaired Glucose and Insulin Metabolism and Progression from Prediabetes to Diabetes in Middle-Aged Americans," *Diabetes Care* 37, no. 2 (February 2014): 419–27, doi: 10.2337/dc13-1397; F. Guerrero-Romero and M. Rodriguez-Morán, "Oral Magnesium Supplementation: An Adjuvant Alternative to Facing the Worldwide Challenge of Type 2 Diabetes?," *Cirugia y Cirujanos* 82, no. 3 (May–June 2014): 282–89; A. Galli-Tsinopoulou et al., "Association between Magnesium Concentration and HbA1c in Children and Adolescents with Type 1 Diabetes Mellitus," *Journal of Diabetes* 6, no. 4 (July 2014): 369–77, doi: 10.1111/1753-0407.12118.

44. G. N. Dakhale, H. V. Chaudhari, and M. Shrivastava, "Supplementation of Vitamin C Reduces Blood Glucose and Improves Glycosylated Hemoglobin in Type 2 Diabetes Mellitus: A Randomized, Double-Blind Study," *Advances in Pharmacological Sciences* 2 (2011): 195271, doi: 10.1155/2011/195271.

45. P. V. Rao and S. H. Gan, "Cinnamon: A Multifaceted Medicinal Plant," *Evidence-Based Complementary and Alternative Medicine* 2014 (2014): 642942, doi: 10.1155/2014/642942; X. Bi, J. Lim, and C. J. Henry, "Spices in the Management of Diabetes Mellitus," *Food Chemistry* 217 (February 15, 2017): 281–93, doi: 10.1016/j.foodchem.2016.08.111.

46. Carly R. Pacanowski and David A. Levitsky, "Frequent Self-Weighing and Visual Feedback for Weight Loss in Overweight Adults," *Journal of Obesity* 2 (June 2015): 1–9, doi: 10.1155/2015/763680.

CHAPTER 15: S IS FOR SLEEP ISSUES

1. K. Yaffe et al., "Sleep-Disordered Breathing, Hypoxia, and Risk of Mild Cognitive Impairment and Dementia in Older Women," *JAMA* 306, no. 6 (August 10, 2011): 613–19, doi: 10.1001/jama.2011.1115; Yo-El S. Ju, Brendan P. Lucey, and David M. Holtzman, "Sleep and Alzheimer Disease Pathology—A Bidirectional Relationship," *Nature Reviews Neurology* 10 (2014): 115–19, doi: 10.1038/nrneurol.2013.269; W. P. Chang et al., "Sleep Apnea and the Risk of Dementia: A Population-Based 5-Year Follow-Up Study in Taiwan," *PLOS One* 8, no. 10 (October 24, 2013): e78655, doi: 10.1371/journal.pone.0078655; R. Sterniczuk et al., "Sleep Disturbance Is Associated with Incident Dementia and Mortality," *Current Alzheimer Research* 10, no. 7 (September 2013): 767–75; R. S. Osorio

et al., "Sleep-Disordered Breathing Advances Cognitive Decline in the Elderly," *Neurology* 84, no. 19 (May 12, 2015): 1964–71, doi: 10.1212/WNL.0000000000001566.

2. R. C. Kessler et al., "Insomnia and the Performance of US Workers: Results from the American Insomnia Survey," *Sleep* 34, no. 9 (September 1, 2011): 1161–71, doi: 10.5665 /SLEEP.1230.

3. C. Hublin et al., "Heritability and Mortality Risk of Insomnia-Related Symptoms: A Genetic Epidemiologic Study in a Population-Based Twin Cohort," *Sleep* 34, no. 7 (July 1, 2011): 957–64, doi: 10.5665/SLEEP.1136.

4. D. F. Kripke, R. D. Langer, and L. E. Kline, "Hypnotics' Association with Mortality or Cancer: A Matched Cohort Study," *BMJ Open* 2, no. 1 (February 27, 2012): e000850, doi: 10.1136/bmjopen-2012-000850.

5. E. J. Van Someren et al., "Disrupted Sleep: From Molecules to Cognition," *Journal of Neuroscience* 35, no. 41 (October 14, 2015): 13889–95, doi: 10.1523/JNEUROSCI.2592 -15.2015; J. C. Chen et al., "Sleep Duration, Cognitive Decline, and Dementia Risk in Older Women," *Alzheimer's & Dementia* 12, no. 1 (January 2016): 21–33, doi: 10.1016/j .jalz.2015.03.004.

6. E. L. Elcombe et al., "Hippocampal Volume in Older Adults at Risk of Cognitive Decline: The Role of Sleep, Vascular Risk, and Depression," *Journal of Alzheimer's Disease* 44, no. 4 (2015): 1279–90, doi: 10.3233/JAD-142016.

7. H. B. Kim et al., "Longer Duration of Sleep and Risk of Cognitive Decline: A Meta-Analysis of Observational Studies," *Neuroepidemiology* 47, nos. 3–4 (2016): 171–80, doi: 10.1159/000454737.

8. AAA Foundation for Driving Safety, "Missing 1-2 Hours of Sleep Doubles Crash Risk," December 6, 2016, *AAA NewsRoom*, http://newsroom.aaa.com/2016/12/missing-1-2 -hours-sleep-doubles-crash-risk/.

9. L. Harmat, L. J. Takács, and R. Bódizs, "Music Improves Sleep Quality in Students," *Journal of Advanced Nursing* 62, no. 3 (May 2008): 327–35, doi: 10.1111/j.1365-2648.2008.04602.x.

10. N. Goel, H. Kim, and R. P. Lao, "An Olfactory Stimulus Modifies Nighttime Sleep in Young Men and Women," *Chronobiology International* 22, no. 5 (2005): 889–904, doi: 10.1080/07420520500263276; M. Hardy et al., "Replacement of Drug Treatment for Insomnia by Ambient Odour," *Lancet* 346, no. 8976 (September 9, 1995): 701.

11. M. S. Majid et al., "The Effect of Vitamin D Supplement on the Score and Quality of Sleep in 20-50 Year-Old People with Sleep Disorders Compared with Control Group," *Nutritional Neuroscience* (May 5, 2017): 1–9, doi: 10.1080/1028415X.2017.1317395.

12. W. R. Pigeon et al., "Effects of a Tart Cherry Juice Beverage on the Sleep of Older Adults with Insomnia: A Pilot Study," *Journal of Medicinal Food* 13, no. 3 (June 2010): 579–83, doi: 10.1089/jmf.2009.0096; G. Howatson et al., "Effect of Tart Cherry Juice (*Prunus Cerasus*) on Melatonin Levels and Enhanced Sleep Quality," *European Journal of Nutrition* 51, no. 8 (December 2012): 909–16, doi: 10.1007/s00394-011-0263-7.

13. T. Traustadóttir et al., "Tart Cherry Juice Decreases Oxidative Stress in Healthy Older Men and Women," *Journal of Nutrition* 139, no. 10 (October 2009): 1896–900, doi: 10.3945 /jn.109.111716.

14. S. M. Chang and C. H. Chen, "Effects of an Intervention with Drinking Chamomile Tea on Sleep Quality and Depression in Sleep Disturbed Postnatal Women: A Randomized Controlled Trial," *Journal of Advanced Nursing* 72, no. 2 (February 2016): 306–15, doi: 10.1111/jan.12836; A. Ngan and R. Conduit, "A Double-Blind, Placebo-Controlled Investigation of the Effects of Passiflora Incarnata (Passionflower) Herbal Tea on Subjective Sleep Quality," *Phytotherapy Research* 25, no. 8 (August 2011): 1153–59, doi: 10.1002/ptr.3400.

CHAPTER 16: THE MEMORY RESCUE DIET

1. Y. Gu et al., "Mediterranean Diet, Inflammatory and Metabolic Biomarkers, and Risk of Alzheimer's Disease," *Journal of Alzheimer's Disease* 22, no. 2 (2010): 483–92; S. Gardener

et al., "Adherence to a Mediterranean Diet and Alzheimer's Disease Risk in an Australian Population," *Translational Psychiatry* 2 (October 2, 2012): e164.

2. Michelle Luciano et al., "Mediterranean-Type Diet and Brain Structural Change from 73 to 76 Years in a Scottish Cohort," *Neurology* 88, no. 5 (January 31, 2017): 449–55.

3. Julie A. Mattison et al., "Caloric Restriction Improves Health and Survival of Rhesus Monkeys," *Nature Communications*, no. 14063 (2017), doi: 10.1038/ncomms14063, https://www.nature.com/articles/ncomms14063.

4. J. A. Luchsinger et al., "Caloric Intake and the Risk of Alzheimer Disease," *Archives of Neurology* 59, no. 8 (August 2002): 1258–63.

5. E. Ravussin et al., "A 2-Year Randomized Controlled Trial of Human Caloric Restriction: Feasibility and Effects on Predictors of Health Span and Longevity," *Journals of Gerontology: Series A, Biological Sciences and Medical Sciences* 70, no. 9 (September 2015): 1097–104.

6. Y. Wang and E. Mandelkow, "Degradation of Tau Protein by Autophagy and Proteasomal Pathways," *Biochemical Society Transactions* 40, no. 4 (August 2012): 644–52; Qian Li, Yi Liu, and Miao Sun, "Autophagy and Alzheimer's Disease," *Cellular and Molecular Neurobiology* 37, no. 3 (April 2017): 377–88.

7. A. Farooq et al., "A Prospective Study of the Physiological and Neurobehavioral Effects of Ramadan Fasting in Preteen and Teenage Boys," *Journal of the Academy of Nutrition and Dietetics* 115, no. 6 (June 2015): 889–97.

8. N. M. Hussin et al., "Efficacy of Fasting and Calorie Restriction (FCR) on Mood and Depression among Ageing Men," *Journal of Nutrition, Health and Aging* 17, no. 8 (2013): 674–80.

9. Tatiana Moro et al., "Effects of Eight Weeks of Time-Restricted Feeding (16/8) on Basal Metabolism, Maximal Strength, Body Composition, Inflammation, and Cardiovascular Risk Factors in Resistance-Trained Males," *Journal of Translational Medicine* 14, no. 1 (October 13, 2016): 290.

10. M. A. Faris et al., "Intermittent Fasting during Ramadan Attenuates Proinflammatory Cytokines and Immune Cells in Healthy Subjects," *Nutrition Research* 32, no. 12 (December 2012): 947–55; A. R. Vasconcelos et al., "Intermittent Fasting Attenuates Lipopolysaccharide-Induced Neuroinflammation and Memory Impairment," *Journal of Neuroinflammation* 11, no. 1 (May 6, 2014): 85.

11. Ben Spencer, "Why You Should NEVER Eat after 7 p.m.: Late Night Meals 'Increases the Risk of Heart Attack and Stroke,'" *Daily Mail*, August 31, 2016, http://www.dailymail.co.uk /health/article-3767231/Why-NEVER-eat-7pm-Late-night-meals-increases-risk-heart -attack-stroke.html; Claudia Tanner, "Why Eating Late at Night Will Do More Than Just Make You Gain Weight—It Also Raises Risk of Diabetes and Heart Disease, Study Reveals," *Daily Mail*, June 6, 2017, http://www.dailymail.co.uk/health/article-4573270/Eating-night -raises-risk-diabetes-heart-disease.html.

12. R. O. Roberts et al., "Relative Intake of Macronutrients Impacts Risk of Mild Cognitive Impairment or Dementia," *Journal of Alzheimer's Disease* 32, no. 2 (2012): 329–39.

13. Y. Gu et al., "Nutrient Intake and Plasma β-Amyloid," *Neurology* 78, no. 23 (June 5, 2012): 1832–40.

14. Mark C. Houston, "Saturated Fats and Coronary Heart Disease," *Annals of Nutritional Disorders & Therapy* 4, no. 2 (2017): 1038.

15. K. A. Page et al., "Medium-Chain Fatty Acids Improve Cognitive Function in Intensively Treated Type 1 Diabetic Patients and Support In Vitro Synaptic Transmission during Acute Hypoglycemia," *Diabetes* 58, no. 5 (May 2009): 1237–44.

16. B. A. Golomb and A. K. Bui, "A Fat to Forget: Trans Fat Consumption and Memory," *PLOS One* 10, no. 6 (June 17, 2015): e0128129.

17. P. Usai et al., "Frontal Cortical Perfusion Abnormalities Related to Gluten Intake and Associated Autoimmune Disease in Adult Coeliac Disease: 99mTc-ECD Brain SPECT Study," *Digestive and Liver Disease* 36, no. 8 (August 2004): 513–18.

18. Megan Anne Arroll, Lorraine Wilder, and James Neil, "Nutritional Interventions for the Adjunctive Treatment of Schizophrenia: A Brief Review," *Nutrition Journal* 13, no. 1 (September 16, 2014): 91.

19. H. Niederhofer, "Association of Attention-Deficit/Hyperactivity Disorder and Celiac Disease: A Brief Report," *Primary Care Companion for CNS Disorders* 13, no. 3 (2011): pii: PCC.10br01104; P. Whiteley et al., "The ScanBrit Randomised, Controlled, Single-Blind Study of a Gluten- and Casein-Free Dietary Intervention for Children with Autism Spectrum Disorders," *Nutritional Neuroscience* 13, no. 2 (April 2010): 87–100.

20. R. Mesnage et al., "Potential Toxic Effects of Glyphosate and Its Commercial Formulations below Regulatory Limits," *Food and Chemical Toxicology* 84 (October 2015): 133–53.

21. Vincent F. Garry et al., "Birth Defects, Season of Conception, and Sex of Children Born to Pesticide Applicators Living in the Red River Valley of Minnesota, USA," *Environmental Health Perspectives* 110, suppl. 3 (June 2002): 441–49, https://www.ncbi.nlm.nih.gov/pmc/articles/PMC1241196/pdf/ehp110s-000441.pdf.

22. "15 Health Problems Linked to Monsanto's Roundup," *EcoWatch*, January 23, 2015, http://ecowatch.com/2015/01/23/health-problems-linked-to-monsanto-roundup/.

23. Elaine Schmidt, "This Is Your Brain on Sugar: UCLA Study Shows High-Fructose Diet Sabotages Learning, Memory," *UCLA Newsroom*, May 15, 2012.

24. Rachel B. Acton et al., "Added Sugar in the Packaged Foods and Beverages Available at a Major Canadian Retailer in 2015: A Descriptive Analysis," *CMAJ Open* 5, no. 1 (January–March 2017): E1.

25. A. Adan, "Cognitive Performance and Dehydration," *Journal of the American College of Nutrition* 31, no. 2 (April 2012): 71–78.

26. R. D. Abbott et al., "Midlife Milk Consumption and Substantia Nigra Neuron Density at Death," *Neurology* 86, no. 6 (February 9, 2015): 512–19; A. Kyrozis et al., "Dietary and Lifestyle Variables in Relation to Incidence of Parkinson's Disease in Greece," *European Journal of Epidemiology* 28, no. 1 (January 2013): 67–77.

27. Andrew Weil, "Does Milk Cause Cancer?" March 30, 2007, http://www.drweil.com/drw/u/QAA400175/Does-Milk-Cause-Cancer.html.

28. Mark Moss and Lorraine Oliver, "Plasma 1,8-Cineole Correlates with Cognitive Performance following Exposure to Rosemary Essential Oil Aroma," *Therapeutic Advances in Psychopharmacology* 2, no. 3 (June 2012): 103–13; M. Moss et al., "Aromas of Rosemary and Lavender Essential Oils Differentially Affect Cognition and Mood in Healthy Adults," *International Journal of Neuroscience* 113, no. 1 (January 2003): 15–38.

29. Mustafa Chopan and Benjamin Littenberg, "The Association of Hot Red Chili Pepper Consumption and Mortality: A Large Population-Based Cohort Study," *PLOS One* 12, no. 1 (2017): e0169876.

30. K. H. Cox, A. Pipingas, and A. B. Scholey, "Investigation of the Effects of Solid Lipid Curcumin on Cognition and Mood in a Healthy Older Population," *Journal of Psychopharmacology* 29, no. 5 (May 2015): 642–51.

31. Chopan and Littenberg, "The Association of Hot Red Chili Pepper Consumption and Mortality: A Large Population-Based Cohort Study," e0169876.

32. L. C. Tapsell et al., "Health Benefits of Herbs and Spices: The Past, the Present, the Future," *Medical Journal of Australia* 185, suppl. 4 (August 21, 2006): S4–24.

33. S. Rastogi, M. M. Pandey, and A. Rawat, "Spices: Therapeutic Potential In Cardiovascular Health," *Current Pharmaceutical Design* (October 21, 2016): [Epub ahead of print].

34. Ibid.

35. Pasupuleti Visweswara Rao and Siew Hua Gan, "Cinnamon: A Multifaceted Medicinal Plant," *Evidence-Based Complementary and Alternative Medicine* 2014 (2014): 642942.

36. T. D. Presley et al., "Acute Effect of a High Nitrate Diet on Brain Perfusion in Older Adults," *Nitric Oxide* 24, no. 1 (January 1, 2011): 34–42; E. L. Wightman et al., "Dietary Nitrate Modulates Cerebral Blood Flow Parameters and Cognitive Performance in

Humans: A Double-Blind, Placebo-Controlled, Crossover Investigation," *Physiology and Behavior* 149 (October 1, 2015): 149–58; Ddos S. Baião et al., "Beetroot Juice Increase Nitric Oxide Metabolites in Both Men and Women Regardless of Body Mass," *International Journal of Food Sciences and Nutrition* 67, no. 1 (2016): 40–46.

37. A. Aleixandre and M. Miguel, "Dietary Fiber and Blood Pressure Control," *Food and Function* 7, no. 4 (April 2016): 1864–71.

38. P. Surampudi et al., "Lipid Lowering with Soluble Dietary Fiber," *Current Atherosclerosis Reports* 18, no. 12 (December 2016): 75.

39. L. Stojanovska et al., "Maca Reduces Blood Pressure and Depression, in a Pilot Study in Postmenopausal Women," *Climacteric* 18, no. 1 (February 2015): 69–78.

40. Rao and Gan, "Cinnamon: A Multifaceted Medicinal Plant," 642942.

41. Anjali Ganjre et al., "Anti-Carcinogenic and Anti-Bacterial Properties of Selected Spices: Implications in Oral Health," *Clinical Nutrition Research* 4, no. 4 (October 2015): 209–15.

42. C. Poly et al., "The Relation of Dietary Choline to Cognitive Performance and White-Matter Hyperintensity in the Framingham Offspring Cohort," *American Journal of Clinical Nutrition* 94, no. 6 (December 2011): 1584–91.

43. T. P. Ng et al., "Curry Consumption and Cognitive Function in the Elderly," *American Journal of Epidemiology* 164, no. 9 (November 1, 2006): 898–906, doi: 10.1093/aje/kwj267; Ganjre et al., "Anti-Carcinogenic and Anti-Bacterial Properties of Selected Spices: Implications in Oral Health," 209–15.

44. Ganjre et al., "Anti-Carcinogenic and Anti-Bacterial Properties of Selected Spices: Implications in Oral Health," 209–15.

45. Rao and Gan, "Cinnamon: A Multifaceted Medicinal Plant," 642942.

46. Ganjre et al., "Anti-Carcinogenic and Anti-Bacterial Properties of Selected Spices: Implications in Oral Health," 209–15.

47. H. R. Schumacher et al., "Randomized Double-Blind Crossover Study of the Efficacy of a Tart Cherry Juice Blend in Treatment of Osteoarthritis (OA) of the Knee," *Osteoarthritis and Cartilage* 21, no. 8 (August 2013): 1035–41, doi: 10.1016/j.joca.2013.05.009; G. Howatson et al., "Influence of Tart Cherry Juice on Indices of Recovery Following Marathon Running," *Scandinavian Journal of Medicine & Science in Sports* 20, no. 6 (December 2010): 843–52, doi: 10.1111/j.1600-0838.2009.01005.x.

48. Y. Kashiwaya et al., "A Ketone Ester Diet Exhibits Anxiolytic and Cognition-Sparing Properties, and Lessens Amyloid and Tau Pathologies in a Mouse Model of Alzheimer's Disease," *Neurobiology of Aging* 4, no. 6 (June 2013): 1530–39, doi: 10.1016/j.neurobiolaging.2012.11.023.

49. F. Samini et al., "Curcumin Pretreatment Attenuates Brain Lesion Size and Improves Neurological Function Following Traumatic Brain Injury in the Rat," *Pharmacology, Biochemistry, and Behavior* 110 (September 2013): 238–44, doi: 10.1016/j.pbb.2013.07.019.

50. T. E. Sullivan et al., "Effects of Olfactory Stimulation on the Vigilance Performance of Individuals with Brain Injury," *Journal of Clinical and Experiential Neuropsychology* 20, no. 2 (April 1998): 227–36, doi: 10.1076/jcen.20.2.227.1175.

51. P. L. Crowell and M. N. Gould, "Chemoprevention and Therapy of Cancer by d-Limonene," *Critical Reviews in Oncogenesis* 5, no. 1 (1994): 1–22, doi: 10.1615/CritRevOncog.v5.i1.10.

52. J. NM et al., "Beyond the Flavour: A De-Flavoured Polyphenol Rich Extract of Clove Buds (Syzygium Aromaticum L) as a Novel Dietary Antioxidant Ingredient," *Food & Function* 6, no. 10 (October 2015): 3373–82, doi: 10.1039/c5fo00682a.

53. E. A. Offord et al., "Mechanisms Involved in the Chemoprotective Effects of Rosemary Extract Studied in Human Liver and Bronchial Cells," *Cancer Letters* 114, nos. 1–2 (March 19, 1997): 275–81.

54. Ganjre et al., "Anti-Carcinogenic and Anti-Bacterial Properties of Selected Spices: Implications in Oral Health," 209–15.

55. A. Ghajar et al., "Crocus Sativus L. versus Citalopram in the Treatment of Major Depressive Disorder with Anxious Distress: A Double-Blind, Controlled Clinical Trial,"

Pharmacopsychiatry (October 4, 2016), doi: 10.1055/s-0042-116159; H. A. Hausenblas et al., "A Systematic Review of Randomized Controlled Trials Examining the Effectiveness of Saffron (*Crocus sativus* L.) on Psychological and Behavioral Outcomes," *Journal of Integrative Medicine* 13, no. 4 (July 2015): 231–40, doi: 10.1016/S2095-4964(15)60176-5.

56. S. K. Kulkarni , M. K. Bhutani, and M. Bishnoi, "Antidepressant Activity of Curcumin: Involvement of Serotonin and Dopamine System," *Psychopharmacology* 201, no. 3 (December 2008): 435–42, doi: 10.1007/s00213-008-1300-y; A. L. Lopresti et al., "Curcumin for the Treatment of Major Depression: A Randomised, Double-Blind, Placebo Controlled Study," *Journal of Affective Disorders* 167 (2014): 368–75, doi: 10.1016/j.jad.2014.06.001.

57. A. L. Lopresti and P. D. Drummond, "Efficacy of Curcumin, and a Saffron/Curcumin Combination for the Treatment of Major Depression: A Randomised, Double-Blind, Placebo-Controlled Study," *Journal of Affective Disorders* 207 (January 1, 2017): 188–96, doi: 10.1016/j.jad.2016.09.047.

58. S. Barker et al., "Improved Performance on Clerical Tasks Associated with Administration of Peppermint Odor," *Perceptual and Motor Skills* 97, no. 3, part 1 (December 2003): 1007–10, doi: 10.2466/pms.2003.97.3.1007.

59. P. R. Zoladz and B. Raudenbush, "Cognitive Enhancement through Stimulation of the Chemical Senses," *North American Journal of Psychology* 7, no. 1 (April 2005): 125–40.

60. H. M. Chen and H. W. Chen, "The Effect of Applying Cinnamon Aromatherapy for Children with Attention Deficit Hyperactivity Disorder," *Journal of Chinese Medicine* 19, no. 112 (2008): 27–34.

61. "Study Finds That Peppermint and Cinnamon Lower Drivers' Frustration and Increase Alertness," Wheeling Jesuit University website, accessed May 30, 2017, http://www.wju.edu/about/adm_news_story.asp?iNewsID=1882&strBack=/about/adm_news_archive.asp.

62. Kulkarni, Bhutani, and Bishnoi, "Antidepressant Activity of Curcumin: Involvement of Serotonin and Dopamine System," 435–42.

63. T. Yamada et al., "Effects of Theanine, r-glutamylethylamide, on Neurotransmitter Release and Its Relationship with Glutamic Acid Neurotransmission," *Nutritional Neuroscience* 8, no. 4 (August 2005): 219–26, doi: 10.1080/10284150500170799.

64. Diana Walcutt, "Chocolate and Mood Disorders," Psych Central, http://psychcentral.com/blog/archives/2009/04/27/chocolate-and-mood-disorders/; A. A. Sunni and R. Latif, "Effects of Chocolate Intake on Perceived Stress; a Controlled Clinical Study," *International Journal of Health Sciences (Qassim)* 8, no. 4 (October 2014): 393–401.

65. University of Warwick, "Fruit and Veggies Give You the Feel-Good Factor," *ScienceDaily*, July 10, 2016, www.sciencedaily.com/releases/2016/07/160710094239.htm.

66. Stojanovska et al., "Maca Reduces Blood Pressure and Depression, in a Pilot Study in Postmenopausal Women," 69–78.

67. Cornell University, "Omega-3 Fatty Acids: Good for the Heart, and (Maybe) Good for the Brain," *ScienceDaily*, November 8, 2004, www.sciencedaily.com/releases/2004/11/041108024221.htm.

68. D. M. Lovinger, "Serotonin's Role in Alcohol's Effects on the Brain," *Alcohol Health and Research World* 21, no. 2 (1997): 114–20.

69. R. P. Sharma and R. A. Coulombe Jr., "Effects of Repeated Doses of Aspartame on Serotonin and Its Metabolite in Various Regions of the Mouse Brain," *Food and Chemical Toxicology* 25, no. 8 (August 1987): 565–68.

70. "Foods That Fight Winter Depression," WebMD, accessed May 30, 2017, http://www.webmd.com/depression/features/foods-that-fight-winter-depression#1.

71. J. Todd et al., "The Antimicrobial Effects of Cinnamon Leaf Oil against Multi-Drug Resistant Salmonella Newport on Organic Leafy Greens," *International Journal of Food Microbiology* 166, no. 1 (August 16, 2013):193–99, doi: 10.1016/j.ijfoodmicro.2013.06.021.

72. H. Hosseinzadeh et al., "Effects of Different Levels of Coriander (*Coriandrum sativum*) Seed Powder and Extract on Serum Biochemical Parameters, Microbiota,

and Immunity in Broiler Chicks," *Scientific World Journal* 2014 (December 28, 2014): 628979, doi: http://dx.doi.org/10.1155/2014/628979.

73. X. Dai et al., "Consuming Lentinula Edodes (Shiitake) Mushrooms Daily Improves Human Immunity: A Randomized Dietary Intervention in Healthy Young Adults," *Journal of the American College of Nutrition* 34, no. 6 (2015): 478–87, doi: 10.1080/07315724.2014.950391; J. M. Gaullier et al., "Supplementation with a Soluble β-glucan Exported from Shiitake Medicinal Mushroom, Lentinus Edodes (Berk.) Singer Mycelium: A Crossover, Placebo-Controlled Study in Healthy Elderly," *International Journal of Medicinal Mushrooms* 13, no. 4 (2011): 319–26.

74. L. C. Chandra et al., "White Button, Portabella, and Shiitake Mushroom Supplementation Up-Regulates Interleukin-23 Secretion in Acute Dextran Sodium Sulfate Colitis C57BL/6 Mice and Murine Macrophage J.744.1 Cell Line," *Nutrition Research* 33, no. 5 (May 2013): 388–96, doi: 10.1016/j.nutres.2013.02.009.

75. I. A. Myles, "Fast Food Fever: Reviewing the Impacts of the Western Diet on Immunity," *Nutrition Journal* 13 (June 17, 2014): 61, doi: 10.1186/1475-2891-13-61.

76. H. L. Bradlow et al., "Indole-3-Carbinol: A Novel Approach to Breast Cancer Prevention," *Annals of the New York Academies of Sciences* 768 (September 30, 1995): 180–200.

77. Rao and Gan, "Cinnamon: A Multifaceted Medicinal Plant," 642942; X. Bi, J. Lim, and C. J. Henry, "Spices in the Management of Diabetes Mellitus," *Food Chemistry* 217 (February 15, 2017): 281–93, doi: 10.1016/j.foodchem.2016.08.111.

78. Bi, Lim, and Henry, "Spices in the Management of Diabetes Mellitus," 281–93.

79. Pigeon et al., "Effects of a Tart Cherry Juice Beverage on the Sleep of Older Adults with Insomnia: A Pilot Study," 579–83; G. Howatson et al., "Effect of Tart Cherry Juice (Prunus Cerasus) on Melatonin Levels and Enhanced Sleep Quality," *European Journal of Nutrition* 51, no. 8 (December 2012): 909–16, doi: 10.1007/s00394-011-0263-7; T. Traustadóttir et al., "Tart Cherry Juice Decreases Oxidative Stress in Healthy Older Men and Women," *Journal of Nutrition* 139, no. 10 (October 2009): 1896–900, doi: 10.3945/jn.109.111716.

CHAPTER 17: SHARPEN YOUR MEMORY

1. Martin Dresler et al., "Mnemonic Training Reshapes Brain Networks to Support Superior Memory," *Neuron* 93, no. 5 (March 8, 2017): 1227–35, doi: http://dx.doi.org/10.1016/j.neuron.2017.02.003.

2. Bruce Goldman, "Memorization Tool Bulks Up Brain's Internal Connections, Scientists Say," press release, Stanford Medicine News Center, March 8, 2017, https://med.stanford.edu/news/all-news/2017/03/memorization-tool-bulks-up-brains-internal-connections.html.

3. J. L. Hardy et al., "Enhancing Cognitive Abilities with Comprehensive Training: A Large, Online, Randomized, Active-Controlled Trial," *PLOS One* 10, no. 9 (September 2, 2015): e0134467, doi: 10.1371/journal.pone.0134467.

4. Rui Nouchi et al., "Brain Training Game Boosts Executive Functions, Working Memory and Processing Speed in the Young Adults: A Randomized Controlled Trial," *PLOS One* 8, no. 2 (February 6, 2013): e55518, doi: 10.1371/journal.pone.0055518; Jessica Skorka-Brown et al., "Playing Tetris Decreases Drug and Other Cravings in Real World Settings," *Addictive Behaviors* 51 (December 2015): 165–70, doi: 10.1016/j.addbeh.2015.07.020; Lotte F. van Dillen and Jackie Andrade, "Derailing the Streetcar Named Desire. Cognitive Distractions Reduce Individual Differences in Cravings and Unhealthy Snacking in Response to Palatable Food," *Appetite* 96 (January 1, 2016): 102–10, doi: 10.1016/j.appet.2015.09.013.

5. Dharma Singh Khalsa et al., "Cerebral Blood Flow Changes during Chanting Meditation," *Nuclear Medicine Communications* 30, no. 12 (December 2009): 956–61, doi: 10.1097/MNM.0b013e32832fa26c; Andrew Newberg et al., "The Measurement of Cerebral Blood Flow during the Complex Cognitive Task of Meditation: A Preliminary SPECT Study," *Psychiatry Research: Neuroimaging* 106 (April 2001): 113–22.

6. Andrew Newberg et al., "Cerebral Blood Flow during Meditative Prayer: Preliminary

Findings and Methodological Issues," *Perceptual and Motor Skills* 97, no. 2 (October 2003): 625–30, doi: 10.2466/pms.2003.97.2.625.

7. Willem J. R. Bossers et al., "A 9-Week Aerobic and Strength Training Program Improves Cognitive and Motor Function in Patients with Dementia: A Randomized, Controlled Trial," *American Journal of Geriatric Psychiatry* 23, no. 11 (November 2015): 1106–16, doi: 10.1016/j.jagp.2014.12.191; Teresa Liu-Ambrose et al., "Resistance Training and Executive Functions: A 12-Month Randomized Controlled Trial," *Archives of Internal Medicine* 170, no. 2 (January 2010): 170–78, doi: 10.1001/archinternmed.2009.494.

8. Gregory D. Clemenson and Craig E. L. Stark, "Virtual Environmental Enrichment through Video Games Improves Hippocampal-Associated Memory," *Journal of Neuroscience* 35, no. 49 (December 9, 2015): 16116–25, doi: https://doi.org/10.1523/JNEUROSCI.2580-15.2015.

9. K. Koch et al., "Extensive Learning Is Associated with Gray Matter Changes in the Right Hippocampus," *NeuroImage* 125 (January 15, 2016): 627–32, doi: 10.1016/j.neuroimage .2015.10.056.

10. Richard A. P. Roche et al., "Prolonged Rote Learning Produces Delayed Memory Facilitation and Metabolic Changes in the Hippocampus of the Ageing Human Brain," *BMC Neuroscience* 10, no. 136 (November 20, 2009): 136, doi: 10.1186/1471-2202-10-136.

11. Martin Dresler et al., "Mnemonic Training Reshapes Brain Networks to Support Superior Memory," *Neuron* 93, no. 5 (March 8, 2017): 1227–35, doi: http://dx.doi.org/10.1016/j .neuron.2017.02.003.

12. Marcus Herdener et al., "Musical Training Induces Functional Plasticity in Human Hippocampus," *Journal of Neuroscience* 30, no. 4 (January 27, 2010): 1377–84, doi: https://doi.org/10.1523/JNEUROSCI.4513-09.2010.

13. Kirk I. Erickson et al., "Exercise Training Increases Size of Hippocampus and Improves Memory," *PNAS* 108, no. 7 (February 15, 2011): 3017–22, doi: 10.1073/pnas.1015950108.

14. P. Gerber et al., "Juggling Revisited—A Voxel-Based Morphometry Study with Expert Jugglers," *NeuroImage* 95 (July 15, 2014): 320–25, doi: http://doi.org/10.1016/j .neuroimage.2014.04.023; J. Boyke et al., "Training-Induced Brain Structure Changes in the Elderly," *Journal of Neuroscience* 28, no. 28 (July 9, 2008): 7031–35, doi: 10.1523 /JNEUROSCI.0742-08.2008.

15. Ladina Bezzola et al., "Training-Induced Neural Plasticity in Golf Novices," *Journal of Neuroscience* 31, no. 35 (August 31, 2011): 12444–48, doi: https://doi.org/10.1523 /JNEUROSCI.1996-11.2011.

16. Steven Brown et al., "The Neural Basis of Human Dance," *Cerebral Cortex* 16, no. 8 (August 2006): 1157–67, doi: 10.1093/cercor/bhj057; K. Sacco et al., "Motor Imagery of Walking Following Training in Locomotor Attention. The Effect of 'The Tango Lesson,'" *NeuroImage* 32, no. 3 (September 2006): 1441–49, doi: 10.1016/j.neuroimage.2006.05.018; Madeleine E. Hackney and Gammon M. Earhart, "Effects of Dance on Movement Control in Parkinson's Disease: A Comparison of Argentine Tango and American Ballroom," *Journal of Rehabilitation Medicine* 41, no. 6 (May 2009): 475–81, doi: 10.2340/16501977-0362.

17. Lauren Stewart et al., "Brain Changes after Learning to Read and Play Music," *NeuroImage* 20, no. 1 (September 2003): 71–83, doi: http://doi.org/10.1016/S1053-8119(03)00248-9.

18. C. Niemann et al., "Exercise-Induced Changes in Basal Ganglia Volume and Cognition in Older Adults," *Neuroscience* 281 (December 5, 2014): 147–63.

19. Sung Park et al., "Experience-Dependent Plasticity of Cerebellar Vermis in Basketball Players," *Cerebellum* 8, no. 3 (September 2009): 334–39, doi: 10.1007/s12311-009-0100-1.

20. George W. Rebok et al., "Ten-Year Effects of the Advanced Cognitive Training for Independent and Vital Elderly Cognitive Training Trial on Cognition and Everyday Functioning in Older Adults," *Journal of the American Geriatrics Society* 62, no. 1 (2014): 16–24, doi: 10.1111/jgs.12607.

21. Kim E. Innes et al., "Meditation and Music Improve Memory and Cognitive Function in Adults with Subjective Cognitive Decline: A Pilot Randomized Controlled Trial," *Journal of Alzheimer's Disease* 56, no. 3 (January 2017): 899–916, doi: 10.3233/JAD-160867.

22. H. J. Trappe and G. Voit, "The Cardiovascular Effect of Musical Genres: A Randomized Controlled Study on the Effect of Compositions by W. A. Mozart, J. Strauss, and ABBA," *Deutsches Ärzteblatt International* 113, no. 20 (May 20, 2016): 347–52, doi: 10.3238 /arztebl.2016.0347.

23. H. P. Lee, Y. C. Liu, and M. F. Lin, "Effects of Different Genres of Music on the Psycho-Physiological Responses of Undergraduates," *Hu Li Za Zhi: The Journal of Nursing* 63, no. 6 (December 2016): 77–88, doi: 10.6224/JN.63.6.77.

24. M. Herdener et al., "Musical Training Induces Functional Plasticity in Human Hippocampus," *Journal of Neuroscience* 30, no. 4 (January 27, 2010): 1377–84, doi: https://doi.org/10.1523/JNEUROSCI.4513-09.2010; Benjamin Rich Zendel, Karen A. Willoughby, and Joanne F. Rovet, "Neuroplastic Effects of Music Lessons on Hippocampal Volume in Children with Congenital Hypothyroidism," *Neuroreport* 24, no. 17 (December 4, 2013): 947–50, doi: 10.1097/WNR.0000000000000031; M. S. Oechslin et al., "Hippocampal Volume Predicts Fluid Intelligence in Musically Trained People," *Hippocampus* 23, no. 7 (July 2013): 552–58, doi: 10.1002/hipo.22120.

25. S. Sheldon and J. Donahue, "More Than a Feeling: Emotional Cues Impact the Access and Experience of Autobiographical Memories," *Memory & Cognition* (February 27, 2017): doi: 10.3758/s13421-017-0691-6.

26. Frances A. Yates, *The Art of Memory* (London: Pimlico, 2007), 64.

CHAPTER 18: MEMORY MEDICATIONS

1. T. Darreh-Shori et al., "Sustained Cholinesterase Inhibition in AD Patients Receiving Rivastigmine for 12 Months," *Neurology* 59, no. 4 (August 27, 2002): 563–72.

2. M. D. Santos et al., "The Nicotinic Allosteric Potentiating Ligand Galantamine Facilitates Synaptic Transmission in the Mammalian Central Nervous System," *Molecular Pharmacology* 61, no. 5 (May 2002): 1222–34.

3. "Alzheimer's Patients Who Fail on Aricept (Donepezil) May Benefit from Exelon (Rivastigmine)," press release, April 24, 2002, Novartis, http://www.evaluategroup .com/Universal/View.aspx?type=Story&id=25015.

4. Birgitta Johansson et al., "Methylphenidate Reduces Mental Fatigue and Improves Processing Speed in Persons Suffered a Traumatic Brain Injury," *Brain Injury* 29, no. 6 (March 2015): 758–65, doi: 10.3109/02699052.2015.1004747; William Breitbart et al., "A Randomized, Double-Blind, Placebo-Controlled Trial of Psychostimulants for the Treatment of Fatigue in Ambulatory Patients with Human Immunodeficiency Virus Disease," *Archives of Internal Medicine* 161, no. 3 (February 12, 2001): 411–20, doi: 10.1001/archinte.161.3.411.

5. S. Rahman et al., "Methylphenidate ('Ritalin') Can Ameliorate Abnormal Risk-Taking Behavior in the Frontal Variant of Frontotemporal Dementia," *Neuropsychopharmacology* 31, no. 3 (March 2006): 651–58, doi: 10.1038/sj.npp.1300886; P. R. Padala et al., "Methylphenidate for Apathy and Functional Status in Dementia of the Alzheimer Type," *American Journal of Geriatric Psychiatry* 18, no. 4 (April 2010): 371–74, doi: 10.1097 /JGP.0b013e3181cabcf6; P. B. Rosenberg et al., "Safety and Efficacy of Methylphenidate for Apathy in Alzheimer's Disease: A Randomized, Placebo-Controlled Trial," *Journal of Clinical Psychiatry* 74, no. 8 (August 2013): 810–16, doi: 10.4088/JCP.12m08099.

6. R. M. Battleday and A. K. Brem, "Modafinil for Cognitive Neuroenhancement in Healthy Non-Sleep-Deprived Subjects: A Systematic Review," *European Neuropsychopharmacology* 25, no. 11 (November 2015): 1865–81, doi: 10.1016/j.euroneuro.2015.07.028.

CHAPTER 19: BRAIN-ENHANCEMENT THERAPIES

1. S. Y. Chen et al., "Reversible Changes of Brain Perfusion SPECT for Carbon Monoxide Poisoning-Induced Severe Akinetic Mutism," *Clinical Nuclear Medicine* 41, no. 5 (May 2016): e221–27, doi: 10.1097/RLU.0000000000001121.

2. R. Boussi-Gross et al., "Hyperbaric Oxygen Therapy Can Improve Post Concussion Syndrome Years after Mild Traumatic Brain Injury—Randomized Prospective Trial," *PLOS*

One 8, no. 11 (November 15, 2013): e79995, doi: 10.1371/journal.pone.007999; S. Tal et al., "Hyperbaric Oxygen May Induce Angiogenesis in Patients Suffering from Prolonged Post-Concussion Syndrome Due to Traumatic Brain Injury," *Restorative Neurology and Neuroscience* 33, no. 6 (2015): 943–51, doi: 10.3233/RNN-150585; P. G. Harch et al., "A Phase I Study of Low-Pressure Hyperbaric Oxygen Therapy for Blast-Induced Post-Concussion Syndrome and Post-Traumatic Stress Disorder," *Journal of Neurotrauma* 29, no. 1 (January 1, 2012): 168–85, doi: 10.1089/neu.2011.1895.

3. S. Efrati et al., "Hyperbaric Oxygen Induces Late Neuroplasticity in Post Stroke Patients—Randomized, Prospective Trial," *PLOS One* 8, no. 1 (2013): e53716, doi: 10.1371/journal.pone.0053716.

4. S. Efrati et al., "Hyperbaric Oxygen Therapy Can Diminish Fibromyalgia Syndrome—Prospective Clinical Trial," *PLOS One* 10, no. 5 (May 26, 2015): e0127012, doi: 10.1371/journal.pone.0127012.

5. C. Y. Huang et al., "Hyperbaric Oxygen Therapy as an Effective Adjunctive Treatment for Chronic Lyme Disease," *Journal of the Chinese Medical Association* 77, no. 5 (May 2014): 269–71, doi: 10.1016/j.jcma.2014.02.001.

6. I. H. Chiang et al., "Adjunctive Hyperbaric Oxygen Therapy in Severe Burns: Experience in Taiwan Formosa Water Park Dust Explosion Disaster," *Burns* (December 2016): doi: 10.1016/j.burns.2016.10.016.

7. M. Löndahl et al., "Relationship Between Ulcer Healing after Hyperbaric Oxygen Therapy and Transcutaneous Oximetry, Toe Blood Pressure and Ankle-Brachial Index in Patients with Diabetes and Chronic Foot Ulcers," *Diabetologia* 54, no. 1 (January 2011): 65–68, doi: 10.1007/s00125-010-1946-y.

8. A. M. Eskes et al., "Hyperbaric Oxygen Therapy: Solution for Difficult to Heal Acute Wounds? Systematic Review," *World Journal of Surgery* 35, no. 3 (March 2011): 535–42, doi: 10.1007/s00268-010-0923-4; J. J. Shaw et al., "Not Just Full of Hot Air: Hyperbaric Oxygen Therapy Increases Survival in Cases of Necrotizing Soft Tissue Infections," *Surgical Infections* 15, no. 3 (June 2014): 328–35, doi: 10.1089/sur.2012.135.

9. Mina Taghizadeh Asl et al., "Brain Perfusion Imaging with Voxel-Based Analysis in Secondary Progressive Multiple Sclerosis Patients with a Moderate to Severe Stage of Disease: A Boon for the Workforce," *BMC Neurology* 16 (May 26, 2016): 79, doi: 10.1186/s12883-016-0605-4.

10. P. S. Dulai et al., "Systematic Review: The Safety and Efficacy of Hyperbaric Oxygen Therapy for Inflammatory Bowel Disease," *Alimentary Pharmacology and Therapeutics* 39, no. 11 (June 2014): 1266–75, doi: 10.1111/apt.12753.

11. D. N. Teguh et al., "Early Hyperbaric Oxygen Therapy for Reducing Radiotherapy Side Effects: Early Results of a Randomized Trial in Oropharyngeal and Nasopharyngeal Cancer," *International Journal of Radiation Oncology, Biology, Physics* 75, no. 3 (November 1, 2009): 711–16, doi: 10.1016/j.ijrobp.2008.11.056; N. A. Schellart et al., "Hyperbaric Oxygen Treatment Improved Neurophysiologic Performance in Brain Tumor Patients after Neurosurgery and Radiotherapy: A Preliminary Report," *Cancer* 117, no. 15 (August 1, 2011): 3434–44, doi: 10.1002/cncr.25874.

12. D. A. Rossignol et al., "The Effects of Hyperbaric Oxygen Therapy on Oxidative Stress, Inflammation, and Symptoms in Children with Autism: An Open-Label Pilot Study," *BMC Pediatrics* 7, no. 36 (November 16, 2007): 36, doi: 10.1186/1471-2431-7-36; D. A. Rossignol et al., "Hyperbaric Treatment for Children with Autism: A Multicenter, Randomized, Double-Blind, Controlled Trial," *BMC Pediatrics* 9, no. 21 (March 13, 2009), doi: 10.1186/1471-2431-9-21.

13. A. Mukherjee et al., "Intensive Rehabilitation Combined with HBO2 Therapy in Children with Cerebral Palsy: A Controlled Longitudinal Study," *Undersea and Hyperbaric Medicine* 41, no. 2 (March–April 2014): 77–85.

14. D. White and S. Tavakoli, "Repetitive Transcranial Magnetic Stimulation for Treatment of Major Depressive Disorder with Comorbid Generalized Anxiety Disorder," *Annals of Clinical Psychiatry* 27, no. 3 (August 2015): 192–96.

15. M. Ceccanti et al., "Deep TMS on Alcoholics: Effects on Cortisolemia and Dopamine Pathway Modulation. A Pilot Study," *Canadian Journal of Physiology and Pharmacology* 93, no. 4 (April 2015): 283–90, doi: 10.1139/cjpp-2014-0188.

16. L. Dinur-Klein et al., "Smoking Cessation Induced by Deep Repetitive Transcranial Magnetic Stimulation of the Prefrontal and Insular Cortices: A Prospective, Randomized Controlled Trial," *Biological Psychiatry* 76, no. 9 (November 1, 2014): 742–49, doi: 10.1016/j.biopsych.2014.05.020.

17. P. S. Boggio et al., "Noninvasive Brain Stimulation with High-Frequency and Low-Intensity Repetitive Transcranial Magnetic Stimulation Treatment for Posttraumatic Stress Disorder," *Journal of Clinical Psychiatry* 71, no. 8 (August 2010): 992–99, doi: 10.4088/JCP.08m04638blu.

18. A. P. Trevizol et al., "Transcranial Magnetic Stimulation for Obsessive-Compulsive Disorder: An Updated Systematic Review and Meta-Analysis," *Journal of ECT* 32, no. 4 (December 2016): 262–66, doi: 10.1097/YCT.0000000000000335.

19. H. L. Drumond Marra et al., "Transcranial Magnetic Stimulation to Address Mild Cognitive Impairment in the Elderly: A Randomized Controlled Study," *Behavioural Neurology* 2015 (2015): 287843, doi: 10.1155/2015/287843; W. M. McDonald, "Neuromodulation Treatments for Geriatric Mood and Cognitive Disorders," *American Journal of Geriatric Psychiatry* 24, no. 12 (December 2016): 1130–41, doi: 10.1016/j.jagp.2016.08.014; J. M. Rabey and E. Dobronevsky, "Repetitive Transcranial Magnetic Stimulation (rTMS) Combined with Cognitive Training Is a Safe and Effective Modality for the Treatment of Alzheimer's Disease: Clinical Experience," *Journal of Neural Transmission (Vienna)* 123, no. 12 (December 2016): 1449–55, doi: 10.1007/s00702-016-1606-6.

20. M. Yilmaz et al., "Effectiveness of Transcranial Magnetic Stimulation Application in Treatment of Tinnitus," *Journal of Craniofacial Surgery* 25, no. 4 (July 2014): 1315–18, doi: 10.1097/SCS.0000000000000782.

21. T. V. Kulishova and O. V. Shinkorenko, "The Effectiveness of Early Rehabilitation of the Patients Presenting with Ischemic Stroke," *Voprosy Kurortologii, Fizioterapii, I Lechebnoi Fizicheskoi Kultury* 6 (November–December 2014): 9–12.

22. H. L. Drumond Marra et al., "Transcranial Magnetic Stimulation to Address Mild Cognitive Impairment in the Elderly: A Randomized Controlled Study," *Behavioural Neurology* 2015 (2015): 287843, doi: 10.1155/2015/287843.

23. J. Guez et al., "Influence of Electroencephalography Neurofeedback Training on Episodic Memory: A Randomized, Sham-Controlled, Double-Blind Study," *Memory* 23, no. 5 (2015): 683–94, doi: 10.1080/09658211.2014.921713; S. Xiong et al., "Working Memory Training Using EEG Neurofeedback in Normal Young Adults," *Bio-Medical Materials and Engineering* 24, no. 6 (2014): 3637–44, doi: 10.3233/BME-141191; J. R. Wang and S. Hsieh, "Neurofeedback Training Improves Attention and Working Memory Performance," *Clinical Neurophysiology* 124, no. 12 (December 2013): 2406–20, doi: 10.1016/j.clinph.2013.05.020.

24. S. E. Kober et al., "Specific Effects of EEG Based Neurofeedback Training on Memory Functions in Post-Stroke Victims," *Journal of Neuroengineering and Rehabilitation* 12 (December 1, 2015): 107, doi: 10.1186/s12984-015-0105-6.

25. V. Meisel et al., "Neurofeedback and Standard Pharmacological Intervention in ADHD: A Randomized Controlled Trial with Six-Month Follow-Up," *Biological Psychology* 94, no. 1 (September 2013): 12–21, doi: 10.1016/j.biopsycho.2013.04.015.

26. J. Kopřivová et al., "Prediction of Treatment Response and the Effect of Independent Component Neurofeedback in Obsessive-Compulsive Disorder: A Randomized, Sham-Controlled, Double-Blind Study," *Neuropsychobiology* 67, no. 4 (2013): 210–23, doi: 10.1159/000347087.

27. E. J. Cheon et al., "The Efficacy of Neurofeedback in Patients with Major Depressive Disorder: An Open Labeled Prospective Study," *Applied Psychophysiology and Biofeedback* 41, no. 1 (March 2016): 103–10, doi: 10.1007/s10484-015-9315-8.

28. T. Surmeli et al., "Quantitative EEG Neurometric Analysis-Guided Neurofeedback Treatment in Postconcussion Syndrome (PCS): Forty Cases. How Is Neurometric Analysis

Important for the Treatment of PCS and as a Biomarker?" *Clinical EEG and Neuroscience* 48, no. 3 (May 2016): 217–30, doi: 10.1177/1550059416654849.

29. R. Rostami and F. Dehghani-Arani, "Neurofeedback Training as a New Method in Treatment of Crystal Methamphetamine Dependent Patients: A Preliminary Study," *Applied Psychophysiology and Biofeedback* 40, no. 3 (September 2015): 151–61, doi: 10.1007/s10484-015-9281-1.

30. P. Kubik et al., "Neurofeedback Therapy Influence on Clinical Status and Some EEG Parameters in Children with Localized Epilepsy," *Przeglad Lekarski* 73, no. 3 (2016): 157–60.

31. M. P. Jensen et al., "Use of Neurofeedback to Enhance Response to Hypnotic Analgesia in Individuals with Multiple Sclerosis," *International Journal of Clinical and Experimental Hypnosis* 64, no. 1 (2016): 1–23, doi: 10.1080/00207144.2015.1099400.

32. A. Azarpaikan et al., "Neurofeedback and Physical Balance in Parkinson's Patients," *Gait and Posture* 40, no. 1 (2014): 177–81, doi: 10.1016/j.gaitpost.2014.03.179.

33. M. Y. Cheng et al., "Sensorimotor Rhythm Neurofeedback Enhances Golf Putting Performance," *Journal of Sport and Exercise Psychology* 37, no. 6 (December 2015): 626–36, doi: 10.1123/jsep.2015-0166.

34. J. Gruzelier et al., "Acting Performance and Flow State Enhanced with Sensory-Motor Rhythm Neurofeedback Comparing Ecologically Valid Immersive VR and Training Screen Scenarios," *Neuroscience Letters* 480, no. 2 (August 16, 2010): 112–16, doi: 10.1016/j .neulet.2010.06.019; N. Rahmati et al., "The Effectiveness of Neurofeedback on Enhancing Cognitive Process Involved in Entrepreneurship Abilities among Primary School Students in District No. 3 Tehran," *Basic and Clinical Neuroscience* 5, no. 4 (October 2014): 277–84.

35. T. L. Huang and C. Charyton, "A Comprehensive Review of the Psychological Effects of Brainwave Entrainment," *Alternative Therapies in Health and Medicine* 14, no. 5 (September 2008): 38–50.

36. J. C. Mazziotta et al., "Tomographic Mapping of Human Cerebral Metabolism: Subcortical Responses to Auditory and Visual Stimulation," *Neurology* 34, no. 6 (June 1984): 825–28.

37. P. T. Fox and M. E. Raichle, "Stimulus Rate Determines Regional Brain Blood Flow in Striate Cortex," *Annals of Neurology* 17, no. 3 (March 1985): 303–5, doi: 10.1002/ana .410170315.

38. H. Y. Tang et al., "A Pilot Study of Audio-Visual Stimulation as a Self-Care Treatment for Insomnia in Adults with Insomnia and Chronic Pain," *Applied Psychophysiology and Biofeedback* 39, nos. 3–4 (December 2014): 219–25, doi: 10.1007/s10484-014-9263-8; V. Abeln et al., "Brainwave Entrainment for Better Sleep and Post-Sleep State of Young Elite Soccer Players—A Pilot Study," *European Journal of Sport Science* 14, no. 5 (2014): 393–402, doi: 10.1080/17461391.2013.819384.

39. Ibid.; C. Gagnon and F. Boersma, "The Use of Repetitive Audio-Visual Entrainment in the Management of Chronic Pain," *Medical Hypnoanalysis Journal* 7 (1992): 462–68.

40. Huang and Charyton, "A Comprehensive Review of the Psychological Effects of Brainwave Entrainment," 38–50.

41. D. Anderson, "The Treatment of Migraine with Variable Frequency Photo-Stimulation," *Headache* 29, no. 3 (March 1989): 154–55.

42. K. Berg and D. Siever, "A Controlled Comparison of Audio-Visual Entrainment for Treating Seasonal Affective Disorder," *Journal of Neurotherapy* 13, no. 3 (2009): 166–75, doi: 10.1080/10874200903107314; D. S. Cantor and E. Stevens, "QEEG Correlates of Auditory-Visual Entrainment Treatment Efficacy of Refractory Depression," *Journal of Neurotherapy* 13, no. 2 (April 2009): 100–108, doi: 10.1080/10874200902887130.

CHAPTER 21: HOW TO START YOUR PERSONAL MEMORY RESCUE PLAN

1. "Making Lifestyle Changes That Last," American Psychological Association, http://www.apa.org/helpcenter/lifestyle-changes.aspx.

2. Phillippa Lally and Benjamin Gardner, "Promoting Habit Formation," *Health Psychology*

Review 7, suppl. 1 (October 2011): S137–58, doi: 10.1080/17437199.2011.603640; Benjamin Gardner, Phillippa Lally, and Jane Wardle, "Making Health Habitual: The Psychology of 'Habit-Formation' and General Practice," *British Journal of General Practice* (December 2012): 664–66, doi: 10.3399/bjgp12X659466.

3. Vanessa M. Patrick and Henrik Hagtvedt, "'I Don't' versus 'I Can't': When Empowered Refusal Motivates Goal-Directed Behavior," *Journal of Consumer Research* 39, no. 2 (August 2012): 371–81, doi: 10.1086/663212; Catherine Clifford, "3 Scientifically Proven Ways to Break Your Bad Habits," CNBC, January 6, 2017, http://www.cnbc.com/2017 /01/06/3-scientifically-proven-ways-to-break-your-bad-habits.html.

4. Tia Ngandu et al., "A 2 Year Multidomain Intervention of Diet, Exercise, Cognitive Training, and Vascular Risk Monitoring versus Control to Prevent Cognitive Decline in At-Risk Elderly People (FINGER): A Randomised Controlled Trial," *Lancet* 385, no. 9984 (June 6, 2015): 2255–63, doi: 10.1016/S0140-6736(15)60461-5.

Index

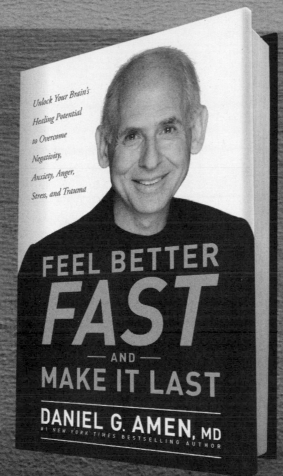

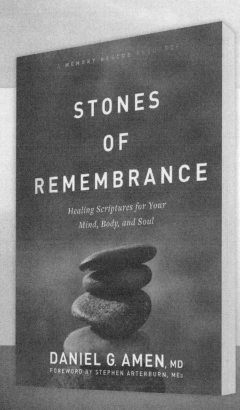

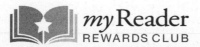